Progress in Biomaterials and Technologies in Dentistry

Progress in Biomaterials and Technologies in Dentistry

Giuseppe Minervini
Gianmarco Abbadessa

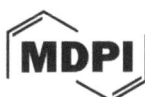

Basel • Beijing • Wuhan • Barcelona • Belgrade • Novi Sad • Cluj • Manchester

Editors

Giuseppe Minervini
Multidisciplinary Department
of Medical-Surgical and
Dental Specialties
University of Campania
"Luigi Vanvitelli"
Naples
Italy

Gianmarco Abbadessa
Division of Neurology
University of Campania
"Luigi Vanvitelli"
Naples
Italy

Editorial Office
MDPI AG
Grosspeteranlage 5
4052 Basel, Switzerland

This is a reprint of articles from the Special Issue published online in the open access journal *Biomedicines* (ISSN 2227-9059) (available at: www.mdpi.com/journal/biomedicines/special_issues/ RG16G9LX28).

For citation purposes, cite each article independently as indicated on the article page online and as indicated below:

Lastname, A.A.; Lastname, B.B. Article Title. *Journal Name* **Year**, *Volume Number*, Page Range.

ISBN 978-3-7258-2172-3 (Hbk)
ISBN 978-3-7258-2171-6 (PDF)
doi.org/10.3390/books978-3-7258-2171-6

© 2024 by the authors. Articles in this book are Open Access and distributed under the Creative Commons Attribution (CC BY) license. The book as a whole is distributed by MDPI under the terms and conditions of the Creative Commons Attribution-NonCommercial-NoDerivs (CC BY-NC-ND) license.

Contents

About the Editors ix

Preface xi

Eugen Bud, Alexandru Vlasa, Mariana Pacurar, Adrian Matei, Anamaria Bud and Andreea-Raluca Szoke et al.
A Retrospective Histological Study on Palatal and Gingival Mucosa Changes during a Rapid Palatal Expansion Procedure
Reprinted from: *Biomedicines* 2023, *11*, 3246, doi:10.3390/biomedicines11123246 1

Md Iqbal Hossain, Abdullah Bin Shams, Shuvashis Das Gupta, Gary J. Blanchard, Ali Mobasheri and Ehsanul Hoque Apu
The Potential Role of Ionic Liquid as a Multifunctional Dental Biomaterial
Reprinted from: *Biomedicines* 2023, *11*, 3093, doi:10.3390/biomedicines11113093 15

Nataly Mory, Rocío Cascos, Alicia Celemín-Viñuela, Cristina Gómez-Polo, Rubén Agustín-Panadero and Miguel Gómez-Polo
Comparison of the Surface Roughness of CAD/CAM Metal-Free Materials Used for Complete-Arch Implant-Supported Prostheses: An In Vitro Study
Reprinted from: *Biomedicines* 2023, *11*, 3036, doi:10.3390/biomedicines11113036 32

Miguel de Araújo Nobre, Carlos Moura Guedes, Ricardo Almeida, António Silva and Nuno Sereno
The All-on-4 Concept Using Polyetheretherketone (PEEK)—Acrylic Resin Prostheses: Follow-Up Results of the Development Group at 5 Years and the Routine Group at One Year
Reprinted from: *Biomedicines* 2023, *11*, 3013, doi:10.3390/biomedicines11113013 47

Horia Opris, Mihaela Baciut, Marioara Moldovan, Stanca Cuc, Ioan Petean and Daiana Opris et al.
Comparison of the Eggshell and the Porcine Pericardium Membranes for Guided Tissue Regeneration Applications
Reprinted from: *Biomedicines* 2023, *11*, 2529, doi:10.3390/biomedicines11092529 64

Emilia Bologa, Simona Stoleriu, Irina Nica, Ionuț Tărăboanță, Andrei Georgescu and Ruxandra Ilinca Matei et al.
The Effect of Three Desensitizing Toothpastes on Dentinal Tubules Occlusion and on Dentin Hardness
Reprinted from: *Biomedicines* 2023, *11*, 2464, doi:10.3390/biomedicines11092464 77

Marcin Stasiak and Paulina Adamska
Should Cone-Beam Computed Tomography Be Performed Prior to Orthodontic Miniscrew Placement in the Infrazygomatic Crest Area?—A Systematic Review
Reprinted from: *Biomedicines* 2023, *11*, 2389, doi:10.3390/biomedicines11092389 87

Javier Echarri-Nicolás, María José González-Olmo, Pablo Echarri-Labiondo and Martín Romero
Changes in Molar Tipping and Surrounding Alveolar Bone with Different Designs of Skeletal Maxillary Expanders
Reprinted from: *Biomedicines* 2023, *11*, 2380, doi:10.3390/biomedicines11092380 109

Hind Mubaraki, Navin Anand Ingle, Mohammad Abdul Baseer, Osamah M AlMugeiren, Sarah Mubaraki and Marco Cicciù et al.
Effect of Silver Diamine Fluoride on Bacterial Biofilms—A Review including In Vitro and In Vivo Studies
Reprinted from: *Biomedicines* 2023, *11*, 1641, doi:10.3390/biomedicines11061641 120

Emil Crasnean, Alina Ban, Raluca Roman, Cristian Dinu, Mihaela Băciuț and Vlad-Ionuț Nechita et al.
The Impact of Benign Jawbone Tumors on the Temporomandibular Joint and Occlusion in Children: A Ten-Year Follow-Up Study
Reprinted from: *Biomedicines* 2023, *11*, 1210, doi:10.3390/biomedicines11041210 133

Ani Belcheva, Elitsa Veneva and Reem Hanna
Effect of Various Protocols of Pre-Emptive Pulpal Laser Analgesia on Enamel Surface Morphology Using Scanning Electron Microscopy: An Ex Vivo Study
Reprinted from: *Biomedicines* 2023, *11*, 1077, doi:10.3390/biomedicines11041077 145

Akiva Elad, Patrick Rider, Svenja Rogge, Frank Witte, Dražen Tadić and Željka Perić Kačarević et al.
Application of Biodegradable Magnesium Membrane Shield Technique for Immediate Dentoalveolar Bone Regeneration
Reprinted from: *Biomedicines* 2023, *11*, 744, doi:10.3390/biomedicines11030744 155

Reiko Tokuyama-Toda, Hirochika Umeki, Shinji Ide, Fumitaka Kobayashi, Shunnosuke Tooyama and Mai Umehara et al.
A New Implantation Method for Orthodontic Anchor Screws: Basic Research for Clinical Applications
Reprinted from: *Biomedicines* 2023, *11*, 665, doi:10.3390/biomedicines11030665 168

Louisa M. Wendorff-Tobolla, Michael Wolgin, Gernot Wagner, Irma Klerings, Anna Dvornyk and Andrej M. Kielbassa
A Systematic Review and Meta-Analysis on the Efficacy of Locally Delivered Adjunctive Curcumin (*Curcuma longa* L.) in the Treatment of Periodontitis
Reprinted from: *Biomedicines* 2023, *11*, 481, doi:10.3390/biomedicines11020481 180

Shanlin Li, Adam Tanner, Georgios Romanos and Rafael Delgado-Ruiz
Heat Accumulation in Implant Inter-Osteotomy Areas—An Experimental In Vitro Study
Reprinted from: *Biomedicines* 2022, *11*, 9, doi:10.3390/biomedicines11010009 197

Inês Cardoso-Martins, Sofia Pessanha, Ana Coelho, Sofia Arantes-Oliveira and Paula F. Marques
Evaluation of the Efficacy of CPP-ACP Remineralizing Mousse in Molar-Incisor Hypomineralized Teeth Using Polarized Raman and Scanning Electron Microscopy—An *In Vitro* Study
Reprinted from: *Biomedicines* 2022, *10*, 3086, doi:10.3390/biomedicines10123086 209

Kamil Górski, Marta Borowska, Elżbieta Stefanik, Izabela Polkowska, Bernard Turek and Andrzej Bereznowski et al.
Application of Two-Dimensional Entropy Measures to Detect the Radiographic Signs of Tooth Resorption and Hypercementosis in an Equine Model
Reprinted from: *Biomedicines* 2022, *10*, 2914, doi:10.3390/biomedicines10112914 220

Davide Foschi, Andrea Abate, Cinzia Maspero, Luca Solimei, Claudio Lanteri and Valentina Lanteri
Method Presentation of a New Integrated Orthodontic-Conservative Approach for Minimally Invasive Full Mouth Rehabilitation: Speed Up Therapy
Reprinted from: *Biomedicines* **2022**, *10*, 2536, doi:10.3390/biomedicines10102536 . . . . **238**

About the Editors

Giuseppe Minervini

Giuseppe Minervini graduated in Dental Medicine in July 2016 with honors. During his undergraduate studies, he participated in the Erasmus project at "Rey Juan Carlos Alcorcon" in Madrid, Spain, from September 2013 to June 2014. He received his Postgraduate Diploma in Orthodontics in December 2020 from the University of Campania, Luigi Vanvitelli, Naples, Italy, and later earned his PhD at the same institution (XXXIV cycle). In 2019, he attended the Tweed Study Course at the Charles H. Tweed International Foundation in Tucson, Arizona. Currently, he serves as an Adjunct Professor at Saveetha Dental College and Hospitals, Saveetha University, Chennai. Dr. Minervini is recognized as one of the top 10 experts worldwide in the field of "Temporomandibular disorders" according to Scopus' rankings. He is a Subject Expert in Dental Materials and a tutor at the Orthodontics Dentistry School at the University of Campania, Luigi Vanvitelli. His contributions include serving as an Editor for numerous dentistry journals (10 editorial boards, 14 Special Issues), and he is an active member of SIDO, EOS, and GSID. With over 188 publications, 70 posters, and an h-index of 32, he is a frequent speaker at national and international conferences. Dr. Minervini has received several awards for his contributions to the field. His research interests include biomedical and biomaterials applications in craniofacial, oral, and temporomandibular districts, as well as orthodontics, orofacial pain, temporomandibular joint disorders, and telemedicine.

Gianmarco Abbadessa

Gianmarco Abbadasse graduated with honors in Medicine and Surgery from the University of Campania "Luigi Vanvitelli" (Naples, Italy) in 2016, achieving 110/110 summa cum laude. He completed his Neurology Residency at the same institution in 2021, also summa cum laude. Since 2021, he has been a PhD student and Research Fellow at the University of Campania, and a Visiting PhD student at Imperial College London since July 2023. He previously held a fellowship at the T-reg cell lab, University of Naples Federico II (2020–2023) and interned at the Athinoula A. Martinos Center for Biomedical Imaging, Harvard Medical School (2019), and at the Division of Neurology, University of Campania (2012–2017). Abbadasse is a Senior Coordinator of the Italian Section of Young Neurologists (SIgN) under the Italian Society of Neurology (SIN). He is a member of the AINI, EAN, and AAN and serves on EAN Scientific Panels for Neuroimmunology and Multiple Sclerosis. He has been a Guest Editor for *Frontiers in Neuroscience*, *Frontiers in Neurology*, and the *Journal of Clinical Medicine*, and he is an Academic Editor for PLOS ONE. His awards include the EAN Research Training Fellowship (2024), AAN International Scholarship (2020, 2023), and the Marco Vergelli Award (2022). He holds certifications in Bioinformatics (University of Toronto), Machine Learning (Stanford University), and Statistics (UCL). His research focuses on neuroimmunology, multiple sclerosis, bioinformatics, and digital technology. Abbadasse has presented at numerous conferences and authored or co-authored 63 publications, with 20 as the first author. His work has been cited 588 times, and he holds an h-index of 13.

Preface

Dear Colleagues,

Dentistry is an interdisciplinary field that combines the principles of medical and material sciences toward the development of therapeutic strategies. Continuous progress in the biomaterials field allows for the development of new studies and methods to treat and rehabilitate patients. The growth of pharmaceutics and biomaterials as a research field has provided a novel set of therapeutic strategies for dental applications. Topics in this Special Issue include, but are not limited to, the following: new restorative materials, new regenerative materials, and translational research in all fields of dentistry.

Giuseppe Minervini and Gianmarco Abbadessa
Editors

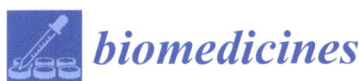

Article

A Retrospective Histological Study on Palatal and Gingival Mucosa Changes during a Rapid Palatal Expansion Procedure

Eugen Bud [1], Alexandru Vlasa [2,*], Mariana Pacurar [1], Adrian Matei [3], Anamaria Bud [4,*], Andreea-Raluca Szoke [5] and Giuseppe Minervini [6]

1. Department of Orthodontics and Dental-Facial Orthopedics, Faculty of Dental Medicine, George Emil Palade University of Medicine and Pharmacy, Science and Technology, 540139 Târgu-Mureș, Romania; eugen.bud@umfst.ro (E.B.); mariana.pacurar@umfst.ro (M.P.)
2. Department of Periodontology and Oral-Dental Diagnosis, Faculty of Dental Medicine, George Emil Palade University of Medicine and Pharmacy, Science and Technology, 540139 Târgu-Mureș, Romania
3. Independent Researcher, 540139 Târgu-Mureș, Romania
4. Department of Pedodontics, Faculty of Dental Medicine, George Emil Palade University of Medicine and Pharmacy, Science and Technology, 540139 Târgu-Mureș, Romania
5. Department of Physiopathology, Faculty of General Medicine, George Emil Palade University of Medicine and Pharmacy, Science and Technology, 540139 Târgu-Mureș, Romania; andreea-raluca.szoke@umfst.ro
6. Multidisciplinary Department of Medical-Surgical and Dental Specialties, University of Campania, Luigi Vanvitelli, 80138 Naples, Italy; giuseppe.minervini@unicampania.it
* Correspondence: alexandru.vlasa@umfst.ro (A.V.); anamaria.bud@umfst.ro (A.B.); Tel.: +40-742825920 (A.V.); +40-744437661 (A.B)

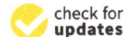

Citation: Bud, E.; Vlasa, A.; Pacurar, M.; Matei, A.; Bud, A.; Szoke, A.-R.; Minervini, G. A Retrospective Histological Study on Palatal and Gingival Mucosa Changes during a Rapid Palatal Expansion Procedure. *Biomedicines* 2023, 11, 3246. https://doi.org/10.3390/biomedicines11123246

Academic Editor: Oliver Schierz

Received: 8 November 2023
Revised: 3 December 2023
Accepted: 5 December 2023
Published: 7 December 2023

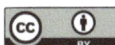

Copyright: © 2023 by the authors. Licensee MDPI, Basel, Switzerland. This article is an open access article distributed under the terms and conditions of the Creative Commons Attribution (CC BY) license (https://creativecommons.org/licenses/by/4.0/).

Abstract: The most common inflammatory reactions in the oral mucosa are found at the gingival level. The treatment of these inflammations requires, first of all, the removal of the causative factor; often, this maneuver is sufficient. The aim of this retrospective study was to evaluate clinical and histopathological changes that occur in terms of gingival and palatal mucosa enlargement during palatal expansion treatment and their evolution during treatment. Twenty-five (*n* = 25) research participants, aged between thirteen and twenty-six years old, were examined in this retrospective study. At the end of the treatment, fragments of tissue from the affected level were obtained via incisional biopsy and sent to the histopathology laboratory for a specialized examination. The changes identified were specific to mechanical traumatic injuries, thus excluding hyperplasia from other etiologies (infectious, tumoral, or non-mechanical traumatic). The examined fragments showed hyperplasia. The histopathological examination revealed the mechanical character of the lesion, strengthening the causal relationship between the insertion of the expander and the occurrence of hyperplasia of the palatal mucosa. The type of palatal expander influenced the degree of inflammation, with the severity of hyperplasia being more pronounced in the case of mini-implant-anchored rapid palatal expander (MARPE) usage than in the case of tooth-borne rapid palatal expander (RPE) usage. The analysis of the distance between the expander and the palatal mucosa did not provide conclusive results; the incidence and severity of the reaction were variable in patients with the same distance between the expander and the palatal or gingival mucosa.

Keywords: rapid palatal expansion; mini-implant-assisted rapid palatal expander; MARPE; gingival overgrowth; hyperplasia

1. Introduction

The mucosa of the oral cavity is in direct contact with the environment and is frequently subjected to multiple sources of damage. Its reduced thickness is a factor that makes it even more susceptible to damage, especially that of traumatic origin (mechanical, physical, or chemical) [1]. The most common inflammatory reactions in the oral mucosa are found at the gingival level. According to etiology and pathological changes, they are classified into inflammatory hyperplasia (chronic or acute), drug-induced hyperplasia, hyperplasia associated with systemic diseases, gingival tumors, and pseudo-hyperplasia [2]. In addition to these forms, hyperplasia of the mucosa can occur at the lingual or palatal level. Regardless of the location, making the differential diagnosis is essential for developing a correct treatment plan [3]. Patients presenting to dental clinics may present with inflammation of the oral mucosa that does not respond to improved oral hygiene or periodontal treatment. This fact indicates the presence of a specific etiological factor [4]. The treatment of these inflammations requires, first of all, the removal of the causative factor; often, this maneuver is sufficient [5]. In cases of severe inflammation of traumatic origin, in addition to removing the cause, surgical excision of the tissue fragment is recommended, and in inflammations of toxic origin, specific drug treatment is indicated [6].

Rapid palatal expansion (RPE) is a treatment method used to correct the reduced size of the jaw. It involves separating the medial palatine suture to widen the maxillary basal bone in young children, adolescents, and adults. The procedure has been used for more than a century in orthodontic therapy, and its effects on dentition and the craniofacial skeleton have been studied and documented by various authors [7–9].

The application of the palatal expander is an invasive maneuver and, as such, may produce secondary reactions at a local level of traumatic origin. Thus, local and regional hyperplasia of the oral mucosa is a frequently encountered effect in palatal expander cases [10]. This depends on the patient's reactivity to mechanical damage and the distance of application of the expander to the mucosa, being favored by the presence of some local factors such as pre-existing carious lesions or tartar deposits [11]. Also, another cause of mucosal lesions in the case of orthodontic expanders is their overfrequent activation, a fact that does not allow the bone structures to adapt. In order to carry out the orthodontic treatment, the expander cannot be removed from the oral cavity, and as a consequence, treating mucosal hyperplasia becomes problematic.

The aim of this retrospective study was to evaluate clinical and histopathological changes that occur at gingival and palatal mucosa levels during palatal expansion treatment and their evolution during treatment. The null hypothesis of the present study was that palatal expanders do not cause mechanical trauma after insertion of this device and that there are no differences between post-therapeutic sites treated with conventional tooth-borne RPE techniques and mini-implant RPE.

2. Materials and Methods

2.1. Specimens and Sampling Technique

The authors chose the PICO framework [12] in order to achieve the objectives of this study, since it is the most commonly used model for structuring clinical questions (Figure 1). A power analysis was conducted to calculate the sample size. Based on previously available literature [6,8,9], using a package (Pwr) in R software (Bioconductor™, version 3.18 for Windows™, Boston, MA, USA) with a 95% confidence interval and 80% power of the study, the sample size was determined. This study was conducted in compliance with the Declaration of Helsinki. Ethical clearance was obtained from the Institutional Review Board of the Sc Algocalm Srl Private Medical Clinic, number 994/01.02.2023. Twenty-five ($n = 25$) research participants, of whom seventeen ($n = 17$) were females and eight ($n = 8$) were males, aged between thirteen and twenty-six years old, were examined for this retrospective study after written informed consent was obtained from them or their legal guardians.

The inclusion criteria for this study were as follows:
- Gingival and palatal mucosa enlargement associated/consecutive with the rapid palatal expansion procedure.
- No medication for associated systemic conditions.
- The exclusion criteria for the study group were:
- Smokers.
- Patients with cardiovascular disease, diabetes, or epilepsy.

- Associated systemic medication, which could induce soft tissue modifications.

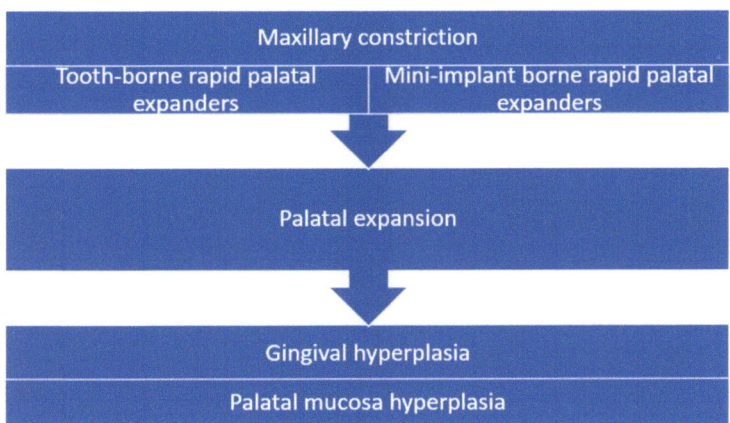

Figure 1. PICO chart followed within study protocol.

2.2. Palatal Expander Placement

After clinical and radiographical examination, the diagnosis of maxillary constriction was confirmed, and the decision for the rapid palatal expansion treatment method was taken. In the study group, sixteen ($n = 16$) patients were treated using tooth-borne palatal expanders (Figure 2). The expanders were inserted into the oral cavity of the patients at the level of the posterior third of the hard palate. The palatal expanders were placed 1–3 mm from the palatal mucosa at the time of insertion.

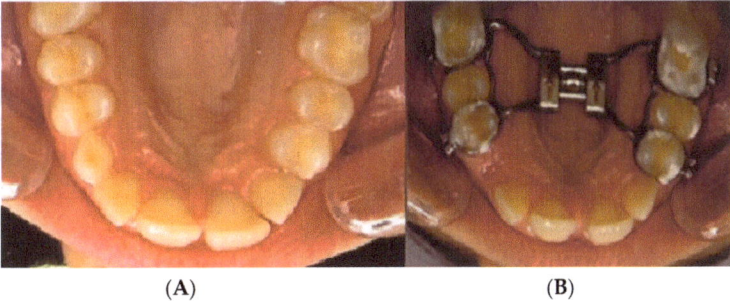

Figure 2. Images of the study group treated with tooth-borne appliances: (**A**) initial situation; (**B**) after RPE insertion.

Nine ($n = 9$) research participants were treated using mini-implant anchorage rapid palatal expanders (MARPE) (Figure 2). The anchorage achieved in these cases was of a hybrid type, made on four mini-implants (Figure 3) inserted into the patient's hard palate and bilaterally on the first molar and/or first premolar by means of metal rings.

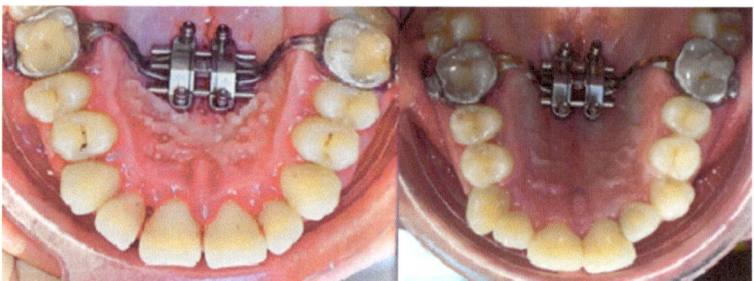

Figure 3. Hybrid anchorage in the study groups; four mini-implants supported RPE.

2.3. Assessment of the Study Group

Following the application of the expander, the research participants presented themselves for regular checks (four- to six-week intervals) or unannounced, in case of emergencies, where the presence or absence of the local inflammatory reaction of the mucosa was observed (Figures 4–7).

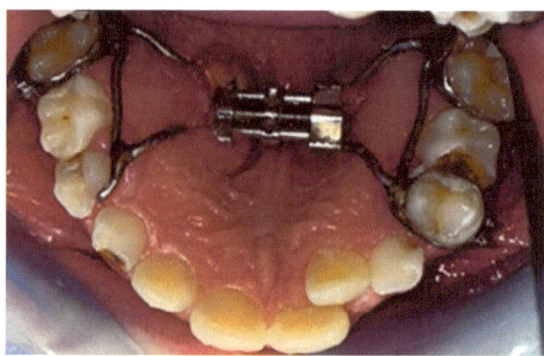

Figure 4. RPE expander inserted into the oral cavity. The presence of mucosal changes at the local-regional level and the presence of favorable factors (carious lesions) were observed.

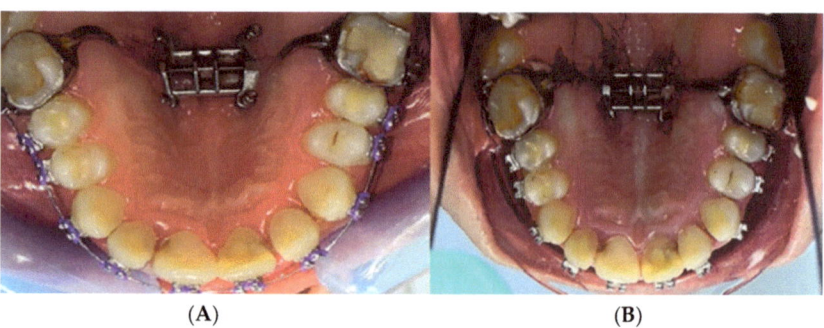

(**A**)   (**B**)

Figure 5. (**A**) MARPE expander with hybrid anchorage inserted into the oral cavity; (**B**) an accentuated vascular pattern was observed at the six-week check-up stage.

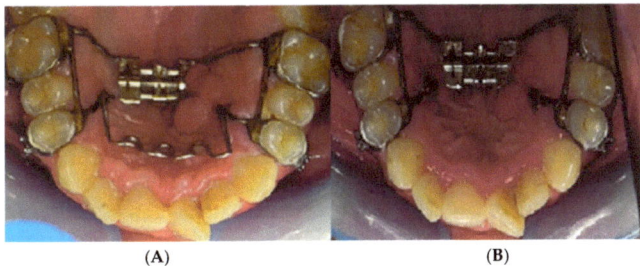

Figure 6. (**A**) RPE-type expander equipped with a tongue crib to combat infantile swallowing; (**B**) clinical aspect after the removal of the tongue crib.

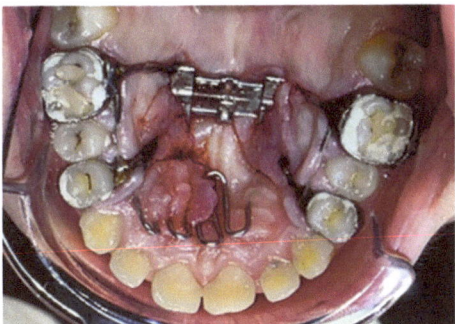

Figure 7. Severe inflammatory reaction of the palatal and gingival mucosa.

At the end of the treatment, following the removal of the expander (Figure 8), in order to examine the cellular changes within the hyperplasia of the palatal mucosa in palatal expander wearers and to confirm the diagnosis, fragments of tissue from the affected level were obtained via incisional biopsy and sent to the histopathology laboratory for a specialized examination. Surgical excision of the lesions was then performed, achieved under local anesthesia with the aid of topical application of lidocaine 2% (Septodont, Creteil, France), followed by intraoral infiltration of the hard palate using a solution of articaine and epinephrine 1:100,000 (ARTICAINE, Septodont), achieved with the aid of a syringe with a thin needle (0.30 × 38 mm). The biological product obtained was stored in a container with formalin and thus transported to the analysis laboratory in order to obtain a histopathological diagnosis.

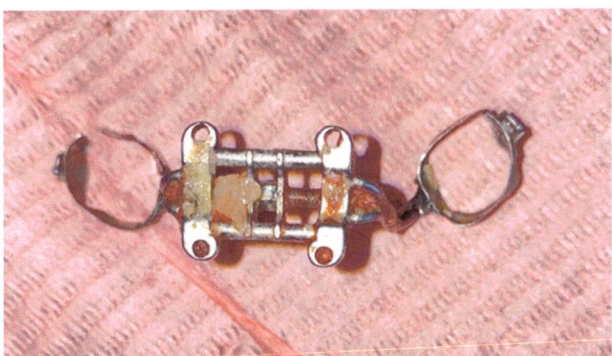

Figure 8. Expander removed from the oral cavity. Fragments of hyperplastic tissue were observed.

2.4. Histopathological Analysis Protocol

The tissues sent for microscopic examination were fixed in formalin and embedded in paraffin. The paraffin blocks were cut with a microtome into 3 μm sections to conduct the Hematoxylin and Eosin (H&E) staining using the Thermo Scientific Gemini AS Automated Slide Stainer. Then, six sections were cut from the paraffin blocks for the immunohistochemical reactions. The primary antibodies used were anti-Pan keratin (AE1/AE3/PCK26) primary antibody and CONFIRM anti-Ki-67 (30-9). Rabbit monoclonal primary antibody, CONFIRM anti-CD3 (2GV6) rabbit monoclonal primary antibody, CONFIRM anti-CD20 (L26) primary antibody, CONFIRM anti-CD68 (KP-1) primary antibody, and CD31 (JC70) mouse monoclonal antibody were also used. All the immunohistochemistry studies were performed using a DAB detection kit on a Ventana BenchMark GX automated slide staining system. The slides were examined under a Carl Zeiss microscope (Carl Zeiss Microimaging GmbH, Jena, Germany) equipped with an AxioCam MRc5 color digital camera. The interpretation was performed by an experienced pathologist.

3. Results

During the histopathological examination (Figures 9–12), all cases (*n*. 25) presented the following characteristics:

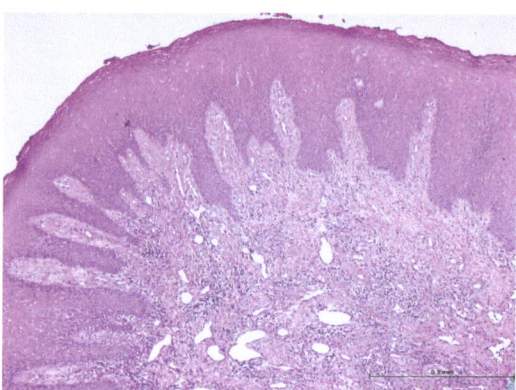

Figure 9. Histologic aspects in H&E staining (magnification ×100); marked acanthosis of the spinous layer was observed in the areas with a pseudo-epitheliomatous appearance.

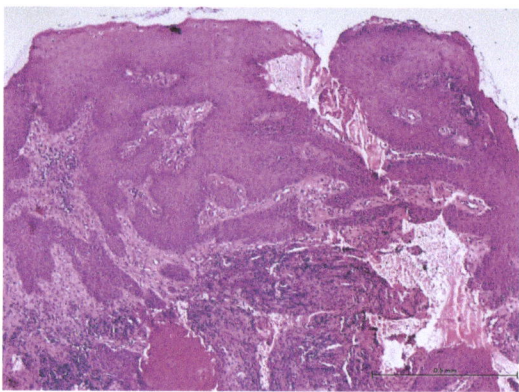

Figure 10. Histologic aspects in H&E staining (magnification ×100); the subepithelial connective tissue showed a moderate, polymorphic inflammatory infiltrate consisting of lymphocytes, histiocytes, plasma cells, and eosinophils.

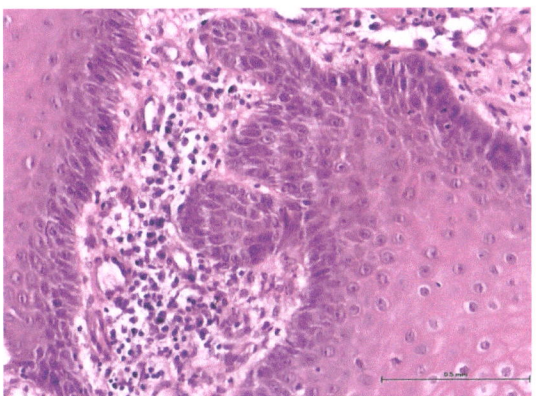

Figure 11. Histologic aspects in H&E staining (magnification ×200); interstitial edema, polymorphic inflammatory infiltrate, numerous small vessels with slightly ballooned endothelium, and red blood cells in the lumen.

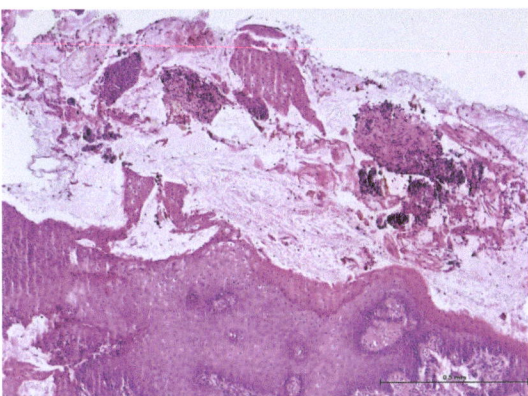

Figure 12. Histologic aspects in H&E staining (magnification ×100); dental plaque deposits were observed.

The palatal mucosa was partially covered by keratinized stratified squamous epithelium with foci of parakeratosis. Marked acanthosis of the spinous layer was observed in the areas with a pseudo-epitheliomatous appearance. Acanthosis with elongation of ridges in the spinous layer was also observed. In the connective tissue of the subepithelial layer, there was edema, a small polymorphic inflammatory infiltrate consisting of rare lymphocytes, rare histiocytes, plasma cells, and eosinophilic granulocytes. Numerous small, thin-walled vessels, some with ballooned endothelium and dilated endothelium, with or without the presence of haematocytes, were also visible, along with dilated lymphatic vessels. In the middle of the fragments, marked acanthosis areas showed a keratinization tendency. In eleven cases ($n = 11$) on the epithelium's surface, mucus deposits, fibrin-hematic material, and bacterial colonies (bacterial plaque) were observed.

After performing immunohistochemical reactions, the final histopathological diagnosis was reactive acanthosis of the palatal epithelium, likely due to mechanical causes, with a tendency for keratinization (Figures 13–18).

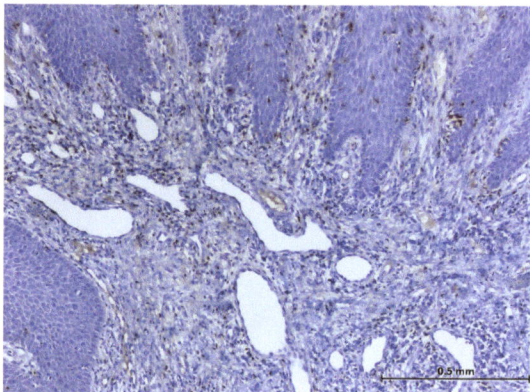

Figure 13. Immunohistochemistry: CD3 reaction highlights rare T lymphocytes (magnification ×100).

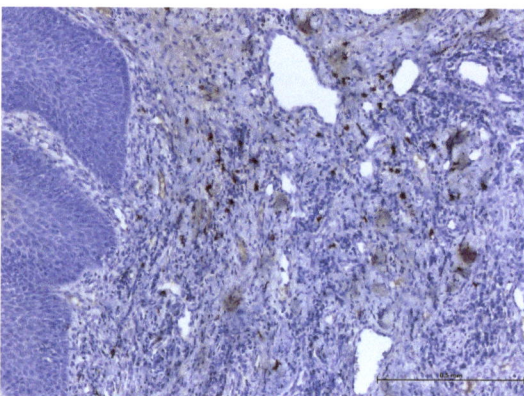

Figure 14. Immunohistochemistry: CD20 reaction highlights rare B lymphocytes (magnification ×100).

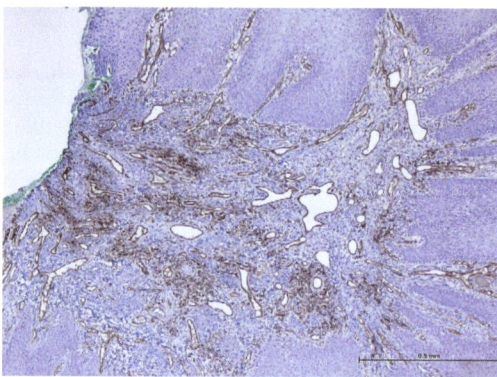

Figure 15. Immunohistochemistry: CD31 reaction marks endothelial cells of blood and lymphatic vessels (magnification ×100).

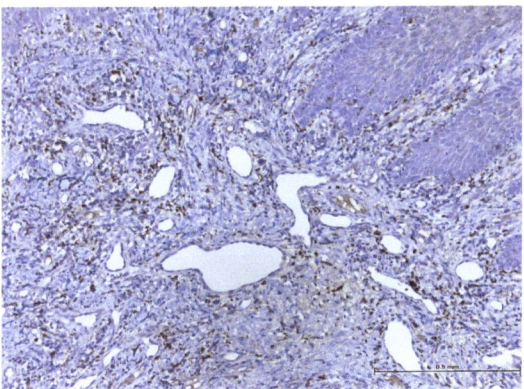

Figure 16. Immunohistochemistry: CD8 reaction shows a moderate number of macrophages (magnification ×100).

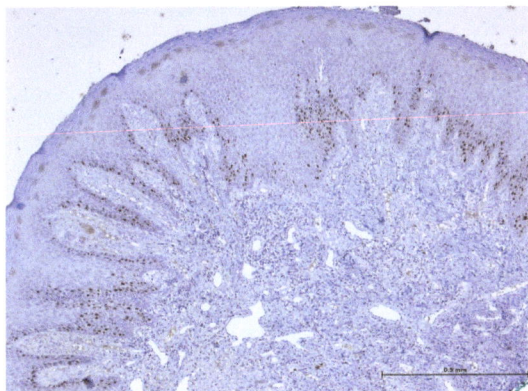

Figure 17. Immunohistochemistry: Ki-67 nuclear proliferation index marks the basal keratinocytes (magnification ×50).

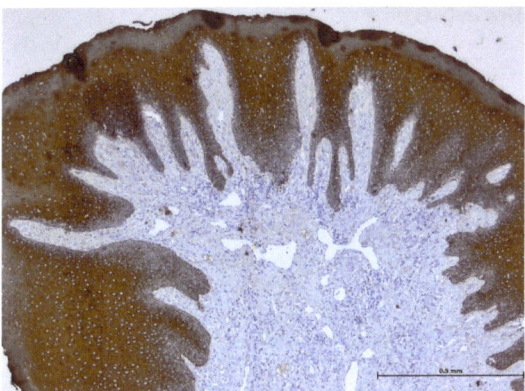

Figure 18. Immunohistochemistry: Anti-Pan Keratin marks the surface epithelium (magnification ×50).

The changes identified were specific to mechanical traumatic injuries, thus excluding hyperplasia from other etiologies (infectious, tumoral, or non-mechanical traumatic). The examined fragments showed hyperplasia, with widening of the spinous layer (acanthosis) without acantholysis and without hyperkeratosis. The elongated ridges showed a slight tendency to merge. The epithelium was mostly destroyed and partially replaced by granular tissue. Around the large vessels, with their partial interest, numerous granulocytes were highlighted, penetrating from the outside towards the middle of the vessel. Histologically, the masticatory mucosa has a partially ortho-keratinized and para-keratinized stratified squamous epithelium. The amount of keratinization of the oral mucosa reflects the amount of stress or mechanical abrasion that the region experiences. An ortho-keratinized epithelium contains keratinocytes with keratin and nuclei, whereas the para-keratinized epithelium lacks nuclei. Differentiating between ortho- and para-keratinized tissue is based on appearance and has no clinical significance. Because this mucosa is generally under higher stress levels, it has more pronounced dermal papillae and rete ridges than the oral lining mucosa. The layer of connective tissue termed lamina propria is located underneath the epithelium and comprises collagen, blood vessels, neurons, fibroblasts, and a small number of inflammatory cells.

Trauma caused by the insertion of an expander into the oral cavity was considered to be the causative factor of the inflammatory reaction. The continuous irritating factor was represented by the presence of the expander, and, in some cases, the tongue crib was considered a contributing factor to the inflammation.

4. Discussion

This study was performed in order to improve our insight into the role of palatal expanders that might induce palatal and gingival overgrowth during orthodontic force application. On average, after six months of expander placement, the authors detected, using clinical and histopathological examinations, a clear diagnosis of mechanically induced hyperplasia. From a total of twenty-five ($n. 25$) cases analyzed, sixteen patients were treated with tooth-borne rapid palatal expanders, and nine ($n. 9$) were treated with mini-implant-assisted rapid palatal expansion devices. The degree of severity varied from one patient to another, especially depending on the distance from the palatal mucosa where the expander was inserted, the reactivity of the patient, compliance with the recommendations related to the expander activation, and the hygiene of the patients. These results are consistent with similar previous studies published in the literature [13–16]. Furthermore, as suggested by previous studies [17–19], although the occurrence of hyperplasia was not directly correlated with the patients' hygiene, patients with inadequate hygiene presented a high degree of severity of inflammation. The presence of bonded fixed orthodontic appliances also had a negative impact on gingival health.

Of the twenty-five cases, the insertion distance between the palatal mucosa and the appliance was less than 2 mm in five patients, 2 mm in twelve patients, and 3 mm in eight patients. On average, patients with an expander inserted at 3 mm presented a lower degree of inflammation of the palatal mucosa without influencing the results, followed by orthodontic treatment. Patients with the expander at a distance of 1.5 mm presented severe mucosal hyperplasia. Patients with an expander inserted at 2 mm showed a variable degree of hyperplasia. Considering these aspects, the authors conclude that the proximity of the expander to the mucosa represents an irritating thorn which has a role as a favoring factor in the occurrence of inflammation. Among the twenty-five cases, only two patients did not fully comply with the indications related to expander activation; overactivation was observed in those cases. In these cases, patients presented a higher degree of hyperplasia, confirming the negative role of overactivation due to the non-adaptation of bone structures to the new clinical situation. These results were also observed by previous researchers like Jeon et al. (2002) [20] and Yacout et al. (2022) [21].

Six of the patients described an increased sensitivity to mechanical trauma, with the rapid appearance of ecchymoses or hematomas even at low intensities of the traumatic factor. However, no significant differences were observed between these patients and the rest in terms of the severity of the inflammatory reaction in the oral mucosa. Schuster et al. [22]

reported medical complications such as pain and decubitae in a third of the inquired offices, but they suggested that side effects of RME are often temporary and permanent damages are rather rare. No significant differences were observed in the degree of hyperplasia in male versus female patients. Related to the age of the patients, the study group between thirteen and sixteen years old showed, in general, more severe forms of hyperplasia compared to patients over sixteen years old. Further studies conducted by Bishara et al. [23] regarding the age of patients concluded that the side effects of RME tend to be smaller in children than they are in adolescence and adults and are associated with the degree of skeletal maturity. Furthermore, Capelozza et al. [24] noticed multiple side effects, such as pain, edema, and ulceration, when using palatal expansion in adult patients. In the present study, although the reactions were more severe, no biological samples were collected to see the blood level of hormones, but the authors suspect this factor to be relevant, considering the results obtained in the mentioned age categories. Future studies can be relevant to support these findings and to observe if there could be a possible relationship between blood hormone levels and the degree of inflammation. As a treatment option for persistent palatal hypertrophy associated with maxillary expansion procedures, Omezli et al. [13] suggest that, under general anesthesia, the hypertrophic areas in the palatal region be excised with the help of a scalpel and electrocautery to smooth the area of the palatal mucosa in order to prevent food retention.

Careful design and application of the MARPE appliance can achieve successful transverse expansion of the maxilla and the surrounding structures in patients beyond the age typically considered acceptable for traditional rapid palatal expansion, with minor buccal tipping but without bone loss or trauma of the palatal mucosa [25]. Tsai et al. [26] conducted a study on twenty-nine patients treated with MARPE and found that 48.3% of the subjects reported swelling or inflammation over the palatal mucosa, 41.4% of the subjects complained of difficulty cleaning around the device, and 37.9% experienced soft tissue impingement during expansion.

The widening of maxillofacial spaces is a significant factor in the improvement of nasal breathing, a major advantage of the use of RPE. In children, the use of RME can reduce tonsillar and adenoidal volume, as reported by Yoon et al. [27]. Some of the most significant results of the use of RPE in the aforementioned study are the reduction in adenoidal volume experienced by 90% of children and the tonsillar volume reduction experienced by 97.5% of children. The average volume decreases were 20.1% and 40.2%, as measured by CBTC. RPE usage shows other significant positive effects, including a reduction in oral breathing, likely associated with enhanced nasal philtrum [28]. This also led to a lower rate of nasal-respiratory infections.

The use of RPE can also have positive implications for reducing the effects of obstructive sleep apnea (OSA) [29]. This is likely due to a combination of factors, including lower tongue collapse incidence associated with persistent oral breathing, adeno-tonsillar volume decreases, and pharyngeal segment stiffening. Another positive impact of the use of RPE is the improvement of Eustachian tube function. It improves the strength of the tensor palatine muscles and the function of the elevator, leading to a reduced occurrence of ear infections, a leading cause of hearing loss.

Previous researchers, like Stasiak et al. [30], demonstrated in a very comprehensive systematic review that it is not possible to establish the generally recommended target site for the placement of the mini-implants in the area. The high variability of bone measurements and the lack of reliable predictors of bone availability justify the use of CBCT for mini-implant trajectory planning.

Although no significant results were found in this study regarding a possible correlation between gingival overgrowth and the age of the patients, some authors, like Guan et al. [31], emphasize the importance of early orthodontic treatment as it helps patients achieve balanced development of masticatory function.

The reduction in bone density through the removal of myeloid HIF1 and impaired Acp5 and Rank1 gene expressions leads to significantly higher induced tooth movement.

This has been demonstrated in recent experiments by Kirschneck et al. [32]. It could be an alternative therapeutic approach to lower treatment-related periodontal hazards.

The strengths of this study reside in the histological examination, which revealed the mechanical character of the lesion, strengthening the causal relationship between the insertion of the expander and the occurrence of hyperplasia. This is based on histological indicators, including acanthosis phenomena and the destruction of epithelial tissue, followed by its replacement with granulation tissue.

This study had several limitations. The suggested methodology is difficult to apply in practice considering the costs of histopathological examination. Moreover, the study needs to be applied to an adequate number of cases to confirm whether the type of design and activation time could influence the results and to follow both the clinical and stability outcomes of the use of palatal expanders. Comparative studies can be conducted to evaluate the efficacy of these devices. Long-term studies assessing this clinical situation could provide valuable insights. Clearly, a more thorough analysis is needed to fully understand the cause of malocclusion and define proper treatment.

5. Conclusions

Following the results of this study, the authors can conclude that the type of palatal expander influences the degree of inflammation, the severity of hyperplasia was more pronounced in the case of MARPE than in the case of RPE usage, the analysis of the distance between the expander and the palatal mucosa did not provide conclusive results, and the incidence and severity of the reaction were variable in patients with the same distance between the expander and the palatal or gingival mucosa. Additionally, overactivation of the expander caused increased hyperplasia of the palatal mucosa. The histopathological examination revealed the mechanical character of the lesion, strengthening the causal relationship between the insertion of the expander and the occurrence of hyperplasia of the palatal mucosa.

Author Contributions: Conceptualization, E.B. and A.V.; methodology, A.B. and A.-R.S.; software, A.M.; validation, M.P., A.V., G.M. and E.B.; investigation, A.B. and A.-R.S.; writing—original draft preparation, A.V.; writing—review and editing, M.P. and E.B.; visualization, A.M.; supervision, M.P., G.M.; project administration, E.B. and A.B. All authors have read and agreed to the published version of the manuscript.

Funding: This work was supported by the George Emil Palade University of Medicine, Pharmacy, Sciences, and Technology of Târgu Mures, Research Grant number 163/1/10.01.2023.

Institutional Review Board Statement: This study was conducted in compliance with the Declaration of Helsinki. Ethical clearance was obtained from the Institutional Review Board of Sc Algocalm Srl Private Medical Clinic, number 994/01.02.2023.

Informed Consent Statement: Informed consent was obtained from all subjects involved in the study.

Data Availability Statement: The supporting information for this research can be checked with the corresponding authors at: alexandru.vlasa@umfst.ro; anamaria.bud@umfst.ro.

Conflicts of Interest: The authors declare no conflict of interest.

List of Abbreviation

RPE	Rapid Palatal expander
MARPE	Mini-implant anchorage rapid palatal expander
PICO	Population, intervention, control, and outcomes
Pwr	Power
H&E	Hematoxylin and Eosin
AE1/AE3/PCK26	Anti-Pan Keratin primary antibody
CONFIRM Anti-Ki-67	Rabbitt Monoclonal Primary Antibody
CD31 (JC70)	Mouse Monoclonal Antibody

References

1. Ozgoz, M.; Arabaci, T. Chronic Inflammatory Gingival Enlargement and Treatment: A Case Report. *Adv. Dent. Oral Health* **2018**, *9*, 555766. [CrossRef]
2. Ferreira, L.; Peng, H.-H.; Cox, D.P.; Chambers, D.W.; Bhula, A.; Young, J.D.; Ojcius, D.M.; Ramos-Junior, E.S.; Morandini, A.C. Investigation of foreign materials in gingival lesions: A clinicopathologic, energy-dispersive microanalysis of the lesions and in vitro confirmation of pro-inflammatory effects of the foreign materials. *Oral Surg. Oral Med. Oral Pathol. Oral Radiol.* **2019**, *128*, 250–267. [CrossRef]
3. O'connell, S.; Davies, J.; Smallridge, J.; Vaidyanathan, M. Amelogenesis imperfecta associated with dental follicular-like hamartomas and generalised gingival enlargement. *Eur. Arch. Paediatr. Dent.* **2013**, *15*, 361–368. [CrossRef]
4. Rosa, E.P.; Murakami-Malaquias-Silva, F.; Schalch, T.O.; Teixeira, D.B.; Horliana, R.F.; Tortamano, A.; Tortamano, I.P.; Buscariolo, I.A.; Longo, P.L.; Negreiros, R.M.; et al. Efficacy of photodynamic therapy and periodontal treatment in patients with gingivitis and fixed orthodontic appliances. *Medicine* **2020**, *99*, e19429. [CrossRef] [PubMed]
5. Cekici, A.; Kantarci, A.; Hasturk, H.; Van Dyke, T.E. Inflammatory and immune pathways in the pathogenesis of periodontal disease. *Periodontol. 2000* **2013**, *64*, 57–80. [CrossRef] [PubMed]
6. Gual-Vaques, P.; Jane-Salas, E.; Egido-Moreno, S.; Ayuso-Montero, R.; Mari-Roig, A.; Lopez-Lopez, J. Inflammatory papillary hyperplasia: A systematic review. *Med. Oral Patol. Oral Cir. Buccal* **2016**, *22*, e36–e42. [CrossRef]
7. Brunetto, D.P.; Sant'Anna, E.F.; Machado, A.W.; Moon, W. Non-surgical treatment of transverse deficiency in adults using Micro implant-assisted Rapid Palatal Expansion (MARPE). *Dent. Press J. Orthod.* **2017**, *22*, 110–125. [CrossRef] [PubMed]
8. Lo Giudice, A.; Barbato, E.; Cosentino, L.; Ferraro, C.M.; Leonardi, R. Alveolar bone changes after rapid maxillary expansion with tooth-born appliances: A systematic review. *Eur. J. Orthod.* **2017**, *40*, 296–303. [CrossRef]
9. Bucci, R.; D'Antò, V.; Rongo, R.; Valletta, R.; Martina, R.; Michelotti, A. Dental and skeletal effects of palatal expansion techniques: A systematic review of the current evidence from systematic reviews and meta-analyses. *J. Oral Rehabil.* **2016**, *43*, 543–564. [CrossRef]
10. Campanile, G.L.; Lotti, T.M.; Orlandini, S.Z. Macroscopic Anatomy, Histology and Electron Microscopy of the Oral Cavity and Normal Anatomic Variants. In *Oral Diseases*; Springer: Berlin/Heidelberg, Germany, 1999; pp. 1–5. [CrossRef]
11. Oh, H.; Park, J.; Lagravere-Vich, M.O. Comparison of traditional RPE with two types of micro-implant assisted RPE: CBCT study. *Semin. Orthod.* **2019**, *25*, 60–68. [CrossRef]
12. Centre for Evidence-Based Medicine (CEBM). Asking Focused Questions. University of Oxford, Oxford, UK. Available online: https://www.cebm.ox.ac.uk/resources/ebm-tools/asking-focused-questions (accessed on 25 October 2023).
13. Ömezli, M.M.; Torul, D.; Avci, T. Persistent Palatal Hypertrophy Associated with Rapid Maxillary Expansion Procedure: Report of a Rare Case. *Biomedicine* **2020**, *10*, 49–51. [CrossRef] [PubMed]
14. Pinto, A.S.; Alves, L.S.; Zenkner, J.E.; Zanatta, A.; Maltz, F.B. Gingival enlargement in orthodontic patients: Effect of treatment duration. *Am. J. Orthod. Dentofac. Orthop.* **2017**, *152*, 477–482. [CrossRef] [PubMed]
15. Manuelli, M.; Marcolina, M.; Nardi, N.; Bertossi, D.; De Santis, D.; Ricciardi, G.; Luciano, U.; Nocini, R.; Mainardi, A.; Lissoni, A.; et al. Oral mucosal complications in orthodontic treatment. *Minerva Dent. Oral Sci.* **2019**, *68*, 84–88. [CrossRef] [PubMed]
16. Awartani, F.; Atassi, F. Oral Hygiene Status among Orthodontic Patients. *J. Contemp. Dent. Pract.* **2010**, *11*, 25–32. [CrossRef]
17. Arab, S.; Malekshah, S.N.; Mehrizi, E.A.; Khanghah, A.E.; Naseh, R.; Imani, M.M. Effect of fixed orthodontic treatment on salivary flow, pH and microbial count. *J. Dent.* **2016**, *13*, 18–22.
18. Türkkahraman, H.; Sayin, M.O.; Bozkurt, F.Y.; Yetkin, Z.; Kaya, S.; Onal, S. Archwireligation techniques, microbial colonization, and periodontal status inorthodontically treated patients. *Angle Orthod.* **2005**, *75*, 231–236.
19. Sukontapatipark, W.; El-Agroudi, M.A.; Selliseth, N.J.; Thunold, K.; Selvig, K.A. Bacterial colonization associated with fixed orthodontic appliances. A scanning electron microscopy study. *Eur. J. Orthod.* **2001**, *23*, 475–484. [CrossRef] [PubMed]
20. Jeon, J.Y.; Choi, S.-H.; Chung, C.J.; Lee, K.-J. The success and effectiveness of miniscrew-assisted rapid palatal expansion are age- and sex-dependent. *Clin. Oral Investig.* **2022**, *26*, 2993–3003. [CrossRef]
21. Yacout, Y.M.; Abdalla, E.M.; El Harouny, N.M. Skeletal and dentoalveolar effects of slow vs rapid activation protocols of miniscrew-supported maxillary expanders in adolescents: A randomized clinical trial. *Angle Orthod.* **2022**, *92*, 579–588. [CrossRef]
22. Schuster, G.; Borel-Scherf, I.; Schopf, P.M. Frequency of and complications in the use of RPE appliances—Results of a survey in the Federal State of Hesse, Germany. *J. Orofac. Orthop.* **2005**, *66*, 148–161. [CrossRef]
23. Bishara, S.E.; Staley, R.N. Maxillary expansion: Clinical implications. *Am. J. Orthod. Dentofac. Orthop.* **1987**, *91*, 3–14. [CrossRef] [PubMed]
24. Capelozza Filho, L.; da Silva Filho, O.G.; Ursi, W.J. Non-surgically assisted rapid maxillary expansion in adults. *Int. J. Adult Orthod. Orthognath. Surg.* **1996**, *11*, 57–70.
25. Carlson, C.; Sung, J.; McComb, R.W.; Machado, A.W.; Moon, W. Microimplant-assisted rapid palatal expansion appliance to orthopedically correct transverse maxillary deficiency in an adult. *Am. J. Orthod. Dentofac. Orthop.* **2016**, *149*, 716–728. [CrossRef] [PubMed]
26. Tsai, H.-R.; Ho, K.-H.; Wang, C.-W.; Wang, K.-L.; Hsieh, S.-C.; Chang, H.-M. Evaluation of Patients' Experiences after Microimplant-Assisted Rapid Palatal Expansion (MARPE) Treatment. *Taiwan. J. Orthod.* **2021**, *33*, 2. [CrossRef]
27. Yoon, A.; Abdelwahab, M.; Bockow, R.; Vakili, A.; Lovell, K.; Chang, I.; Ganguly, R.; Liu, S.Y.-C.; Kushida, C.; Hong, C. Impact of rapid palatal expansion on the size of adenoids and tonsils in children. *Sleep Med.* **2022**, *92*, 96–102. [CrossRef] [PubMed]

28. Compadretti, G.C.; Tasca, I.; Alessandri-Bonetti, G.; Peri, S.; D'addario, A. Acoustic rhinometric measurements in children undergoing rapid maxillary expansion. *Int. J. Pediatr. Otorhinolaryngol.* **2006**, *70*, 27–34. [CrossRef] [PubMed]
29. Cerritelli, L.; Hatzopoulos, S.; Catalano, A.; Bianchini, C.; Cammaroto, G.; Meccariello, G.; Iannella, G.; Vicini, C.; Pelucchi, S.; Skarzynski, P.H.; et al. Rapid Maxillary Expansion (RME): An Otolaryngologic Perspective. *J. Clin. Med.* **2022**, *11*, 5243. [CrossRef]
30. Stasiak, M.; Adamska, P. Should Cone-Beam Computed Tomography Be Performed Prior to Orthodontic Miniscrew Placement in the Infrazygomatic Crest Area?—A Systematic Review. *Biomedicines* **2023**, *11*, 2389. [CrossRef]
31. Guan, H.; Yonemitsu, I.; Ikeda, Y.; Ono, T. Reversible Effects of Functional Mandibular Lateral Shift on Masticatory Muscles in Growing Rats. *Biomedicines* **2023**, *11*, 2126. [CrossRef]
32. Kirschneck, C.; Straßmair, N.; Cieplik, F.; Paddenberg, E.; Jantsch, J.; Proff, P.; Schröder, A. Myeloid HIF1α Is Involved in the Extent of Orthodontically Induced Tooth Movement. *Biomedicines* **2021**, *9*, 796. [CrossRef]

Disclaimer/Publisher's Note: The statements, opinions and data contained in all publications are solely those of the individual author(s) and contributor(s) and not of MDPI and/or the editor(s). MDPI and/or the editor(s) disclaim responsibility for any injury to people or property resulting from any ideas, methods, instructions or products referred to in the content.

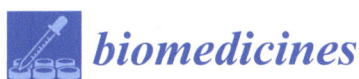

Review

The Potential Role of Ionic Liquid as a Multifunctional Dental Biomaterial

Md Iqbal Hossain [1], Abdullah Bin Shams [2], Shuvashis Das Gupta [3], Gary J. Blanchard [1], Ali Mobasheri [3,4,5,6] and Ehsanul Hoque Apu [3,7,8,9,10,*]

1. Department of Chemistry, Michigan State University, East Lansing, MI 48824, USA; hossai13@chemistry.msu.edu (M.I.H.); blanchard@chemistry.msu.edu (G.J.B)
2. The Edward S. Rogers Sr. Department of Electrical Computer Engineering, University of Toronto, Toronto, ON M5S 3G4, Canada; abdullahbinshams@gmail.com
3. Research Unit of Health Science and Technology, Faculty of Medicine, University of Oulu, 90220 Oulu, Finland; shuvashis.dasgupta@oulu.fi (S.D.G.); ali.mobasheri@oulu.fi (A.M.)
4. Division of Public Health, Epidemiology and Health Economics, WHO Collaborating Center for Public Health Aspects of Musculo-Skeletal Health and Ageing, University of Liège, 4000 Liège, Belgium
5. State Research Institute Centre for Innovative Medicine, 08410 Vilnius, Lithuania
6. Department of Joint Surgery, The First Affiliated Hospital of Sun Yat-sen University, Guangzhou 510080, China
7. Department of Biomedical Sciences, College of Dental Medicine, Lincoln Memorial University, Knoxville, TN 37923, USA
8. Institute for Quantitative Health Science and Engineering, Department of Biomedical Engineering, Michigan State University, East Lansing, MI 48824, USA
9. Division of Hematology and Oncology, Department of Internal Medicine, Michigan Medicine, University of Michigan, Ann Arbor, MI 48109, USA
10. Centre for International Public Health and Environmental Research, Bangladesh (CIPHER,B), Dhaka 1207, Bangladesh
* Correspondence: ehsanul.hoqueapu@oulu.fi or ehsanul.hoqueapu@lmunet.edu

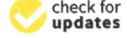

Citation: Hossain, M.I.; Shams, A.B.; Das Gupta, S.; Blanchard, G.J.; Mobasheri, A.; Hoque Apu, E. The Potential Role of Ionic Liquid as a Multifunctional Dental Biomaterial. *Biomedicines* **2023**, *11*, 3093. https://doi.org/10.3390/biomedicines11113093

Academic Editors: Gianluca Gambarini, Giuseppe Minervini and Gianmarco Abbadessa

Received: 6 September 2023
Revised: 27 October 2023
Accepted: 14 November 2023
Published: 20 November 2023

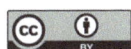

Copyright: © 2023 by the authors. Licensee MDPI, Basel, Switzerland. This article is an open access article distributed under the terms and conditions of the Creative Commons Attribution (CC BY) license (https://creativecommons.org/licenses/by/4.0/).

Abstract: In craniofacial research and routine dental clinical procedures, multifunctional materials with antimicrobial properties are in constant demand. Ionic liquids (ILs) are one such multifunctional intelligent material. Over the last three decades, ILs have been explored for different biomedical applications due to their unique physical and chemical properties, high task specificity, and sustainability. Their stable physical and chemical characteristics and extremely low vapor pressure make them suitable for various applications. Their unique properties, such as density, viscosity, and hydrophilicity/hydrophobicity, may provide higher performance as a potential dental material. ILs have functionalities for optimizing dental implants, infiltrate materials, oral hygiene maintenance products, and restorative materials. They also serve as sensors for dental chairside usage to detect oral cancer, periodontal lesions, breath-based sobriety, and dental hard tissue defects. With further optimization, ILs might also make vital contributions to craniofacial regeneration, oral hygiene maintenance, oral disease prevention, and antimicrobial materials. This review explores the different advantages and properties of ILs as possible dental material.

Keywords: biomaterials; dental materials; ionic liquids (ILs); tissue regeneration and multifunctional

1. Introduction

The first ionic liquid (IL), ethylammonium nitrate, was reported in 1914 by Paul Walden [1]. In 1992, Wilkes and Zaworotko [2] reported the first 1-ethyl-3-methylimidazolium-based air and moisture-stable imidazolium-based ILs, garnering the attention of the research community. To date, this compound class has been used in most science and technology spheres. ILs are salts of relatively large organic cations and inorganic or organic anions. Generally, at least one of the ions is voluminous, asymmetric, and contains nonpolar tails or combinations of these properties. The bulky and asymmetric ions of ILs, compared to simple ions of classical inorganic salts, such as NaCl, prevent crystallization at ambient temperature, with melting points below 100 °C. When the melting points are near or below room temperature, the ILs are termed as room-temperature ionic liquids (RTILs) [3].

ILs have drawn attention due to their attractive properties, including low vapor pressure, high chemical and thermal stability, wide electrochemical window, nonflammability, and the ability to dissolve various organic and inorganic materials. The properties of ILs, such as density, viscosity, and hydrophilicity/hydrophobicity, can be modified by judicious selection of cations and anions, by fine-tuning the lengths of the cation alkyl chain, or by the covalent tethering of task-specific functionalities to one or both of the constituent ions [4–10]. Hence, ILs are frequently referred to as task-specific or designer solvents. Cations and anions of some of the discussed ionic liquids are shown in Figure 1.

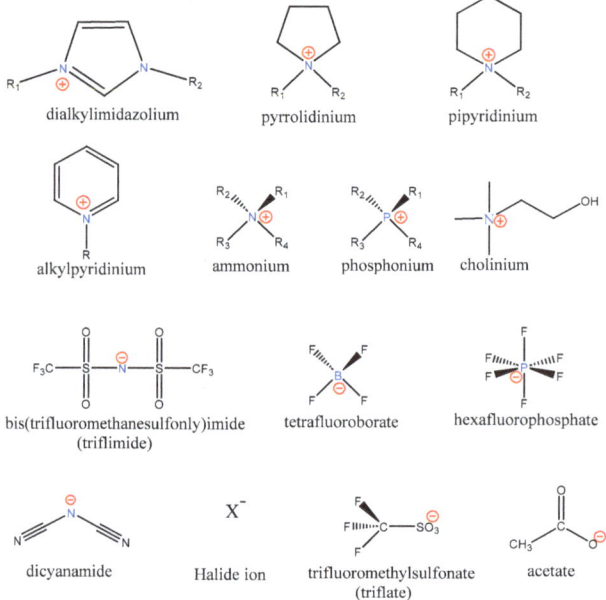

Figure 1. Chemical structures of some typical Ionic Liquid cations and anions [11].

The unique properties of ILs make them particularly promising candidates as environmentally benign or "green" alternatives to organic solvents for chemical synthesis [12], catalysis [13], separation [14], and extraction [15]. Moreover, they represent safe and versatile electrolytes for electrochemical applications (lithium batteries, supercapacitors, and fuel cells) and photovoltaics (dye-sensitized solar cells (DSSCs) [16]). They are also novel functional materials [17] for lubrication [18], microfluidics [19], and sensors [20]. Additionally, the antimicrobial properties of ILs, discovered two decades ago, have facilitated their use in numerous biomedical applications as novel biomaterials.

Although few reviews have explained the potentiality of ILs in biomedical applications, none have discussed the potential role of ILs in dentistry and craniofacial sciences in details. This comprehensive review is a pioneering study in dentistry and craniofacial engineering, exploring the different functionalities and applications of ILs in this field.

2. Ionic Liquids as Antimicrobial Agents

According to the Centers for Disease Control and Prevention (CDC) of the United States (U.S.) [21,22], more than 3 million people become infected with antimicrobial-resistant pathogens, resulting in 48,000 deaths annually in the U.S. These infections are associated with a more than $4.6 billion annual burden on the health care system. These numbers will increase unless action is taken. Therefore, antimicrobial resistance is a pressing issue that must be overcome in global health. While overuse and misuse of antibiotics are growing concerns, the lack of novel antibiotics for resistant bacteria is the main challenge. Therefore, the search for next-generation antibiotics is a race against time. With high tunability and task-specificity, ILs have been envisaged as a promising next-generation antibiotic for resistant microorganisms [23].

Cell membranes, both plasma membranes or internal membranes are made of glycerophospholipids: a glycerol, phosphate group, and two fatty acid chains. Glycerol is a three-carbon poly alcohol that acts as the connector and attaches the phosphate polar (hydrophilic) head group and two nonpolar, hydrophobic hydrocarbon fatty acid tails [24]. The different components of a model lipid bilayer are shown in Figure 2. Cholesterols (not present in the bacterial cell membrane) regulate cell membrane fluidity (stiffness). Cholesterol also plays an essential role in maintaining the integrity of lipid membranes. Xiao-Lei et al. used an egg sphingomyelin (SM)-cholesterol model membrane to show that, in the absence of cholesterol, the meager molar IL: SM ratio can disrupt the model membrane [25]. Transmembrane proteins are embedded into the cell membrane and are responsible for the controlled transportation of materials into and out of the cell [26].

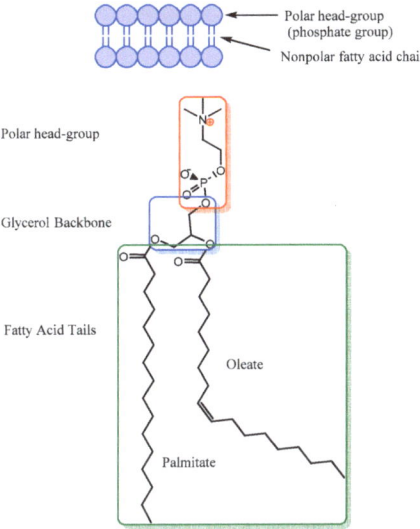

Figure 2. Different components of a model lipid bilayer (Phospholipid) [25].

Due to the surface charge (phosphate head group) of the lipid bi-layer, the cationic moiety of the ILs adsorbed on the lipid membrane interacts with the transdermal protein and disorganizes the bi-layer with the penetration of its long alkyl chain, which ultimately changes the regular properties of a cell membrane [27–29]. The longer the alkyl chain, the higher the antibacterial activity [30]. Fluidity (stiffness) and membrane potential changes affect the biochemical gradients and interrupt the controlled exchange of intercellular and extracellular materials by affecting standard diffusion rates and transdermal protein stability. ILs sometimes initiate irreversible cell wall damage by creating permanent pores, another critical cause of the sub-cellular imbalance [31–33]. Overall, the antimicrobial activity of ILs can be divided into several steps. First, ILs are absorbed into cell membranes due to the electrostatic interactions of the polar head group. Second, they interact with the transmembrane protein. Third, they penetrate the phospholipid bilayer with their hydrophobic tails, disrupting the layer, causing intracellular cytoplasm leakage, and leading to cell lysis [34] (Figure 3). RTILs, based on imidazolium cation with a long alkyl chain and hydrophobic anion bis(trifluoromethansulfonyl)imide (NTf2), show antibacterial activity.

The positive charge of the imidazolium ion is electrostatically attracted to the membrane's negatively charged phosphate head groups while its alkyl long chain can easily penetrate the bacterial cell wall [35]. In particular, the hydrophobic anion (NTf2) of ILs may increase their antibacterial properties by disorganizing membranes.

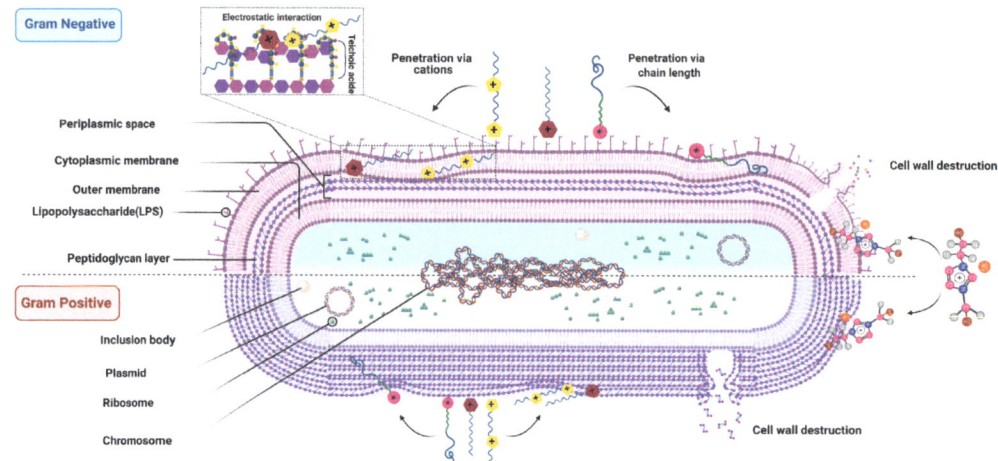

Figure 3. Illustration of how ionic liquids interact with the bacterial cell membrane (both Grampositive and Gram-negative) and ultimately cause cell lysis. Reproduced with permission [34].

Parameters to Control Antimicrobial Properties

Antimicrobial properties can be enhanced by increasing the alkyl chain length. In a recent study, replacing an alkyl group with a phenolic group and increasing the other alkyl chain length of an imidazolium-based IL exhibited minimal inhibitory concentrations (MICs) < 7.81 µM against *Pseudomonas aeruginosa*, *Escherichia coli*, and *Staphylococcus aureus* [30]. ILs become absorbed into the cell membrane by electrostatic interactions between ILs and the polar head groups. Therefore, increasing the number of cations in per-ionic liquids can enhance the efficacy of ILs as antimicrobial agents [29,31]. Polymeric ionic liquids (PILs) are more effective than monomers as one can tune the hydrophobicity and charge density (number of cations) in PILs. Therefore, PILs with better efficacy and lower MIC values than their monomers are better antimicrobial agents for resistant bacteria [23].

3. Biomedical Applications of Ionic Liquids

A series of experimental and computational studies [36–41] have proven that when the ILs' alkyl chain length becomes longer than four carbons, they aggregate and form a nonpolar domain. These nonpolar domains permeate the three-dimensional ionic networks. While the chain length increases, these nonpolar domains become larger and more connected, exhibiting microphase segregation. Ionic liquids show this property even in mixtures with water or other molecular solvents like DMSO, propylene carbonate, acetonitrile, and short-chain primary alcohol [9,10]. This unique property of ILs and their binary mixture with molecular solvents make them universal drug solubilizing agents. The limiting factor for different drug molecules is their poor solubility in biological media and cellular matrices mainly composed of water. RTILs are superior drug delivery materials compared to commonly used salts in pharmaceuticals since they do not possess crystal polymorphism problems and can dissolve organic and inorganic materials. Therefore, turning most drugs into ILs will enhance their therapeutic utility [42–44], making them an active pharmaceutical ingredient ionic liquid (API-IL). Targeted drug delivery encompasses drug packaging, transport to the targeted area, and controlled release. ILs can play a significant role in all areas as they circumvent biological barriers without hampering biological activity [45–47]. Different approaches, such as micelles, inverted micelles, vesicles, liposomes, nanoparticles, emulsions (micro or nano), hydrogels, etc., load drugs and carry them to the targeted area, then control release by photo or thermal sensitivity. ILs can be tailored easily to form emulsions (ILs-in-water and ILs-in-oil). ILs can be used as polar media in IL-in-oil or nonpolar media with a significant alkyl chain length in IL-in-water emulsions. By replacing one of the alkyl groups with task-specific functionality and a large alkyl chain in the other, ILs can form micelles without surfactants. Studies have found the highest drug loading and targeted drug delivery [48–50]. Properties of hydrogel, ionogels, and thermoresponsive gels can be tuned using task-specific ILs and can be used for controlled drug release [51,52].

The long-term stability of proteins is essential in terms of dealing with proteins. Generally, proteins are folded to avoid loss due to aggregation. Instead of aqueous buffers, ILs help prevent aggregation and reverse aggregation or refolding (only 3% loss) for many cycles [53–55]. Controlled manipulations of the polar and nonpolar regions of ILs and their binary mixture enable them to offer low toxicity and thermal and conformational stability [56]. Although it is unclear how ILs interact with proteins, combinations of experimental and theoretical approaches are needed.

4. Ionic Liquid-Based Applications in Craniofacial Engineering and Dentistry
4.1. ILs in Dental Implants

According to the American Academy of Implant Dentistry (AAID) and the American College of Prosthodontists, approximately 36 million U.S. citizens have lost all their teeth, and 120 million are missing at least one. These numbers are expected to grow over the next two decades. People can lose their teeth irrespective of age to numerous causes, including decay, gum disease, injury, accident, cancer, etc. Loss of a single tooth worsens overall oral health by weakening the jawbone. Dental implants are the most common treatment for dental loss. An implant consists of three components: an implant post, a cylindrical screw-shaped device anchored into the mandibular bone that provides necessary support for a dental prosthesis (crown), and an abutment that connects dentures to dental posts (Figure 4). Endo-osseous implants are made of metal, which must be biocompatible, non-corrosive, and flexible with high strength. Pure titanium and different titanium alloys are common materials for endo-osseous implants. Their long-term clinical survival rate has made them the gold standard. Zirconium ceramics have been introduced as an alternative to titanium due to drawbacks reported in the literature, such as allergies, hypersensitivity, metal degradation, and discoloration in the peri-implant regions [57–59].

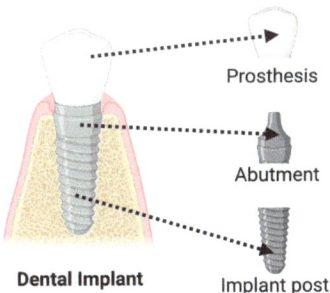

Figure 4. Components of a dental implant. Created with BioRender.com.

A successful dental implant is associated with the osseointegration of surrounding soft and bone tissues with the dental implant surface [60–63]. However, many factors, such as microbial biofilm formation, stress during insertion and mastication of the implant, corrosion, and systematic health and host immune-inflammatory responses, may affect the implant's long-term stability [62]. Therefore, implants are subjected to different processes, including sandblasting, selective ion etching, and bioactive coating to minimize surface roughness, formation of an anti-bacterial biofilm, etc. [64]. Implant surfaces are prone to bacterial colonization, resulting in a "race for the surface" between host tissues and bacteria. Therefore, anti-bacterial biofilm is a determining factor for the long-term stability of the dental implant and is considered a major determining factor of implant failure [65,66]. Zhao et al. have shown how the "race for the surface" occurs using human gingival fibroblasts and different supragingival bacterial strains [66]. Within the first hour, a protective soft tissue seal must form around the implant's neck to prevent bacterial colonization. If this does not occur (i.e., bacteria form a biofilm), fibroblasts lose the battle, and the implants must be replaced. ILs, especially dicationic ILs, have been used to prepare anti-bacterial biofilms, providing essential lubrication, corrosion resistance, and wear performance while maintaining compatibility with the host cells [67,68]. Since ILs act as antimicrobial agents, creating an IL layer can help provide conditions for fibroblast and pre-osteoblast growth and proliferation to form a seal, preventing bacterial growth [67,69,70]. Wheelis et al. evaluated the biocompatibility of dicationic IL coatings on commercially pure titanium disk (cpTi) in a subcutaneous implantation rat model [71]. They used two dicationic ionic liquids with two amino acid anions (IonL-Phe, IonL-Met) and three doses to investigate the interference of coatings in the osteointegration process during the early healing period (Figure 5). They did not observe significant interference in the early healing timeline or tissue regeneration. They also showed in separate studies [67,70] that dicationic IL film remains on the implant surface for more than seven days, maintaining growth conditions for human gingival fibroblasts and pre-osteoblasts while posing severe toxicity to bacterial cells, thus helping the host cells to commandeer the surface.

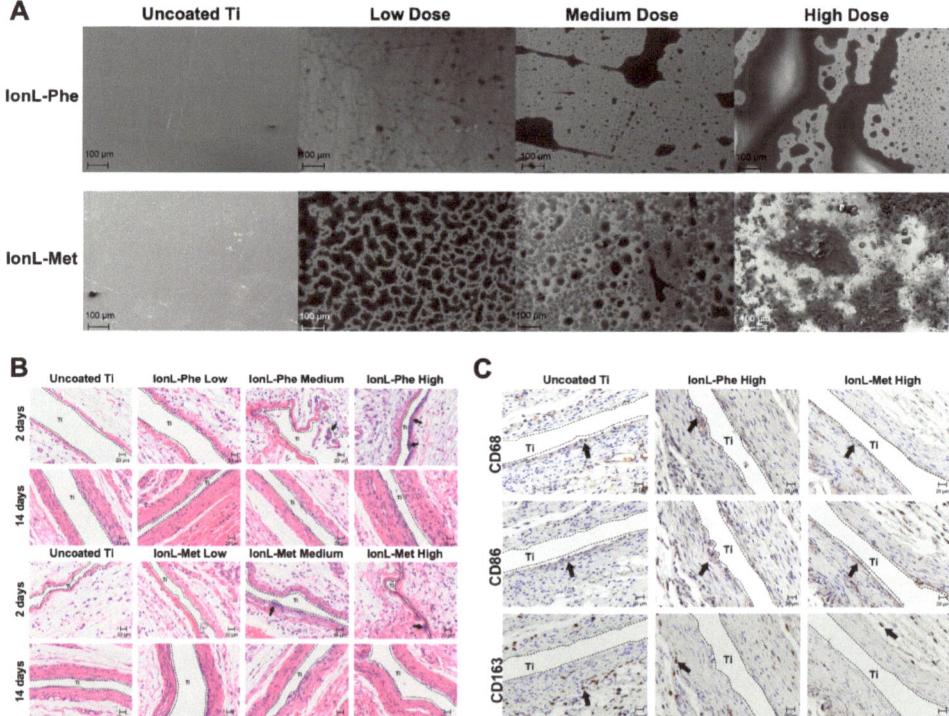

Figure 5. Ionic liquid-coated titanium implant. (**A**) SEM images of titanium surfaces coated and uncoated with ionic liquids at different doses (Scale bar 100 μm). (**B**) Hematoxylin and eosin staining

of titanium implants (coated and uncoated). Images show the healing representation (pointed with arrows) of post-implantation at 2 and 14 days (Scale bar 20 µm). (**C**) Areas marked with arrows showing inflammatory responses of surrounding tissues at 14 days (post-implantation) in coated and uncoated titanium implants (Scale bar 20 µm). Reproduced with permission [71].

4.2. ILs as Dental Infiltrant Materials

Non-cavitated carious lesions near dental surfaces are a prevalent dental disease [72]. To protect dental hard tissues, restorative materials are placed directly into a tooth cavity to prevent further expansion of lesions and restore dental functions and aesthetics. The American Dental Association (ADA) classified restorative materials into four categories in 2003: amalgam, resin-based composites, glass ionomer, and resin-modified glass ionomer. Proper diet, patient education on oral hygiene, and topical fluoride application are the primary treatments for incipient enamel caries lesions [73,74]. The next step is to apply biocompatible materials as resin infiltrates for superficial carious lesions. These infiltrates are light-curable resins that inhibit carious progression by sealing the lesion's body and pores in proximal dental surfaces [75–77].

Designing highly active antimicrobial surfaces or coatings is a significant challenge for public health. Resins are inert methacrylate monomers, such as triethylene glycol dimethacrylate (TEGDMA) and bisphenol A-glycidyl methacrylate (Bis-GMA), that lack antimicrobial activity. Hence, efforts are being made to endow resin infiltrates with antimicrobial properties. Cuppini et al. developed microcapsules loaded with 2.5wt%, 5wt%, or 10wt% ionic liquid as resin infiltrates [78] (Figure 6).

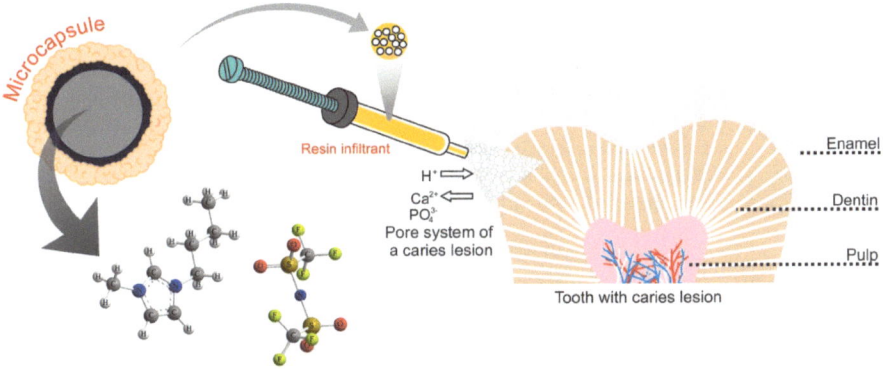

Figure 6. Microcapsules loaded with ionic liquids as dental resin infiltrates. Reproduced with permission [78].

Microcapsule-loaded RTILs show excellent antibacterial properties without changing other physicochemical properties or eliciting cytotoxicity (cell viability > 90%). In recent studies [79,80], three thermally stable epoxy-amine networks were synthesized using imidazolium-based ionic liquid monomers with similar thermomechanical properties to conventional diglycidyl ether (DGEBA) epoxy prepolymers. They further tested antimicrobial properties against *Escherichia coli* (*E. coli*) and found potent biofilm inhibition of ~92%. Importantly, imidazolium ionic liquids can replace carcinogenic bisphenol A. Recently, an RTIL (BMIMTFSI) was successfully used as an antibacterial experimental orthodontic adhesive against *Streptococcus mutans* [81] and resin infiltrate [78].

Nanoparticles, especially silver (AgNP), zinc oxide, titanium dioxide nanoparticles, quaternary ammonium, and cationic nanoparticles, have been incorporated into resin as antibacterial agents, showing promising results [82–84]. Each of these methods has challenges. For example, the primary concern of AgNPs is adverse effects on human health and the dispersion of nanoparticles into solvents. RTILs are used to stabilize nanoparticles and act as antimicrobial agents for dental resins [81,85,86]. Although microorganisms can rapidly develop resistance against nanomaterials, such as AgNP, the infinite tunability of RTILs makes them the ultimate solution for antimicrobial resistance [35,87].

4.3. Ionic Liquids (ILs) as Oral Hygiene Products

Efforts have been made to develop IL-based oral hygiene products, such as dental toothpaste and mouthwash/mouth rinse. Madhusudan et al. proposed an oral care composition for removing or reducing plaque comprising an IL formulated with choline salicylate and tris-(2-hydroxyethyl) methylammonium methylsulfate. They developed 74 prototype formulations; in vivo experimental results suggested several formulations might provide clinical efficacy to disrupt, dissolve, and remove bacterial plaque. The function of ionic liquid-based oral care compositions will also prevent different gingivitis and oral cavity diseases, such as dental caries, calculus, erosion, periodontitis, halitosis, and even salivary gland disorders, including xerostomia/dry mouth [88].

4.4. Ionic Liquids (ILs) as Dental Restorative Materials in Clinics

In clinics, dental cement selection is vital in achieving successful restoration and significantly increases the duration of teeth restoration [89]. Kajimoto et al. explored the possibility of utilizing ILs to mix with dental cement, converting them to multifunctional smart (intelligent) adhesives [90]. Due to the bonding strength of the dental cement, removal from the oral cavity can require excessive force or vibration to the tooth by electrical appliances, which might generate heat. Heating adhesives in the oral cavity have possible drawbacks and risks damaging the surrounding oral mucosa [90]. The group experimented with a specific electric current to trigger and control the heating process by implementing IL-based dental cement. They developed a prototype resin-modified glass-ionomer cement (RMGIC) with an IL and validated the use of an electric current trigger to control the properties of an IL-based smart cement [90]. In a more recent study, the same research team reported that after immersion and decreasing the bonding strength via electrical current application, the electrical conductivity was greater for the RMGIC with IL [91]. Thus, combining dental cement and ILs might represent an effective multifunctional smart material with antimicrobial properties.

5. Biosensor Prospects in Dental Applications

5.1. Interleukin-6 Sensor to Detect Oral Cancer

Researchers have shown that interleukin-6 (IL-6) promotes tumor growth by causing DNA methylation changes, which can lead to changes in the oral cancer cell gene expression [92]. Higher levels of IL-6 have been reported in the serum and saliva of patients with oral cancer than in control subjects, demonstrating a possible relationship between IL-6 and oral cancer [93].

In the future, oral health care could utilize ionic liquids (ILs) as a strategy for early oral cancer diagnosis. IL with menthol can be used to mass-screen patients for early oral cancer diagnosis. The IL's chemical structure can affect the menthol release rate [94]. Complexes can be formed comprising IL with a menthol moiety [94] and IL-6 antibodies [95]. This complex can bind IL-6 and release a proportional amount of menthol. As menthol triggers TRPM8 and induces a cooling sensation, the intensity of this sensation will notify the patient if IL-6 has been released and the amount of IL-6 in the mouth.

5.2. Gingivitis Sensor

A common condition in many oral diseases, such as gingivitis, is inflammation. Microorganisms cause an inflammatory immune response mediated by changes in the vascular network and the exudation of gingival crevicular fluid (GCF), which contains inflammatory and plasma cells, ultimately resulting in tissue death. Gingivitis is the primary cause of bleeding gums that allows plaque to accumulate at the gum line. Tartar will form if plaque is left untreated. This results in bleeding as well as periodontitis, a severe form of gum and jawbone disease [96]. Functionalized IL can be used for early diagnosis of gingivitis and to highlight the damaged gum area. A possible option would be to synthesize fluorescent IL with light intensity that becomes amplified or quenched upon illumination in the presence of hemoglobin [97]. Hemoglobin is the oxygen-carrying protein in red blood cells [98]. Therefore, after rinsing the mouth with the IL complex, fluorescent light would reveal the bleeding sites in the gum. An alternative option would be to make menthol-based IL functionalized for hemoglobin. In this case, the IL can be synthesized to release menthol when in contact with hemoglobin, causing a cooling sensation in the areas affected by gingivitis.

5.3. Tooth Caries and Cracks Sensor

The most prevalent cause of cracked tooth syndrome is chewing on hard foods, which causes an incomplete tooth fracture. This is the third most frequent cause of tooth loss [99], with no suitable diagnosis method. Transillumination and radiographic approaches, traditional dental crack identification methods, are inaccurate and offer subpar imaging resolution [100]. Light-induced fluorescence dental imaging Field [100–102] has recently gained considerable attention as a useful tool for diagnosing small cracks and cracked teeth at an early stage. For real-time diagnosis, fluorescent IL can be used [103]. Here, after rinsing the mouth with the liquid complex, the dyes will fill all possible cracks and, upon illumination, will reveal the location and size of the cracks. It is important to note that the illumination angle is essential to correctly identify the position and depth of the cracks [101]. This method provides a low-cost visual diagnostic tool for occlusal dental caries, proximal dental caries, and tooth cracks. With the recently emerging telemedicine, this technique will make clinical practice more accessible, especially in rural areas of developing countries.

5.4. Breath-Based Sobriety Sensors

Drinking too much alcohol can result in overdose, car accidents, intoxication of athletes/pilots, etc. According to studies, the blood and saliva alcohol levels are consistent [104]. A driver's sobriety can be evaluated using a saliva alcohol test. The main component of alcoholic drinks is ethanol, and saliva typically lacks alcohol subtypes, such as methyl, propyl, or allyl. Ethanol concentration can be identified using ILs [105]. This can be paired with the colorimetric IL to form an ethanol sensor. This hybrid liquid can be used to rinse the mouth for a few seconds. Depending upon the alcohol concentration in the saliva, the color of the liquid would change accordingly and provide a visual indicator of the blood alcohol level. This method can be used as a fast, low-cost, and scalable technique to monitor sobriety.

5.5. Oral Hygiene Sensor

A person's oral cavity contains more than 70 different species of bacteria. Although most are harmless, some bacteria are dangerous and can lead to dental problems, including tooth decay and gum disease [106]. Oral health can be improved, and the risk of dental problems can be decreased by minimizing the number of harmful germs in the mouth. Fluorescent IL (excitation in the visible spectrum) functionalized for harmful bacteria can be synthesized as a toothpaste [107]. This can be used by individuals at home to monitor the effectiveness of brushing based on the number of fluorescent areas. This will significantly help to improve personal hygiene.

6. Toxic Effects of Ionic Liquids (ILs)

Ionic liquids (ILs) have long been considered environmentally friendly and ecologically benign solvents. Nevertheless, concerns have recently arisen regarding their potential toxicity to human health and environmental impact, necessitating a thorough investigation. ILs are engineered to possess low volatility and stability, which, unfortunately, reduces their biodegradability [108]. The toxicity of ILs is contingent upon their chemical composition, including the types of cations, anions, and the alkyl chain length. ILs were found to be toxic or highly toxic toward cells and living organisms [109,110]. Besides hampering the growth rate of microbes, their antibacterial activity also interferes with their productivity [111].

Notably, ILs featuring choline-based components exhibit lower toxicity than the commonly used imidazolium, pyridinium, and pyrrolidinium variants [112–115]. This underscores a clear relationship between IL structure and toxicity, offering prospects for developing less harmful ILs. Even appropriate anions can reduce the half-maximal effective concentration (EC50) values by three orders of magnitude [116]. It is worth noting that when ILs encounter water or other polar solvents, they may undergo ion exchange, forming new substances with potentially different toxic properties. Research endeavors have been undertaken to assess the cytotoxic effects of various piperidinium and pyrrolidinium ILs on the MCF7 human breast cancer cell line. Results suggest that toxicity tends to increase with longer alkyl chain lengths. Furthermore, the nature of the anions also plays a role, with Tf2N appearing to be more toxic than Br- [117]. Similar findings have been observed in studies involving *Escherichia coli*, *Staphylococcus aureus*, *Bacillus subtilis*, *Pseudomonas flurescens*, and *Saccharomyces cerevisiae*, reinforcing the trend that higher alkyl chain lengths are associated with greater toxicity [118,119]. However, further studies are needed to establish the precise molecular mechanism underlying the toxic effects of ILs.

With proper optimization, ILs can be incorporated into drug formulations to avoid the development of cancer treatment resistance. Adequate knowledge of the toxicity will provide vital information for anti-cancer drug development, as apoptosis-related drug resistance is challenging for different cancer types. Additionally, there is an interest in identifying other means of inducing cytotoxicity [120]. This information will improve the efficacy of drugs against cancer progression and neurodegenerative disease.

7. Prospects and Future Directions

Room temperature ionic liquids (RTILs) have high potential in advanced tissue engineering applications, including craniofacial engineering and dental procedures. They can be easily incorporated with self-healing materials [121], magnetoelectric nanoparticles (MENPs) [122,123], and electroconductive materials [124], through advanced tissue engineering applications, such as three-dimensional (3D) cell cultures [125] and 3D bioprinting techniques [126]. They can also be easily combined or used to control multi-functional material-based applications. For example, they can influence applications based on MENPs and electroconductive materials [122], and can be used for implant sensing [127].

7.1. ILs with Electroconductive Material for Dental Tissue Regeneration

Most cell types respond to electrical stimuli, which control the healing and regeneration of skin wounds, spinal cord injury, bone fractures, and neural growth [128]. The combined usage of electroconductive materials and ILs has huge potentiality for guided cell and tissue regeneration and may enable new directions for guided oral tissue regeneration [124]. One of the challenges of dental hard tissue regeneration is the variable growth rate, resulting in its under- or over-growth. The ILs can easily solve this issue by providing better tissue regeneration control. ILs play a vital role in neural degeneration [129] and could be an ideal root canal material to revitalize the dental pulps. By combining multifunctional magnetoelectric nanoparticles (MENPs) with electroconductive and biodegradable materials, ILs will have a potential role in the formulation of smart dental materials [130].

7.2. A Critical Component for Preventive Dental Care and Oral Hygiene

Oral hygiene maintenance is critical for a healthy oral cavity and lifestyle. However, unfortunately, due to musculoskeletal disorders such as osteoarthritis, rheumatoid arthritis, and other conditions, many elders find it challenging to maintain good oral hygiene [131]. Also, those who have arthritis cannot correctly grip a toothbrush [131,132], representing a primary concern for poor oral hygiene, which leads to microbial accumulation and dental plaque formation. Also, Niesten et al. reported that elders residing in institutions generally discontinue oral hygiene maintenance mainly due to inadequate social support and disorientation [132]. Therefore, a need exists to provide improved methods and oral care products, such as toothpaste and mouthwash, for plaque removal/prevention to overcome some of these inefficiencies arising from poor brushing and flossing techniques. In the future, ILs can minimize the gap by improving the antimicrobial properties of toothpaste and mouthwash. This could effectively remove plaque usually unnoticed between teeth, in the teeth cavities and fissures, and in gum pockets. Madhusudan and colleagues with Colgate-Palmolive Company (New York, NY, USA) invented such a concept to integrate ILs in oral care compositions [88].

With advanced 3D bioprinting techniques, there are enormous opportunities for combining various amounts of ILs in toothpaste/mouthwash compositions to enhance the protective environment within the oral cavities. Hayashi et al. recently explored a technique enabling ILs to formulate fluoridated toothpaste. They reported preparing a new class of hybrid ILs, called "fluoride ion-encapsulated germoxane cages", containing a fluoride ion inside [133].

Breath-based sensors could be another area for future bench-side applications of ILs in clinical dentistry. There is evidence that the presence of chronic disease and cancer alters cellular metabolic processes, and these alterations are recorded in the released volatile organic compound (VOC) compositions of cancer cells. We have shown the potential of using VOC sensors as a biomedical engineering approach for oral cancer detection. Due to their multifunctional nature, ILs could be used for such breath-based early detection systems [134].

7.3. As a Routine Anti-Microbial Material for Dental Clinics

Like any healthcare facility, dental clinics pose a risk of spreading coronavirus disease (COVID-19) via cross-infection among patients, dentists, and community members. In clinical dental settings, the instruments produce aerosols, droplets of saliva, secretions, saliva, and blood, which can rapidly transmit viruses between dental practitioners, assistants, and patients and their attendants [135,136]. Due to their antimicrobial properties and chemical characteristics, RTILs could be used for coating the walls, appliances, and surfaces in dental clinics to provide an infection-free environment [137].

A denture appliance resides in the oral cavity and is highly prone to microbial growth, bacterial biofilm formation, and contamination. Many antimicrobial agents are commonly used for denture preparation, such as titanium dioxide, methacrylic acid monomers, silica, and MPDB/12-methacryloyloxy dodecylpyridinium bromide. Due to their multifunctional properties and antimicrobial nature, RTILs can be incorporated as routine agents to fabricate anti-viral dentures [137].

Further studies are required to accurately assess the toxicity at the cellular and molecular levels. Experiments should be conducted utilizing flat two-dimensional (2D) cultures and more advanced three-dimensional (3D) in vitro models (i.e., spheroids, sandwich cultures) with cells embedded in extracellular matrices, such as rat tail-derived collagen type 1 and mice sarcoma tissue-derived basement membrane mimicking matrices [125,138]. After successfully conducting biological characterization with in vitro models, in vivo studies are required to complete the picture of IL toxicity prior to biomedical applications.

8. Conclusions

Ionic liquids (ILs) have a unique multifunctional property that might allow researchers to explore the potentiality of remote sensing and controlling cellular growth in the craniofacial region. ILs are antimicrobial and easy to characterize, enhancing the functionality of dental cement, 3D bioprinting, and implants with sensing capabilities. However, further in vitro and in vivo studies are required to evaluate the cytotoxicity of ILs and optimized their formulations.

Author Contributions: Conceptualization, E.H.A. and M.I.H.; software, E.H.A. and S.D.G.; formal analysis, M.I.H. and E.H.A.; investigation, M.I.H. and A.B.S.; writing—original draft preparation, M.I.H., A.B.S., S.D.G. and E.H.A.; writing—review and editing, M.I.H., E.H.A., A.M. and G.J.B.; supervision, E.H.A.; project administration, E.H.A.; funding acquisition, E.H.A. All authors have read and agreed to the published version of the manuscript.

Funding: This research received no external funding.

Institutional Review Board Statement: Not applicable.

Informed Consent Statement: Not applicable.

Data Availability Statement: Data are contained within the article.

Conflicts of Interest: The authors declare no conflict of interest.

References

1. Walden, P. Molecular Weights and Electrical Conductivity of Several Fused Salts. *Bull. Acad. Imper. Sci.* **1914**, *1800*.
2. Wilkes, J.S.; Zaworotko, M.J. Air and Water Stable 1-Ethyl-3-Methylimidazolium Based Ionic Liquids. *J. Chem. Soc. Chem. Commun.* **1992**, 965–967. [CrossRef]
3. Benedetto, A. Room-Temperature Ionic Liquids Meet Bio-Membranes: The State-of-the-Art. *Biophys. Rev.* **2017**, *9*, 309–320. [CrossRef]
4. Podgorsek, A.; Jacquemin, J.; Pádua, A.A.H.; Costa Gomes, M.F. Mixing Enthalpy for Binary Mixtures Containing Ionic Liquids. *Chem. Rev.* **2016**, *116*, 6075–6106. [CrossRef] [PubMed]
5. Bonhote, P.; Dias, A.P.; Papageorgiou, N.; Kalyanasundaram, K.; Gratzel, M. Hydrophobic, Highly Conductive Ambient-Temperature Molten Salts. *Inorg. Chem.* **1996**, *35*, 1168–1178. [CrossRef] [PubMed]
6. Seddon, K.R.; Stark, A.; Torres, M.-J. Influence of Chloride, Water, and Organic Solvents on the Physical Properties of Ionic Liquids. *Pure Appl. Chem.* **2000**, *72*, 2275–2287. [CrossRef]
7. Earle, M.J.; Seddon, K.R. Ionic Liquids. Green Solvents for the Future. *Pure Appl. Chem.* **2000**, *72*, 1391–1398. [CrossRef]
8. Wang, Y.; Parvis, F.; Hossain, M.I.; Ma, K.; Jarošová, R.; Swain, G.M.; Blanchard, G.J. Local and Long-Range Organization in Room Temperature Ionic Liquids. *Langmuir* **2021**, *37*, 605–615. [CrossRef]
9. Hossain, M.I.; Blanchard, G.J. The Effect of Dilution on Induced Free Charge Density Gradients in Room Temperature Ionic Liquids. *Phys. Chem. Chem. Phys* **2022**, *24*, 3844–3853. [CrossRef]
10. Hossain, M.I.; Blanchard, G.J. Dilution-Induced Changes in Room Temperature Ionic Liquids. Persistent Compositional Heterogeneity and the Importance of Dipolar Interactons. *J. Mol. Liq.* **2022**, *367*, 120447–120455. [CrossRef]
11. Yoo, C.G.; Pu, Y.; Ragauskas, A.J. Ionic Liquids: Promising Green Solvents for Lignocellulosic Biomass Utilization. *Curr. Opin. Green Sustain. Chem.* **2017**, *5*, 5–11. [CrossRef]
12. Miao, W.; Chan, T.H. Ionic-Liquid-Supported Synthesis: A Novel Liquid-Phase Strategy for Organic Synthesis. *Acc. Chem. Res.* **2006**, *39*, 897–908. [CrossRef] [PubMed]
13. Welton, T. Room-Temperature Ionic Liquids. Solvents for Synthesis and Catalysis. *Chem. Rev.* **1999**, *99*, 2071–2084. [CrossRef] [PubMed]
14. Pei, Y.; Wang, J.; Wu, K.; Xuan, X.; Lu, X. Ionic Liquid-Based Aqueous Two-Phase Extraction of Selected Proteins. *Sep. Purif. Technol.* **2009**, *64*, 288–295. [CrossRef]
15. Sun, X.; Luo, H.; Dai, S. Ionic Liquids-Based Extraction: A Promising Strategy for the Advanced Nuclear Fuel Cycle. *Chem. Rev.* **2012**, *112*, 2100–2128. [CrossRef]
16. Zhao, C.; Burrell, G.; Torriero, A.A.; Separovic, F.; Dunlop, N.F.; MacFarlane, D.R.; Bond, A.M. Electrochemistry of Room Temperature Protic Ionic Liquids. *J. Phys. Chem. B* **2008**, *112*, 6923–6936. [CrossRef]
17. Smiglak, M.; Pringle, J.M.; Lu, X.; Han, L.; Zhang, S.; Gao, H.; Macfarlane, D.R.; Rogers, R.D. Ionic Liquids for Energy, Materials, and Medicine. *Chem. Commun.* **2014**, *50*, 9228–9250. [CrossRef]
18. Zhou, F.; Liang, Y.; Liu, W. Ionic Liquid Lubricants: Designed Chemistry for Engineering Applications. *Chem. Soc. Rev.* **2009**, *38*, 2590–2599. [CrossRef]
19. Zhao, C.; Bond, A.M. Photoinduced Oxidation of Water to Oxygen in the Ionic Liquid BMIMBF4 as the Counter Reaction in the Fabrication of Exceptionally Long Semiconducting Silver-Tetracyanoquinodimethane Nanowires. *J. Am. Chem. Soc.* **2009**, *131*, 4279–4287. [CrossRef]
20. Rehman, A.; Zeng, X. Ionic Liquids as Green Solvents and Electrolytes for Robust Chemical Sensor Development. *Acc. Chem. Res.* **2012**, *45*, 1667–1677. [CrossRef]
21. Murray, C.J.; Ikuta, K.S.; Sharara, F.; Swetschinski, L.; Aguilar, G.R.; Gray, A.; Han, C.; Bisignano, C.; Rao, P.; Wool, E. Global Burden of Bacterial Antimicrobial Resistance in 2019: A Systematic Analysis. *Lancet* **2022**, *399*, 629–655. [CrossRef] [PubMed]
22. US CDC. *Antibiotic Resistance Threats in the United States*; US Department of Health and Human Services: Washington, DC, USA, 2019; pp. 1–150.

23. Song, X.; Tian, R.; Liu, K. Recent Advances in the Application of Ionic Liquids in Antimicrobial Material for Air Disinfection and Sterilization. *Front. Cell. Infect. Microbiol.* **2023**, *13*, 1186117. [CrossRef]
24. Nelson, D.L.; Cox, M.M. *Lehninger Principles of Biochemistry*, 6th ed.; W.H. Freeman (U.S.): New York, NY, USA, 2013.
25. Hao, X.-L.; Cao, B.; Dai, D.; Wu, F.-G.; Yu, Z.-W. Cholesterol Protects the Liquid-Ordered Phase of Raft Model Membranes from the Destructive Effect of Ionic Liuqids. *J. Phys. Chem. Lett.* **2022**, *13*, 7386–7391. [CrossRef] [PubMed]
26. Alberts, B.; Bray, D.; Hopkin, K.; Johnson, A.D.; Lewis, J.; Raff, M.; Roberts, K.; Walter, P. *Essential Cell Biology*; Garland Science: New York, NY, USA, 2015; ISBN 1-317-80627-1.
27. Wang, H.; Shi, X.; Yu, D.; Zhang, J.; Yang, G.; Cui, Y.; Sun, K.; Wang, J.; Yan, H. Antibacterial Activity of Geminized Amphiphilic Cationic Homopolymers. *Langmuir* **2015**, *50*, 13469–13477. [CrossRef] [PubMed]
28. Locock, K.E.S.; Michl, T.D.; Stevens, N.; Hayball, J.D.; Vasilev, K.; Postma, A.; Griesser, H.J.; Meagher, L.; Haeussler, M. Antimicrobial Polymethacrylates Synthesized as Mimics of Tryptophan-Rich Cationic Peptides. *ACS Macro Lett.* **2014**, *4*, 319–323. [CrossRef] [PubMed]
29. Qin, J.; Guo, J.; Xu, Q.; Zheng, Z.; Mao, H.; Yan, F. Synthesis of Pyrrolidinium-Type Poly(Ionic Liquid) Membranes for Antibacterial Applications. *ACS Appl. Mater. Interfaces* **2017**, *12*, 10504–10511. [CrossRef]
30. Guzman, L.; Parra-Cid, C.; Cuerrero-Munoz, E.; Pena-Varas, C.; Polo-Cuadrado, E.; Duarte, Y.; Carstro, R.I.; Nerio, L.S.; Araya-Maturana, R.; Asefa, T.; et al. Antimicrobial Properties of Novel Ionic Liquids Derived from Imidazolium Cation with Phenolic Functional Groups. *Bioorganic Chem.* **2021**, *115*, 105289–105299. [CrossRef]
31. Zheng, Z.; Xu, Q.; Guo, J.; Qin, J.; Mao, H.; Wang, B.; Yan, F. Structure-Antibacterial Activity Relationships of Imidazolium-Type Ionic Liquid Monomers, Poly(Ionic Liquids) and Poly (Ionic Liuqid) Membranes: Effect of Alkyl Chain Length and Cations. *ACS Appl. Mater. Interfaces* **2016**, *20*, 12684–12692. [CrossRef]
32. Yang, C.; Ding, X.; Ono, R.J.; Lee, H.; Hsu, L.Y.; Tong, Y.W.; Hedrich, J.; Yang, Y. Brush-Like Polycarbonates Containing Dopamine, Cations, and PEG Providing a Borad-Spectrum, Antibacterial, Adn Antifouling Surface via One-Step Coating. *Adv. Mater.* **2014**, *26*, 7346–7351. [CrossRef]
33. Ibsen, K.N.; Ma, H.; Banerjee, A.; Tanner, E.E.L.; Nangia, S.; Mitragotri, S. Mechanism of Antibacterial Activity of Cholin-Based Ionic Liquids (CAGE). *ACS Biomater. Sci. Eng.* **2018**, *4*, 2370–2379. [CrossRef]
34. Fallah, Z.; Zare, E.N.; Khan, M.A.; Iftekhar, S.; Ghomi, M.; Sharifi, E.; Tajbakhsh, M.; Nikfarjam, N.; Makvandi, P.; Lichtfouse, E.; et al. Ionic Lquid-Based Antimicrobial Materials for Water Treatment, Air Filtration, Food Packaging and Anticorrosion Coatings. *Adv. Colloid Interface Sci.* **2021**, *294*, 102454. [CrossRef]
35. Pendleton, J.N.; Gilmore, B.F. The Antimicrobial Potential of Ionic Liquids: A Source of Chemical Diversity for Infection Andbiofilm Control. *Int. J. Antimicrob. Agents* **2015**, *46*, 131–139. [CrossRef]
36. Canongia Lopes, J.N.; Pádua, A.A. Nanostructural Organization in Ionic Liquids. *J. Phys. Chem. B* **2006**, *110*, 3330–3335. [CrossRef]
37. Xiao, D.; Rajian, J.R.; Li, S.; Bartsch, R.A.; Quitevis, E.L. Additivity in the Optical Kerr Effect Spectra of Binary Ionic Liquid Mixtures: Implications for Nanostructural Organization. *J. Phys. Chem. B* **2006**, *110*, 16174–16178. [CrossRef]
38. Triolo, A.; Russina, O.; Bleif, H.-J.; Di Cola, E. Nanoscale Segregation in Room Temperature Ionic Liquids. *J. Phys. Chem. B* **2007**, *111*, 4641–4644. [CrossRef]
39. Macchiagodena, M.; Gontrani, L.; Ramondo, F.; Triolo, A.; Caminiti, R. Liquid Structure of 1-Alkyl-3-Methylimidazolium-Hexafluorophosphates by Wide Angle X-Ray and Neutron Scattering and Molecular Dynamics. *J. Chem. Phys.* **2011**, *134*, 114521. [CrossRef]
40. Wang, Y.; Voth, G.A. Unique Spatial Heterogeneity in Ionic Liquids. *J. Am. Chem. Soc.* **2005**, *127*, 12192–12193. [CrossRef]
41. Jiang, W.; Wang, Y.; Voth, G.A. Molecular Dynamics Simulation of Nanostructural Organization in Ionic Liquid/Water Mixtures. *J. Phys. Chem. B* **2007**, *111*, 4812–4818. [CrossRef]
42. Bica, K.; Rodríguez, H.; Gurau, G.; Cojocaru, O.A.; Riisager, A.; Fehrmann, R.; Rogers, R.D. Pharmaceutically Active Ionic Liquids with Solids Handling, Enhanced Thermal Stability, and Fast Release. *Chem. Commun.* **2012**, *48*, 5422–5424. [CrossRef]
43. Yan, Z.; Ma, L.; Shen, S.; Li, J. Studies on the Interactions of Some Small Biomolecules with Antibacterial Drug Benzethonium Chloride and Its Active Pharmaceutical Ingredient Ionic Liquid (API-IL) Benzethonium L-Proline at Varying Temperatures. *J. Mol. Liq.* **2018**, *255*, 530–540. [CrossRef]
44. Shekaari, H.; Zafarani-Moattar, M.T.; Mirheydari, S.N.; Faraji, S. Thermophysical Properties of 1-Hexyl-3-Methylimidazolium Sallicylate as an Active Pharmaceutical Ingredient Ionic Liquid (API-IL) in Aqueous Solutions of Glycine Adn L-Aalanine. *J. Chem. Eng. Data* **2019**, *64*, 124–134. [CrossRef]
45. Zhang, Y.; Chen, X.; Lan, J.; You, J.; Chen, L. Synthesis and Biological Applications of Imidazolium-Based Polymerized Ionic Liquid as a Gene Delivery Vector. *Chem. Biol. Drug Des.* **2009**, *74*, 282–288. [CrossRef] [PubMed]
46. Dobler, D.; Schmidts, T.; Klingenhofer, I.; Runkel, F. Ionic Liquids as Ingredients in Topical Drug Delivery Systems. *Int. J. Pharm.* **2013**, *441*, 620–627. [CrossRef] [PubMed]
47. Zakrewsky, M.; Lovejoy, K.S.; Kern, T.L.; Mitragotri, S. Ionic Liquids as a Class of Materials for Transdermal Delivery and Pahtogen Neutralization. *Proc. Natl. Acad. Sci. USA* **2014**, *111*, 13313–13318. [CrossRef] [PubMed]
48. Pyne, A.; Kuchlyan, J.; Maiti, C.; Dhara, D.; Sarkar, N. Cholesterol Based Surface Active Ionic Liquid That Can Form Microemulsions and Spontaneous Vesicles. *Langmuir* **2017**, *33*, 5891–5899. [CrossRef] [PubMed]
49. Poh, Y.; Ng, S.; Ho, K. Formulation and Characterisation of 1-Ethyl-3-Methylimidazolium Acetate-in-Oil Microemulsions as the Potential Vehicle for Drug Delivery across the Skin Barrier. *J. Mol. Liq.* **2019**, *273*, 339–345. [CrossRef]

50. Vashishat, R.; Chabba, S.; Aswal, V.K.; Mahajan, R.K. Probing Molecular Interactions of Tetracaine with Surface Active Ionic Liquid and Subsequent Formation of Vesicle in Aqueous Medium. *J. Mol. Liq.* **2017**, *243*, 503–512. [CrossRef]
51. Viau, L.; Tourné-Péteilh, C.; Devoisselle, J.-M.; Vioux, A. Ionogels as Drug Delivery System: One-Step Sol–Gel Synthesis Using Imidazolium Ibuprofenate Ionic Liquid. *Chem. Commun.* **2009**, *46*, 228–230. [CrossRef]
52. Ziotkowski, B.; Diamond, D. Thermoresponsive Poly(Ionic Liquid) Hydrogels. *Chem. Commun.* **2013**, *49*, 10308–10310. [CrossRef]
53. Byrne, N.; Wang, L.-M.; Belieres, J.-P.; Angell, C.A. Reversible Folding–Unfolding, Aggregation Protection, and Multi-Year Stabilization, in High Concentration Protein Solutions, Using Ionic Liquids. *Chem. Commun.* **2007**, 2714–2716. [CrossRef] [PubMed]
54. Fujita, K.; MacFarlane, D.R.; Forsyth, M. Protein Solubilising and Stabilising Ionic Liquids. *Chem. Commun.* **2005**, 4804–4806. [CrossRef] [PubMed]
55. Attri, P.; Venkatesu, P.; Kumar, A. Activity and Stability of Alpha-Chymotrypsin in Biocompatible Ionic Liquids: Enzyme Refolding by Triethyl Ammonium Acetate. *Phys. Chem. Chem. Phys.* **2011**, *13*, 2788–2796. [CrossRef] [PubMed]
56. Chen, S.; Dong, Y.; Sun, J.; Gu, P.; Wang, J.; Zhang, S. Ionic Liquids Membranes for Liquid Separation: Status and Challenges. *Green Chem.* **2023**, *25*, 5813–5835. [CrossRef]
57. Webber, L.P.; Chan, H.-L.; Wang, H.-L. Will Zirconia Implants Replace Titanium Implants? *Appl. Sci.* **2021**, *11*, 6776. [CrossRef]
58. Duraccio, D.; Mussano, F.; Faga, M.G. Biomaterials for Dental Implants: Current and Future Trends. *J. Mater. Sci.* **2015**, *50*, 4779–4812. [CrossRef]
59. Torres, Y.; Trueba, P.; Pavón, J.J.; Chicardi, E.; Kamm, P.; García-Moreno, F.; Rodríguez-Ortiz, J.A. Design, Processing and Characterization of Titanium with Radial Graded Porosity for Bone Implants. *Mater. Des.* **2016**, *110*, 179–187. [CrossRef]
60. Chehroudi, B.; Gould, T.R.L.; Brunette, D.M. The Role of Connective Tissue in Inhibiting Epithelial Downgrowth on Titanium-Coated Percutaneous Implants. *J. Biomed. Mater. Res.* **1992**, *26*, 493–515. [CrossRef]
61. Chai, W.L.; Brook, I.M.; Palmquist, A.; van Noort, R.; Moharamzadeh, K. The Biological Seal of the Implant–Soft Tissue Interface Evaluated in a Tissue-Engineered Oral Mucosal Model. *J. R. Soc. Interface* **2012**, *9*, 3528–3538. [CrossRef]
62. Chrcanovic, B.R.; Kisch, J.; Albrektsson, T.; Wennerberg, A. Factors Influencing Early Dental Implant Failures. *J. Dent. Res.* **2016**, *95*, 995–1002. [CrossRef]
63. Branemark, P.-I. Osseointegation and Its Experimental Background. *J. Prosthet. Dent.* **1983**, *50*, 399–410. [CrossRef]
64. Mishra, S.K.; Ferreira, J.M.F.; Kannan, S. Mechanically Stable Antimicrobial Chitosan-PVA-Silver Nanocomposite Coatings Deposited on Titanium Implants. *Carbohydr. Polym.* **2015**, *121*, 37–48. [CrossRef] [PubMed]
65. Frandsen, C.J.; Brammer, K.S.; Noh, K.; Johnston, G.; Jin, S. Tantalum Coating on TiO₂ Nanotubes Induces Superior Rate of Matrix Mineralization and Osteofunctionality in Human Osteoblasts. *Mater. Sci. Eng. C* **2014**, *37*, 332–341. [CrossRef] [PubMed]
66. Zhao, B.; Van der Mei, H.C.; Subbiahdoss, G.; de Vries, J.; Rustema-Abbing, M.; Kuijer, R.; Ren, Y. Soft Tissue Integration versus Early Biofilm Formation on Different Dental Implant Materials. *Dent. Mater.* **2014**, *30*, 716–727. [CrossRef] [PubMed]
67. Gindri, I.M.; Siddiqui, D.A.; Bhardwaj, P.; Rodriguez, L.C.; Palmer, K.L.; Frizzo, C.P.; Martins, M.A.P.; Rodrigues, D.C. Dicationic Imidazolium-Based Ionic Liquids: A New Strategy for Non-Toxic and Antimicrobial Materials. *RSC Adv.* **2014**, *4*, 62594–62602. [CrossRef]
68. Gindri, I.M.; Frizzo, C.P.; Bender, C.R.; Tier, A.Z.; Martins, M.A.P.; Villetti, M.A.; Machado, G.; Rodriguez, L.C.; Rodrigues, D.C. Preparation of TiO₂ Nanoparticles Coated with Ionic Liquids: A Supramolecular Approach. *ACS Appl. Mater. Interfaces* **2014**, *6*, 11536–11543. [CrossRef]
69. Gindri, I.M.; Siddiqui, D.A.; Frizzo, C.P.; Martins, M.A.P.; Rodrigues, D.C. Ionic Liquid Coatings for Titanium Surfaces: Effect of IL Structure on Coating Profile. *ACS Appl. Mater. Interfaces* **2015**, *7*, 27421–27431. [CrossRef]
70. Gindri, I.M.; Palmer, K.L.; Siddiqui, D.A.; Aghyarian, S.; Frizzo, C.P.; Martins, M.A.; Rodrigues, D.C. Evaluation of Mammalian and Bacterial Cell Activity on Titanium Surface Coated with Dicationic Imidazolium-Based Ionic Liquids. *RSC Adv.* **2016**, *6*, 36475–36483. [CrossRef]
71. Wheelis, S.E.; Biguetti, C.C.; Natarajan, S.; Guida, L.; Hedden, B.; Garlet, G.P.; Rodrigues, D.C. Investigation of the Early Healing Response to Diacationic Imidazolium-Based Ionic Liquids: A Biocompatible Coating for Titanium Implants. *ACS Biomater. Sci. Eng.* **2020**, *6*, 984–994. [CrossRef]
72. GBD 2017 Oral Disorders Collaborators; Bernabe, E.; Marcenes, W.; Hernandez, C.R.; Bailey, J.; Abreu, L.G.; Alipour, V.; Amini, S.; Arabloo, J.; Arefi, Z.; et al. Global, Regional, and National Levels and Trends in Burden of Oral Conditions from 1990 to 2017: A Systematic Analysis for the Global Burden of Disease 2017 Study. *J. Dent. Res.* **2020**, *99*, 362–373. [CrossRef]
73. Cury, J.A.; Tenuta, L.M. Enamel Remineralizaiton: Controlling the Caries Disease or Treating Early Caries Lesions? *Braz. Oral. Res.* **2009**, *23*, 23–30. [CrossRef]
74. Cumerlato, C.; Demarco, F.F.; Barros, A.J.D.; Peres, M.A.; Peres, K.G.; Cascaes, A.M. Reasons for Direct Restoration Failure from Childhood to Adolescence: A Birth Cohort Study. *J. Dent.* **2019**, *89*, 103183. [CrossRef] [PubMed]
75. Meyer-Lueckel, H.; Paris, S. Progression of Artificial Enamel Caries Lesions after Infiltration with Experimental Light Curing Resins. *Caries Res.* **2008**, *42*, 117–124. [CrossRef] [PubMed]
76. Paris, S.; Bitter, K.; Krois, J.; Meyer-Lueckel, H. Seven-Year-Efficacy of Proximal Caries Infiltration—Randomized Clinical Trial. *J. Dent.* **2020**, *93*, 103277. [CrossRef] [PubMed]
77. Paris, S.; Soviero, V.M.; Chatzidakis, A.J.; Meyer-Lueckel, H. Penetration of Experimental Infiltrants with Different Penetration Coefficients and Ethanol Addition into Natural Caries Lesions in Primary Molars. *Caries Res.* **2012**, *56*, 113–117. [CrossRef]

78. Cuppini, M.; Garcia, I.M.; de Souza, V.S.; Zatta, K.C.; Visioli, F.; Leitune, V.C.B.; Guterres, S.S.; Scholten, J.D.; Collares, F.M. Ionic Liquid-Loaded Microcapsules Doped into Dental Resin Infiltrants. *Bioact. Mater.* **2021**, *6*, 2667–2675. [CrossRef]
79. Livi, S.; Lins, L.C.; Capeletti, L.B.; Chardin, C.; Halawani, N.; Baudoux, J.; Cardoso, M.B. Antibacterial Surface Based on New-Epoxy-Amine Networks Form Ionic Liquid Monomers. *Eur. Polym. J.* **2019**, *116*, 56–64. [CrossRef]
80. Livi, S.; Baudoux, J.; Gerard, J.-F.; Duchet-Rumeau, J. Ionic Liquids: A Versatile Platform for the Design of a Multifunctional Epoxy Networks 2.0 Generation. *Prog. Polym. Sci.* **2022**, *132*, 101581. [CrossRef]
81. Garcia, I.M.; Ferreira, C.J.; de Souza, V.S.; Leitune, V.C.B.; Samuel, S.M.W.; de Souza Balbinot, G.; da Motta, A.D.S.; Visioli, F.; Scholten, J.D.; Collares, F.M. Ionic Liquid as Antibacterial Agent for an Experimental Orthodontic Adhesive. *Dent. Mater.* **2019**, *35*, 1155–1165. [CrossRef]
82. Kielbassa, A.M.; Leimer, M.R.; Hartmann, J.; Harm, S.; Pasztorek, M.; Ulrich, I.B. Ex Vivo Investigation on Internal Tunnel Approach/Internal Resin Infiltration and External Nanosilver-Modified Resin Infiltration of Proximal Caries Exceeding into Dentin. *PLoS ONE* **2020**, *15*, e0228249. [CrossRef]
83. Yu, J.; Huang, X.; Zhou, X.; Han, Q.; Zhou, W.; Liang, J. Anti-Caries Effect of Resin Infiltrant Modified by Quaternary Ammonium Monomers. *J. Dent.* **2020**, *97*, 103355. [CrossRef]
84. Collares, F.M.; Garcia, I.M.; Bohns, F.R.; Motta, A.; Melo, M.A.; Leitune, V.C.B. Guanidine Hydrochloride Polymer Additive to Undertake Ultraconservative Resin Infiltrant against Streptococcus Mutans. *Eur. Polym. J.* **2020**, *133*, 109746. [CrossRef]
85. Garcia, I.M.; Souza, V.S.; Hellriegel, C.; Scholten, J.D.; Collares, F.M. Collares Ionic Liquid-Stabilized Titania Quantum Dots Applied in Adhesive Resin. *J. Dent. Res.* **2019**, *98*, 682–688. [CrossRef] [PubMed]
86. Garcia, I.M.; Souza, V.S.; Scholten, J.D.; Collares, F.M. Quantum Dots of Tantalum Oxide with an Imidazolium Ionic Liquid as Antibacterial Agent for Adhesive Resin. *J. Adhesive Dent.* **2020**, *22*, 207–214.
87. Ferraz, R.; Branco, L.C.; Prudencio, C.; Noronha, J.P.; Petrovski, Ž. Ionic Liquids as Active Pharmaceutical Ingredients. *ChemMedChem* **2011**, *6*, 975–985. [CrossRef] [PubMed]
88. Patel, M.; Picquet, C.; Vandeven, M.; Hassan, M.; Paredes, R. Oral Care Composition Containing Ionic Liquids. U.S. Patent 97117667B2, 1 August 2017.
89. Yu, H.; Zheng, M.; Chen, R.; Cheng, H. Proper Selection of Contemporary Cements. *Oral Health Dent. Manag.* **2014**, *13*, 54–59.
90. Kajimoto, N.; Yuama, E.; Sekine, K.; Hamada, K. Electrical Shear Bonding Strength Reduction of Resin-Modified Glass-Ionomercement Containing Ionic-Liquid: Concept and Validation of a Smart Dental Cement Debonding-on-Demand. *Dent. Mater. J.* **2018**, *37*, 768–774. [CrossRef]
91. Sato, H.; Matsuki, Y.; Kajimoto, N.; Uyama, E.; Horiuchi, S.; Sekine, K.; Tanaka, E.; Hamada, K. Effects of Water Immersion on Shear Bond Strength Reduction after Current Application of Resin-Modified Glass-Ionomer-Cements with and without an Ionic Liquid. *Dent. Mater.* **2021**, *40*, 35–43. [CrossRef]
92. Sun, A.; Chia, J.-S.; Chang, Y.-F.; Chiang, C.-P. Serum Interleukin-6 Level Is a Useful Marker in Evaluating Therapeutic Effects of Levamisole and Chinese Medicinal Herbs on Patients with Oral Lichen Planus. *J. Oral Pathol. Med.* **2002**, *31*, 196–203. [CrossRef]
93. Bigbee, W.L.; Grandis, J.R.; Siegfried, J.M. Multiple Cytokine and Growth Factor Serum Biomarkers Predict Therapeutic Response and Survival in Advanced-Stage Head and Neck Cancer Patients. *Clin. Cancer Res.* **2007**, *13*, 3107–3108. [CrossRef]
94. Blesic, M.; Gunaratne, H.Q.N.; Nockemann, P.; McCarron, P.; Seddon, K.R. Controlled Fragrance Delivery in Functionalised Ionic Liquid-Enzyme Systems. *RSC Adv.* **2013**, *3*, 329–333. [CrossRef]
95. Munje, R.D.; Muthukumar, S.; Jagannath, B.; Prasad, S. A New Paradigm in Sweat Based Wearable Diagnostics Biosensors Using Room Temperature Ionic Liquids (RTILs). *Sci. Rep.* **2017**, *7*, 1950. [CrossRef] [PubMed]
96. Abusleme, L.; Hoare, A.; Hong, B.-Y.; Diaz, P.I. Microbial Signatures of Health, Gingivitis, and Periodontitis. *Periodontology 2000* **2021**, *86*, 57–78. [CrossRef] [PubMed]
97. Chen, X.-W.; Liu, J.-W.; Wang, J.-H. A Highly Fluorescent Hydrophilic Ionic Liquid as a Potential Probe for the Sensing of Biomacromolecules. *J. Phys. Chem. B* **2011**, *115*, 1524–1530. [CrossRef]
98. Giardina, B.; Messana, I.; Scatena, R.; Castagnola, M. The Multiple Functions of Hemoglobin. *Crit. Rev. Biochem. Mol. Biol.* **1995**, *30*, 165–196. [CrossRef]
99. Hasan, S.; Singh, K.; Salati, N. Cracked Tooth Syndrome: Overview of Literature. *Int. J. Appl. Basic Med. Res.* **2015**, *5*, 164. [CrossRef]
100. Kim, H.J.; Ji, S.; Han, J.Y.; Cho, H.B.; Park, Y.-G.; Choi, D.; Cho, H.; Park, J.-U.; Im, W.B. Detection of Cracked Teeth Using a Mechanoluminescence Phosphor with a Stretchable Photodetector Array. *NPG Asia Mater.* **2022**, *14*, 26. [CrossRef]
101. Li, Z.; Holamoge, Y.V.; Li, Z.; Zaid, W.; Osborn, M.L.; Ramos, A.; Miller, J.T.; Li, Y.; Yao, S.; Xu, J. Detection and Analysis of Enamel Cracks by Icg-Nir Fluorescence Dental Imaging. *Ann. N. Y. Acad. Sci.* **2020**, *1475*, 52–63. [CrossRef] [PubMed]
102. Oh, S.H.; Lee, S.R.; Choi, J.Y.; Choi, Y.S.; Kim, S.H.; Yoon, H.C.; Nelson, G. Detection of Dental Caries and Cracks with Quantitative Light-Induced Fluorescence in Comparison to Radiographic and Visual Examination: A Retrospective Case Study. *Sensors* **2021**, *21*, 1741. [CrossRef] [PubMed]
103. Gan, L.; Guo, J.; Che, S.; Xiao, Q.; Wang, M.; You, J.; Wang, C. Design of Functionalized Fluorescent Ionic Liquid and Its Application for Achieving Significant Improvements in Al^{3+} Detecting. *Green Energy Environ.* **2020**, *5*, 195–202. [CrossRef]
104. Gubala, W.; Zuba, D. Comparison of Ethanol Concentrations in Saliva and Blood. *Can. Soc. Forensic Sci. J.* **2002**, *35*, 229–235. [CrossRef]
105. Lee, Y.G.; Chou, T.-C. Ionic Liquid Ethanol Sensor. *Biosens. Bioelectron.* **2004**, *20*, 33–40. [CrossRef] [PubMed]

106. Deo, P.N.; Deshmukh, R. Oral Microbiome: Unveiling the Fundamentals. *J. Oral Maxillofac. Pathol.* **2019**, *23*, 122–128. [CrossRef] [PubMed]
107. Wang, M.; Shi, J.; Mao, H.; Sun, Z.; Siyu, J.; Guo, J.; Yan, F. Fluorescent Imidazolium-Type Poly(Ionic Liquid)s for Bacterial Imaging and Biofilm Inhibition. *Biomacromolecules* **2019**, *20*, 3161–3170. [CrossRef]
108. Flieger, J.; Flieger, M. Ionic Liquids Toxicity—Benefits and Threats. *Int. J. Mol. Sci.* **2020**, *21*, 6267. [CrossRef] [PubMed]
109. Zhao, D.; Liao, Y.; Zhang, Z. Toxicity of Ionic Liquids. *CLEAN—Soil Air Water* **2007**, *35*, 42–48. [CrossRef]
110. Egorova, K.S.; Ananikov, V.P. Toxicity of Ionic Liquids: Eco(Cyto)Activity as Complicated, but Unavoidable Parameter for Task-Specific Optimization. *ChemSusChem* **2014**, *7*, 336–360. [CrossRef]
111. Thuy Pham, T.P.; Cho, C.-W.; Yun, Y.-S. Environmental Fate and Toxicity of Ionic Liquids: A Review. *Water Res.* **2010**, *44*, 352–372. [CrossRef]
112. Łuczak, J.; Hupka, J.; Thöming, J.; Jungnickel, C. Self-Organization of Imidazolium Ionic Liquids in Aqueous Solution. *Colloids Surf. A Physicochem. Eng. Asp.* **2008**, *329*, 125–133. [CrossRef]
113. Łuczak, J.; Jungnickel, C.; Łącka, I.; Stolte, S.; Hupka, J. Antimicrobial and Surface Activity of 1-Alkyl-3-Methylimidazolium Derivatives. *Green Chem.* **2010**, *12*, 593–601. [CrossRef]
114. Kumar, R.A.; Papaïconomou, N.; Lee, J.-M.; Salminen, J.; Clark, D.S.; Prausnitz, J.M. In Vitro Cytotoxicities of Ionic Liquids: Effect of Cation Rings, Functional Groups, and Anions. *Environ. Toxicol.* **2009**, *24*, 388–395. [CrossRef]
115. Amde, M.; Liu, J.-F.; Pang, L. Environmental Application, Fate, Effects, and Concerns of Ionic Liquids: A Review. *Environ. Sci. Technol.* **2015**, *49*, 12611–12627. [CrossRef] [PubMed]
116. Sioriki, E.; Gaillard, S.; Nahra, F.; Imad, R.; Ullah, K.; Wajid, S.; Sharif, D.; Fayyaz, S.; Arshad, F.; Choudhary, M.I. Investigating the Biological Activity of Imidazolium Aurate Salts. *ChemistrySelect* **2019**, *4*, 11061–11065. [CrossRef]
117. Salminen, J.; Papaiconomou, N.; Kumar, R.A.; Lee, J.-M.; Kerr, J.; Newman, J.; Prausnitz, J.M. Physicochemical Properties and Toxicities of Hydrophobic Piperidinium and Pyrrolidinium Ionic Liquids. *Fluid Phase Equilibria* **2007**, *261*, 421–426. [CrossRef]
118. Docherty, K.M.; Kulpa, C.F., Jr. Toxicity and Antimicrobial Activity of Imidazolium and Pyridinium Ionic Liquids. *Green Chem.* **2005**, *7*, 185–189. [CrossRef]
119. Tian, T.; Hu, X.; Guan, P.; Ding, X. Research on Solubility and Bio-Solubility of Amino Acids Ionic Liquids. *J. Mol. Liq.* **2017**, *225*, 224–230. [CrossRef]
120. Rahman, M.A.; Bishayee, K.; Sadra, A.; Huh, S.-O. Oxyresveratrol Activates Parallel Apoptotic and Autophagic Cell Death Pathways in Neuroblastoma Cells. *Biochim. Biophys. Acta Gen. Subj.* **2017**, *1861*, 23–36. [CrossRef] [PubMed]
121. Ashammakhi, N.; Hoque Apu, E.; Caterson, E.J. Self-Healing Biomaterials to Heal Tissues. *J. Carniofacial Surg.* **2021**, *32*, 819–820. [CrossRef]
122. Hoque Apu, E.; Nafiujjaman, M.; Sandeep, S.; Makela, A.V.; Khaleghi, A.; Vainio, S.; Contag, C.H.; Li, J.; Balasingham, I.; Kim, T.; et al. Biomedical Applicaitons of Multifunctional Magnetoelectric Nanoparticles. *Mater. Chem. Front.* **2022**, *6*, 1368–1390. [CrossRef]
123. Ashmmakhi, N.; Hernandez, A.L.; Unluturk, B.D.; Quintero, S.A.; de Barros, N.R.; Hoque Apu, E.; Shams, A.B.; Ostrovidov, S.; Li, J.; Contag, C.H.; et al. Biodegradable Implantable Sensors: Materials Design, Fabrication, and Application. *Adv. Funct. Mater.* **2021**, *31*, 2104149. [CrossRef]
124. Alizadeh, P.; Soltani, M.; Tutar, R.; Hoque Apu, E.; Maduka, C.V.; Unluturk, B.D.; Contag, C.H.; Ashammakhi, N. Use of Electroconductive Biomaterials for Engineering Tissues by 3D Printing and 3D Bioprinting. *Essays Biochem.* **2021**, *65*, 441–466.
125. Hoque Apu, E.; Akram, S.U.; Rissanen, J.; Wan, H.; Salo, T. Desmoglein 3-Influence on Oral Carcinoma Cell Migration and Invasion. *Exp. Cell Res.* **2018**, *370*, 353–364. [CrossRef] [PubMed]
126. Ashammakhi, N.; GhavamiNejad, A.; Tutar, R.; Fricker, A.; Roy, I.; Chatzistavrou, X.; Hoque Apu, E.; Nguyen, K.-L.; Ahsan, T.; Pountos, I.; et al. Highlights on Advancing Frontiers in Tissue Engineering. *Tissue Eng. Part B Rev.* **2022**, *28*, 633–664. [CrossRef] [PubMed]
127. Veletic, M.; Hoque Apu, E.; Simic, M.; Bergsland, J.; Balasingham, I.; Contag, C.H.; Ashammakhi, N. Implants with Sensing Capabilities. *Chem. Rev.* **2022**, *122*, 16329–16363. [CrossRef] [PubMed]
128. Chen, C.; Bai, X.; Ding, Y.; Lee, I.-S. Electrical Stimulation as a Novel Tool for Regulating Cell Behavior in Tissue Engineering. *Biomater. Res.* **2019**, *23*, 25. [CrossRef]
129. Manousiouthakis, E.; Park, J.; Hardy, J.G.; Lee, J.Y.; Schmidt, C.E. Towards the Translation of Electroconductive Organic Materials for Regeneration of Neural Tissues. *Acta Biomater.* **2022**, *139*, 22–42. [CrossRef]
130. Correia, D.M.; Fernandes, L.C.; Fernandes, M.M.; Hermenegildo, B.; Meira, R.M.; Ribeiro, C.; Ribeiro, S.; Reguera, J.; Lanceros-Méndez, S. Ionic Liquid-Based Materials for Biomedical Applications. *Nanomaterials* **2021**, *11*, 2401. [CrossRef]
131. Kelsey, J.L.; Lamster, I.B. Influence of Musculoskeletal Conditions on Oral Health Among Older Adults. *Am. J. Public Health* **2008**, *98*, 1177–1183. [CrossRef]
132. Niesten, D.; van Mourik, K.; Sanden, W. van der The Impact of Frailty on Oral Care Behavior of Older People: A Qualitative Study. *BMC Oral Health* **2013**, *13*, 61–73. [CrossRef]
133. Hayashi, T.; Murase, N.; Sato, N.; Fujino, K.; Sugimura, N.; Wada, H.; Kuroda, K.; Shimojima, A. Fluoride Ion-Encapsulated Germoxane Cages Modified with Organosiloxane Chains as Anionic Components of Ionic Liquids. *Organometallics* **2022**, *41*, 1454–1463. [CrossRef]

134. Farnum, A.; Parnas, M.; Hoque Apu, E.; Cox, E.; Lefevre, N.; Contag, C.H.; Saha, D. Harnessing Insect Olfactory Neural Circuits for Detecting and Discriminating Human Cancers. *Biosens. Bioelectron.* **2023**, *219*, 114814. [CrossRef]
135. Shaikh, M.S.; Lone, M.A.; Kabir, R.; Hoque Apu, E. Periodontal Connections to the Coronavirus Disease 2019: An Unexplored Novel Path? *Adv. Hum. Biol.* **2020**, *10*, 197–198.
136. Isha, S.N.; Ahmad, A.; Kabir, R.; Hoque Apu, E. Dental Clinic Architecture Prevents COVID-19-Like Infectious Diseases. *HERD Health Environ. Res. Des. J.* **2020**, *13*, 240–241. [CrossRef]
137. Rahman, F.; Jahan, S.S.; Shaikh, M.H.; Hoque Apu, E. Use of Antivirals in Denture: A Potential Approach in Dental Practice. *J. Adv. Oral Res.* **2021**, *12*, 5–6. [CrossRef]
138. Salo, T.; Sutinen, M.; Hoque Apu, E.; Sundquist, E.; Cervigne, N.K.; de Oliveira, C.E.; Akram, S.U.; Ohlmeier, S.; Suomi, F.; Eklund, L.; et al. A Novel Human Leiomyoma Tissue Derived Matrix for Cell Culture Studies. *BMC Cancer* **2015**, *15*, 981. [CrossRef] [PubMed]

Disclaimer/Publisher's Note: The statements, opinions and data contained in all publications are solely those of the individual author(s) and contributor(s) and not of MDPI and/or the editor(s). MDPI and/or the editor(s) disclaim responsibility for any injury to people or property resulting from any ideas, methods, instructions or products referred to in the content.

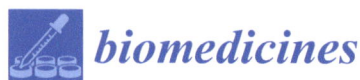

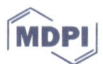

Article

Comparison of the Surface Roughness of CAD/CAM Metal-Free Materials Used for Complete-Arch Implant-Supported Prostheses: An In Vitro Study

Nataly Mory [1], Rocío Cascos [1,2,3,*], Alicia Celemín-Viñuela [1], Cristina Gómez-Polo [4], Rubén Agustín-Panadero [5] and Miguel Gómez-Polo [1]

1. Department of Conservative Dentistry and Orofacial Prosthodontics, Faculty of Dentistry, Complutense University of Madrid, 28040 Madrid, Spain; natmory@ucm.es (N.M.); acelemin@ucm.es (A.C.-V.); mgomezpo@ucm.es (M.G.-P.)
2. Department of Nursing and Estomatology, Faculty of Health Sciences, Rey Juan Carlos University, 28922 Madrid, Spain
3. Department of Prosthetic Dentistry, School of Dentistry, European University of Madrid, 28670 Madrid, Spain
4. Department of Surgery, Faculty of Medicine, University of Salamanca, 37007 Salamanca, Spain; crisgodent@usal.es
5. Prosthodontic and Occlusion Unit, Department of Stomatology, Faculty of Medicine and Dentistry, Universitat de València, 46010 Valencia, Spain; ruben.agustin@uv.es
* Correspondence: rcascos@ucm.es; Tel.: +34-91-394-2029

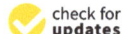

Citation: Mory, N.; Cascos, R.; Celemín-Viñuela, A.; Gómez-Polo, C.; Agustín-Panadero, R.; Gómez-Polo, M. Comparison of the Surface Roughness of CAD/CAM Metal-Free Materials Used for Complete-Arch Implant-Supported Prostheses: An In Vitro Study. *Biomedicines* 2023, 11, 3036. https://doi.org/10.3390/biomedicines11113036

Academic Editor: Giuseppe Minervini

Received: 1 October 2023
Revised: 2 November 2023
Accepted: 6 November 2023
Published: 13 November 2023

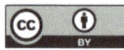

Copyright: © 2023 by the authors. Licensee MDPI, Basel, Switzerland. This article is an open access article distributed under the terms and conditions of the Creative Commons Attribution (CC BY) license (https://creativecommons.org/licenses/by/4.0/).

Abstract: The roughness of the intra-oral surfaces significantly influences the initial adhesion and the retention of microorganisms. The aim of this study was to analyze the surface texture of four different CAD-CAM materials (two high-performance polymers and two fifth-generation zirconia) used for complete-arch implant-supported prostheses (CAISPs), and to investigate the effect of artificial aging on their roughness. A total of 40 milled prostheses were divided into 4 groups ($n = 10$) according to their framework material, bio.HPP (B), bio.HPP Plus (BP), zirconia Luxor Z Frame (ZF), and Luxor Z True Nature (ZM). The areal surface roughness "Sa" and the maximum height "Sz" of each specimen was measured on the same site after laboratory fabrication (lab as-received specimen) and after thermocycling (5–55 °C, 10,000 cycles) by using a noncontact optical profilometer. Data were analyzed using SPSS version 28.0.1. One-way ANOVA with multiple comparison tests ($p = 0.05$) and repeated measures ANOVA were used. After thermocycling, all materials maintained "Sa" values at the laboratory as-received specimen level ($p = 0.24$). "Sz" increased only for the zirconia groups ($p = 0.01$). B-BP exhibited results equal/slightly better than ZM-ZF. This study provides more realistic surface texture values of new metal-free materials used in real anatomical CAISPs after the manufacturing and aging processes and establishes a detailed and reproducible measurement workflow.

Keywords: surface roughness; surface texture; CAD/CAM; high-performance polymers; PEEK; zirconia; thermocycling; complete-arch implant-supported prostheses

1. Introduction

The surface roughness of dental materials which are in contact with soft tissues plays a crucial role in the accumulation and adhesion of biofilm. Rough surfaces promote increased bacterial adhesion due to their larger surface area and cleaning difficulties [1]. Therefore, materials with low surface roughness are essential to minimize bio-adhesion. Previous articles have reported that the clinical acceptability threshold of roughness for dental materials is 0.2 µm (Ra). Below this level, surface roughness does not significantly impact biofilm formation [2]. The microbiota around dental implants differ from the periodontal microbiota [3]. Consequently, one of the main objectives of surface finishing is to achieve a surface roughness below 0.2 mm by utilizing polishing techniques, devices, and materials [4]. Changes in surface roughness can be caused by a complex and changing humid oral environment, changes in temperature [5], manufacturing process (milling, sintering, sandblasting) [6], or modifications performed with rotatory instruments [7]. Furthermore, surface roughness presents significant implications across various crucial aspects for prosthetic dentistry, including bacterial proliferation [8,9], strength [10], optical properties [11,12], and adhesion [13].

The high demands of aesthetic and biocompatible materials have increased the popularity of metal-free materials in prosthetic dentistry and the main emphasis of developers has been on enhancing their optical and mechanical properties. The gold standard for the manufacturing of complete-arch implant-supported prostheses (CAISPs) involved a metal framework and ceramic veneering. However, in recent years, the evolution of digital technologies and cad/cam materials has led to the development of alternative materials such as high-performance polymers like bio.HPP and new generations of zirconia to improve their aesthetics and mechanical properties [14].

Nowadays, high-performance polymer (HPP) materials have gained significant interest in the field of prosthodontics. This attention is attributed to their advantageous mechanical and biocompatible properties, which enhance their possibility to replace traditional metal frameworks in implant-supported prostheses [15]. BioHPP is a modified PEEK with 20–30% of ceramic fillers, and is a semi-crystalline biopolymer characterized by non-allergenic properties, good biocompatibility, low plaque affinity, excellent stability, and high temperature and chemical resistance, as well as resistance to corrosion [16,17]. It also exhibits high mechanical strength [18], high hardness, low water absorption, and low solubility [5]. Furthermore, PEEK-based materials have a low modulus of elasticity like human bone (4 Gpa) [19], which improves the transmission of chewing pressure, reduces stress, and stimulates the bone modeling around the implants. Additionally, advantages include good polishing properties, good esthetics, low weight, and wear resistance [20]. However, PEEK restorations have a white/dentin opaque color and require veneering with composite resin. Considering the mechanical strength [21] and biocompatibility [22], HPP represent a promising alternative for use as framework material in implant-supported rehabilitations [23].

New generations of zirconia have been introduced to combine the advantages of esthetics and translucency with mechanical properties [24]. Zirconia is a polymorphic material with three crystallographic phases: monoclinic, tetragonal, and cubic [25]. It is present in the monoclinic form at room temperature and when heated its phase transformation occurs to its tetragonal form, and further heating leads to its cubic form. Y-TZP (yttria-stabilized tetragonal zirconia polycrystal) can be of three types based on the yttria content: 3Y-TZP (3 mol%), 4Y-TZP (4 mol%), and 5Y-TZP (5 mol%) [26]. The 3Y-TZP (tetragonal zirconia) is the strongest and 5Y-TZP is the most translucent [27]. Recent developments in Y-TZP materials with a higher yttria content (4–6 mol% yttria) have provided a high translucency and adequate strength. Consequently, clinical indications of monolithic zirconia restorations have expanded to avoid interface fractures in veneer-core structures [28,29]; Luxor Z Frame and Luxor Z True Nature (both 5th generation) represent two new brands of these emerging zirconia materials.

The surface roughness of a material results from marks and grooves left by various factors during fabrication, including tools, abrasive particles, and chemical processes [30]. The areal surface roughness parameter "Sa" calculates average surface roughness and is widely used due to its reliability in minimizing the impact of surface defects. It is a 3D surface parameter analogous to "Ra", a 2D parameter which measures linear roughness. Additionally, "Sz" represents the maximum height of the selected area and is the sum of the highest peak height and the deepest valley depth. While useful, "Sz" can be influenced by surface flaws like scratches and contamination, as it relies on peak values. Therefore, using both parameters is essential to assess the surface texture of dental prostheses [6]. There is limited information available about the surface roughness of these CAD/CAM materials when comparing laboratory as-received prostheses and their roughness values after artificial aging. Moreover, there is a lack of studies evaluating surface roughness in CAISPs.

While PEEK was previously used as a long-term provisional material in complete-arch implant restorations, the emergence of modified PEEK materials, as well as the introduction of new translucent zirconia, has significantly enhanced their mechanical properties. Consequently, their clinical indications have expanded to include definitive complete rehabilitations. Therefore, it is clinically relevant to evaluate a critical property like surface roughness due to its significant implications across various essential aspects for implant prosthetic dentistry.

The main objective of this in vitro study was to evaluate the surface roughness of four CAD/CAM materials used for complete-arch implant-supported prostheses (CAISPs) after manufacturing laboratory procedures and to investigate the effect of thermocycling on their surface roughness. The following null hypotheses were evaluated: 1. There are no statistically significant differences in surface roughness among all the studied materials after the manufacturing of CAISDP frameworks. 2. No differences are found on the roughness of the aged specimens among the groups. 3. Thermocycling does not affect the surface roughness of the investigated materials.

2. Materials and Methods

2.1. Sample Size Calculation

A previous pilot study ($n = 3$) was conducted to determine the appropriate sample size. Based on the difference between two independent means (BP and ZF groups) using Sa means and SD values, an effect size of 1.4 was calculated. A sample size of ($n = 10$) specimens per group was calculated using G-power software version 3.1.9.6 (Heinrich-Heine University, Düsseldorf, Germany). A two-tailed analysis with a power of 0.80 and a significance level of $\alpha = 0.05$ was performed. This sample size was consistent with that used in previous studies [1,4,24,31].

2.2. Specimen Preparation: Materials, Design, and Laboratory Manufacturing

The high-performance polymers selected for this study were bioHPP dentin shade A2 and bio.HPP Plus White (Bredent GmbH & Co, Senden, Germany). The zirconia materials chosen included fifth-generation zirconia Luxor Z Frame and zirconia Luxor Z True Nature, both in shade A3 (Bredent GmbH & Co, Senden, Germany), which are translucent multilayer zirconia materials developed for the CAD/CAM milling of full-contour restorations. The compositions of the experimental materials are detailed in Table 1.

Table 1. Summary of experimental materials, abbreviations groups, compositions, and brand names.

Framework Material	Groups	Chemical Composition	Brand Name
Polyether ether ketone	B	Polyether ether ketone with 20 wt.% inorganic fillers *	Bio.hpp
Polyether ether ketone	BP	Polyether ether ketone with 25 wt.% inorganic fillers *	Bio.hpp Plus
Zirconia frame	ZF	94–95% ZrO_2, 4.5–5.5% Y_2O_3, <0.5% Al_2O_3, <0.5% other oxide	Luxor Z Frame
Zirconia monolithic	ZM	90–95% ZrO_2, 4–10% Y_2O_3, $\leq$0.5% Al_2O_3, <0.5% other oxide	Luxor Z True Nature

* TiO_2 and inorganic pigment.

The Bio.HPP materials present a High Fracture Strength of around 1000–1500 N [18]. Additionally, as specified by the manufacturer, the Luxor Z frame zirconia material exhibits a Fracture Strength of >1050 MPa (previously colored disc) and >1100 MPa (white disc version), while the Luxor Z True Nature features a Flexural Strength of 1100 MPa in the cervical region and 750 MPa in the incisal area.

In the present in vitro study, two computer-aided designs for mandibular complete-arch implant-supported prostheses (CAISPs) were employed: one with a total volume STL, and another with a reduced volume framework STL. These STLs were designed using exocad software version 2.4 (Exocad Plovdiv GmbH, Darmstadt, Germany). A total of 40 specimens (CAISPs) were divided into four groups, with $n = 10$ per group, according to their framework material: group B (bioHPP), group BP (bioHPP Plus), group ZF (Luxor Z-Frame zirconia), and group ZM (Monolithic zirconia, Luxor Z True Nature).

For the zirconia rehabilitations, the designs were created with approximately 20% enlarged dimensions to compensate for sintering shrinkage. Subsequently, the samples were milled from pre-sintered zirconium oxide discs using computer-aided machining techniques. Following the milling process, the zirconia frameworks were sintered in a furnace Programat P510 (Ivoclar Vivadent, Schaan, Liechtenstein) according to the manufacturer recommendations. The sintering protocol for bridges above 7 units involved heating at 5 °C/min to 900 °C and then at 2 °C/min to 1500 °C, with a 120-min hold time, and then cooling at 3 °C/min to 900 °C and 7 °C/min to 300 °C. The total time was 13–15 h. In group ZF, a veneering ceramic was applied using a layering technique, with low-fusing glass–ceramic IPS e.max® Ceram (Ivoclar Vivadent, Schaan, Liechtenstein) in shade A2. Then, ZF and ZM samples were glazed, and no mechanical polishing was performed.

Peek-based rehabilitations were milled from bioHPP and bioHPP Plus Bre.cam disks (98.5 mm diameter and 20 mm thickness) using a dental laboratory milling unit (CORiTEC 350i; imes-icore). Group B and BP specimens were veneered with composite resin crea.lign (Bredent GmbH & Co, Senden, Germany), except in the basal area. Finally, the finishing of specimens was completed with the visio.lign toolkit (Bredent GmbH & Co, Senden, Germany) for bioHPP. All procedures were conducted following the manufacturer's specifications (Figure 1). The specimens were subject to ultrasonic cleaning in distilled water for 5 min and then dried with compressed air.

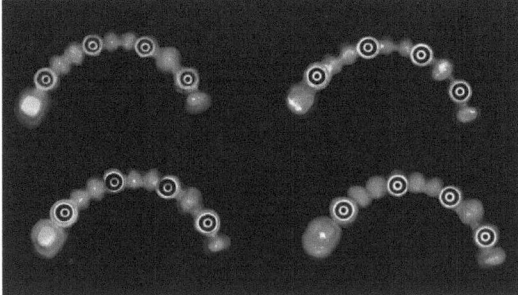

Figure 1. Experimental samples: B (**lower left**); BP (**upper left**); ZF (**lower right**); ZM (**upper right**).

2.3. Surface Texture Analysis

The surface texture of each specimen was measured using a non-contact optical profilometer Alicona Infinite Focus XL200 G5 (Alicona Imaging GmbH, Raaba/Graz, Austria) equipped with a measurement software program (MeasureSuite v. 5.3.1; Alicona Imaging GmbH, Raaba/Graz, Austria). For each specimen, an area of 1.62×1.62 mm^2 was analyzed at the center of the basal side of the 4.6 first molar (non-veneered area). This area corresponds to the maximum field of view achievable using the $10\times$ magnification objective. The same point was observed on each specimen with the use of a silicon mold to allow for comparable results (Figure 2).

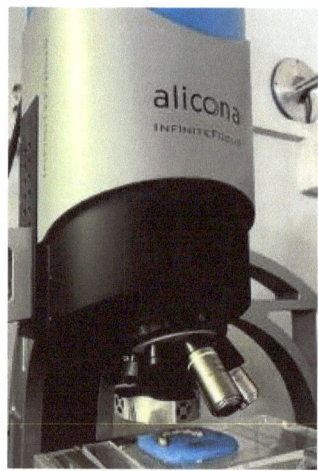

Figure 2. Optical measuring equipment.

A focus variation microscope was chosen as one of the most suitable instruments to perform high-precision three-dimensional surface texture measurements. The surface area was examined in 3D images at 10× magnification. Two tridimensional roughness parameters "Sa" (average areal surface roughness) and "Sz" (maximum height) were evaluated. Specimens were initially measured after laboratory manufacturing "lab as-received specimen". These measurements were considered as baseline values (Sa, Sz). After the artificial aging procedure, the same parameters were measured for the "aged specimens" (Sa tmcl, Sz tmcl), and values were registered in microns. The measurement workflow applied was conducting following the manufacturer's instruction for surface texture measurement. This involved the initial form removal, adjustment of the reference plane, application of the roughness filter to separate roughness from waviness, and using a 0.8 mm cutoff, according to ISO 25178 standards [32,33] (Figure 3). A Gaussian filter was used to eliminate tilt from every surface analysis. Color topographic map images represent the height variations on the surface of the samples (Figure 4). Changes in Sa (Sa-Sa tmcl) and Sz (Sz-Sz tmcl) were analyzed to assess the effect of thermocycling on material roughness.

The accuracy of the profilometer was calibrated for every 10 measurements and all measurements were carried out by a single trained operator. The specimens were codified with an ID number prior to the roughness measurements. The operator conducting the measurements and the statistician performing the data analysis did not have information about the material being evaluated, ensuring a double-blind test.

2.4. Hydrothermal Aging Process of Specimens

To simulate artificial aging, all the specimens were thermocycled for 10,000 cycles, equivalent to one year of clinical function [1]. Thermocycling was performed using a thermal cycler device (VA55, Euroortodoncia, Madrid, Spain) in distilled water at temperatures of $5 \pm 5\ °C$ and $55 \pm 5\ °C$, with an immersion time of 20 s in each bath and a transfer time of 10 s. After the process, the thermocycled (tmcl) specimens were cleaned ultrasonically in distilled water for 5 min and dried.

2.5. Microscopic Observation

A microscopic analysis of two randomly selected samples for each group was conducted (basal side of the 4.6) before and after thermocycling using an optical microscope (VE4, Euroortodoncia, Madrid, Spain) at a magnification of 10×. Images of the samples were captured and subsequently subjected to visual inspection.

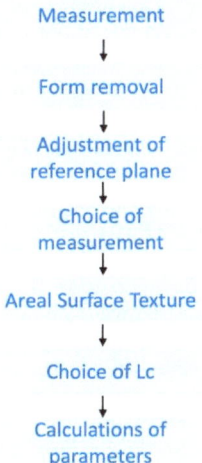

Figure 3. Surface texture measurement workflow.

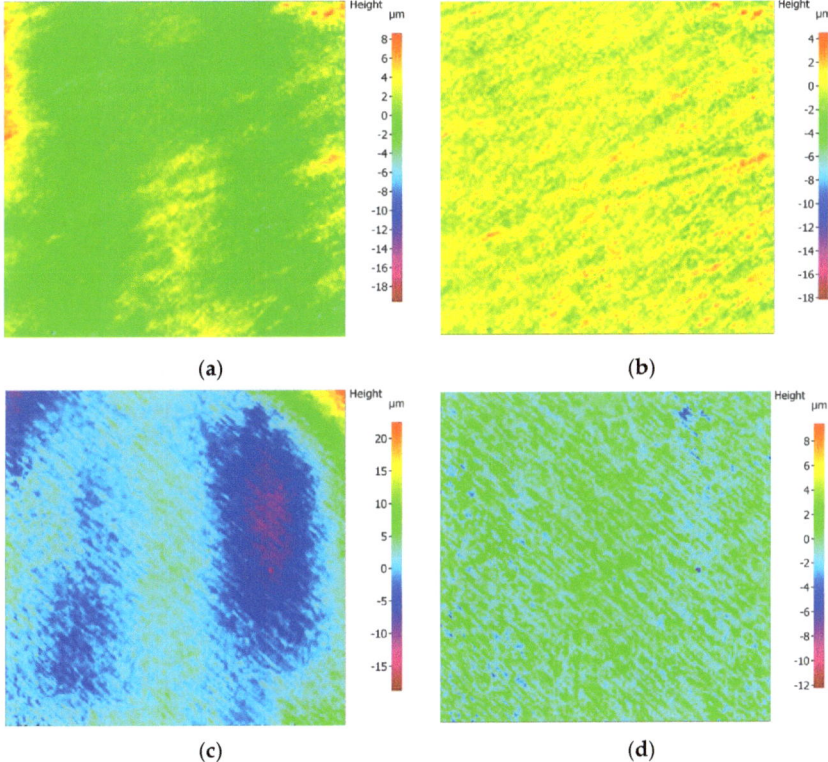

Figure 4. Surface texture measurement: images of the B group (**a**) original dataset; (**b**) filtered roughness dataset; and ZF group (**c**) original dataset; (**d**) filtered roughness dataset at 10× magnification.

2.6. Statistical Analysis

All statistical analyses were performed using a statistical software program SPSS Statistics version 28.0.1.1 (IBM Corporation, Armonk, NY, USA). Descriptive statistics, including mean, median, and standard deviation, were calculated. The normality of the data was assessed using the Shapiro–Wilk test, and parametric statistics were applied. Data were analyzed using a two-sided one-way ANOVA, followed by the Bonferroni corrected test for multiple comparisons to determine the effect of material types. A repeated measures ANOVA was employed to assess the effect of the aging process on surface roughness. A significance level of "$p < 0.05$" was stablished.

3. Results

3.1. Surface Roughness Measurements

The areal surface texture was determined using two commonly used tridimensional roughness parameters: Sa (average areal surface roughness) and Sz (maximum peak-to-valley height). All the samples were measured before and after thermocycling.

The descriptive statistics, mean surface roughness values, and standard deviations for the "Sa" and "Sz" parameters are displayed in Table 2.

Table 2. Mean surface roughness values ± SD (μm) for "Sa" (on the left) and "Sz" (on the right), and after manufacturing (baseline) and after thermocycling (tmcl).

Experimental Group	Sa		Sa	
	Baseline	tmcl	Baseline	tmcl
B	0.66 ± 0.07 [aA]	0.65 ± 0.13 [aA]	16.13 ± 5.84 [aA]	16.56 ± 11.48 [aA]
BP	0.75 ± 0.09 [aA]	0.75 ± 0.14 [aA]	15.08 ± 3.27 [aA]	15.19 ± 4.01 [aA]
ZF	0.75 ± 0.15 [aA]	0.81 ± 0.14 [aA]	33.63 ± 23.91 [bA]	56.55 ± 23.92 [bB]
ZM	0.70 ± 0.09 [aA]	0.75 ± 0.14 [aA]	18.98 ± 9.29 [abA]	33.85 ± 14.90 [aB]

The same superscript lowercase letters in the same column and uppercase letters in the same row indicate no significant differences ($p < 0.05$). See Table 1 for group abbreviations.

3.1.1. Baseline Data

After the manufacturing laboratory procedure, the Sa highest values were observed in the ZF (0.75 ± 0.15) and BP (0.75 ± 0.09) groups, followed by the ZM and the B group with (0.70 ± 0.09) and (0.66 ± 0.07), respectively. Regarding the Sz parameter, the highest value was also obtained in the ZF group (33.63 ± 23.91), followed by the ZM (18.98 ± 9.29), B (16.13 ± 5.84), and BP (15.08 ± 3.27) groups.

At the initial Sa values, there were no statistically significant differences among the groups ($p = 0.21$). However, significant differences were found for the Sz parameter ($p = 0.01$). These differences were specific between the ZF group and the B and BP groups, while no significant difference was noted with the ZM group. The results of the Sz measurements are presented in Figure 5.

3.1.2. Data after Aging Process

Thermocycled specimens (5–55 °C, 10,000 cycles) were analyzed. For the Sa tmcl variable, the ZF group had the highest value (0.81 ± 0.14) and the B group (0.65 ± 0.13) the lowest value. However, no significant differences were detected among the four groups ($p = 0.09$). Regarding the Sz tmcl parameter, the highest value was also obtained in the ZF group (56.55 ± 23.92), followed by the ZM (33.85 ± 14.90), B (16.56 ± 11.48), and BP (15.19 ± 4.01) groups. A one-way ANOVA followed by the Bonferroni post-hoc test revealed significant differences between the ZF group and the rest of the groups (B, BP, and ZM) ($p < 0.05$).

3.1.3. Effect of Thermocycling

A repeated measures ANOVA test was used to assess the influence of thermocycling on the initial surface roughness. Thermocycling exhibited a minimal effect on the "Sa" parameter in relation to the studied materials. No statistically significant differences were found between Sa and Sa tmcl among the four groups. However, significant differences between Sz and Sz tmcl were observed, exclusively in the zirconia groups (ZF and ZM). Hence, the both Sa and Sz values for HPP groups (B and BP) after aging remained similar to those of the lab as-received specimens. The results of measurements for both 3D roughness parameters, before and after thermocycling, are presented in Figure 6.

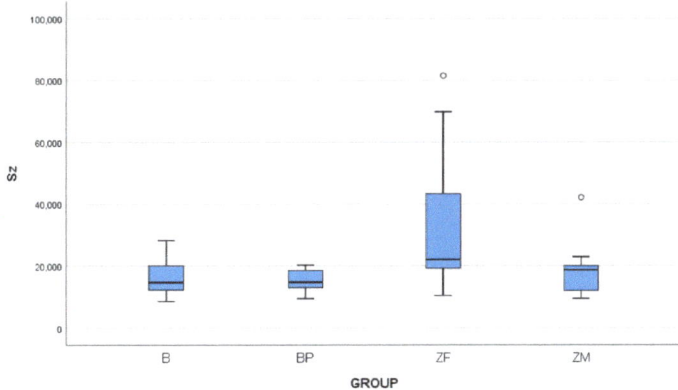

Figure 5. Representative box plot for Sz (μm) baseline data according to total values per group. White dot represents the outlier values.

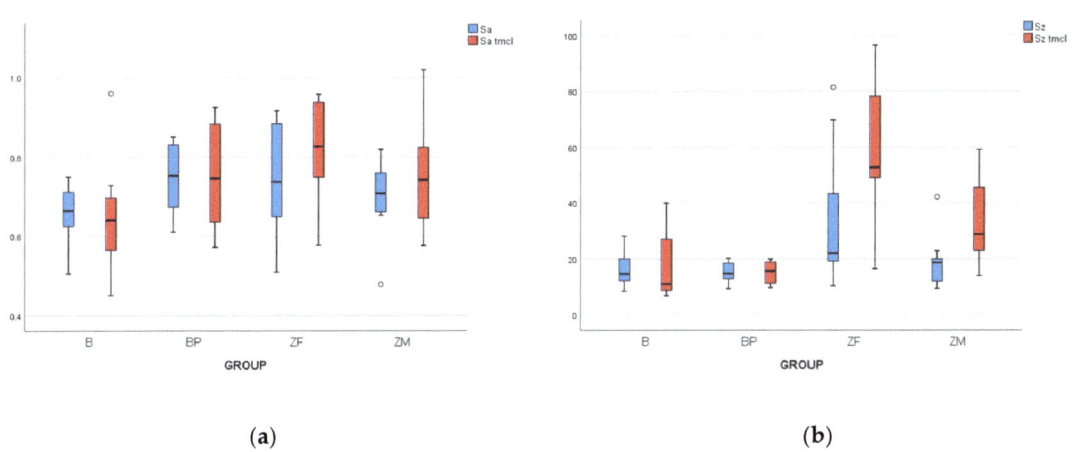

(a) (b)

Figure 6. Representative boxplots of the surface parameters (μm) among studied groups. (**a**) Sa (baseline data) and Sa tmcl (after tmcl data); (**b**) Sz (baseline data) and Sz tmcl (after tmcl data). White dot represents the outlier values.

3.2. Surface Microscopic Analysis

Microscopic assessment at 10× magnification revealed that thermocycling did not induce significant alterations in the modified PEEK-based materials. No cracks were observed, and only small pores and milling lines were detected before and after artificial aging in both the B and BP groups (Figure 7).

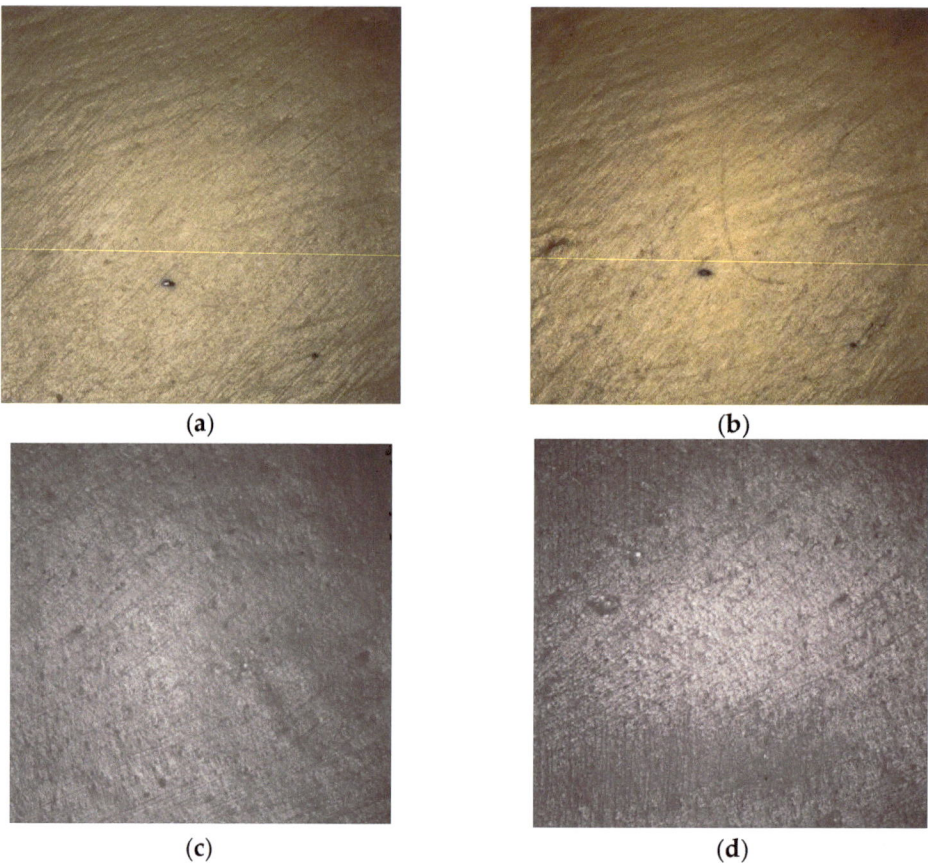

Figure 7. Microscopic images of the B (**a**,**b**) and BP (**c**,**d**) groups at 10× magnification. (**left**) Baseline; (**right**) after tmcl. Small pores and milling lines were observed.

On the other hand, the zirconia groups exhibited surfaces with minor irregularities, including scratches of the milling bur, pre-existing flaws, and small cracks that became more pronounced after artificial aging (Figure 8).

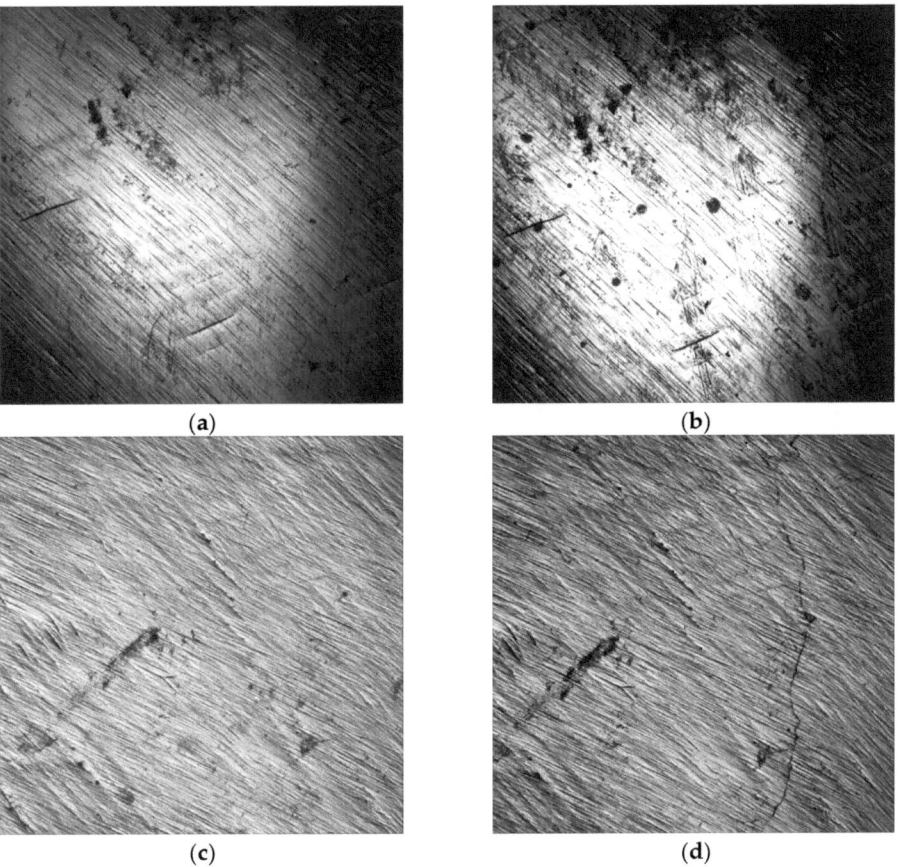

Figure 8. Microscopic images of the ZF (**a**,**b**) and ZM (**c**,**d**) groups at 10× magnification. (**left**) Baseline; (**right**) after tmcl. Scratches and flaws more visible after tmcl.

4. Discussion

In this study, we provide novel insights into surface roughness measurement and its significance in prosthetic dentistry. The main objective of this research is to assess the effect of thermocycling on the surface roughness of state-of-the-art materials, including the latest developments in high-performance polymers (bio.HPP Plus) and translucent zirconia materials (Luxor Z Frame and Luxor Z True Nature). Additionally, we aim to introduce a comprehensive method detailing the essential steps for achieving accurate surface roughness measurements within a determined area, with the goal of reducing inaccuracies associated with conventional linear measurements.

Surface roughness is the most important parameter for describing surface texture and plays a crucial role in various clinical aspects. Its assessment is essential due to its direct influence on microbial adhesion and biofilm formation [1]. This study aimed to compare the surface roughness of framework materials for CAISPs. Previous studies have reported similar results for average roughness in bioHPP [4] and 5Y-ZP zirconia specimens [24]. However, this current research explored differences in specific 3D parameters, "Sa" (average roughness) and "Sz" (highest peak to valley) to achieve a better understanding of surface texture.

Initially, our results indicated that there were no significant differences in the baseline data among the groups for the Sa parameter, suggesting that the materials exhibited similar surface properties. However, we found statistically significant differences for the Sz parameter between the ZF group and the B-BP groups, but not with the ZM group. As a result, the first null hypothesis was partially rejected. These statistical differences between the ZF and B-BP groups can be attributed to the different composition of polymers and ceramics [9].

Moreover, manufacturing procedures can influence surface roughness. Notably, only the ZF group showed significant differences in Sz value, which can be partly attributed to an additional firing process for ceramic veneering during the fabrication of dental prostheses [7], while the ZM group lacks such a coating. It is also possibly due to increased milling complexity and greater flexural strength and hardness compared to the ZM group [34]. Standard deviations (SD) in Sz are notably higher, displaying considerable variability, as is commonly observed in studies evaluating Sz [35]. The zirconia groups showed higher SD compared to the PEEK groups, with the ZF group registering the highest value.

Additionally, the microscopic analysis revealed that ZF exhibited different surface characteristics compared to B and BP, showing more surface defects. These defects may be a result of larger grains within the material, which are removed during the milling or adjustment process [36].

In the aged specimens, Sa tmcl values showed no differences, but significant differences in Sz tmcl were observed for the ZF group in comparison to the other groups. This could be because the ZF group had a composition that differs from the B-BP group, as well as the ZM group. ZF has a higher ZrO_2 content and lower yttria content compared to ZM. These slight variations may make it more susceptible to a phenomenon known as low-temperature degradation (LTD), a chemical property of zirconia that results in surface degradation, microcracking, and reduced strength in the presence of humidity [37].

Considering the effect of thermocycling (TMCL), the results of Sa confirm that it does not increase average roughness for PEEK-based and zirconia materials. In contrast, both zirconia groups (ZF-ZM) showed intra-group differences between initial and post-TMCL values. This can be explained by the zirconia's susceptibility to LTD, which involves a slow transformation from the tetragonal (t) to monoclinic (m) phase, induced by thermal or mechanical stress, and exacerbated in the presence of water, causing a surface deterioration [38]. The presence of Al_2O_3 stabilizes the tetragonal phase and improves hydrothermal ageing resistance; therefore, when the alumina content decreases (≤ 0.05 wt.%), zirconia is more translucent but more susceptible to LTD [39]. Conversely, a higher yttria content reduces LTD by producing a less monoclinic phase and providing greater structural stability. Consequently, translucent zirconia (5Y-ZP) exhibits lower susceptibility to LTD than tetragonal zirconia (3Y-TZP); however, 3Y-TZP still has an adequate durability in oral conditions [40,41]. Theoretically, the aging process should lead to an increase in surface roughness. However, when comparing the initial and final roughness of the bioHPP samples, it became evident that the B-BP groups did not show significant changes in the Sa and Sz parameters, and their values for Sa-Sa tmcl and Sz-Sz tmcl remained unaltered. Notably, the aging process in the zirconia groups ZF-ZM led to significant differences in the Sz-Sz tmcl parameters, with both groups also displaying the highest initial Sz values. These variations in Sz are indicative of the presence of pores, cracks, and flaws, making it a valuable parameter for assessing surface irregularities and specific defects.

In recent years, numerous studies have evaluated surface roughness in PEEK and zirconia materials [2,4,5,7–9,24]. However, only one has been conducted on samples with real anatomies (monolithic zirconia 3-unit bridges) [11]. These studies reveal two distinct trends: some report more favorable results for zirconia materials [22,42], while another opposing trend observes lower roughness in PEEK materials [8]. In thermocycling-induced artificial aging, most studies do not report significant differences in average roughness values (Sa, Ra) before and after TMCL for the two main material types assessed in this study: HPP [1] and translucent zirconia [26].

In most literature reports [4,7,22,24,31], surface texture is typically assessed using simple profile surface measures like Ra or Rz, while areal parameters have proven to be more informative [6]. However, despite using the same parameter, results vary widely, possibly due to the use of different measurement equipment. Some studies use contact profilometers, which provide R values (a line), while others use non-contact optical systems (interferometric, focus variation, or confocal microscopes, AFM), which offer S values (an area). Non-contact optical systems can also calculate bidimensional parameters but may not fully represent the surface. The methodological differences and the wide range of parameter values are mainly attributed to the measurement methods and procedures selected. The absence of standardized measurement methods and failure to specify key factors, such as the length of the profile path for Ra or the cutoff filter, further complicate their reproducibility. In our research, measurements were conducted at a $10\times$ magnification using a Gaussian filter and a cutoff length of 0.8 mm, following ISO 25178 standards. While numerous methods are available for measuring surface roughness, there is a lack of standardized procedures for conducting comparisons across different studies. ISO 4287:1999 [43] measures linear roughness "Ra", which is limited to 2D measurement, while the more recent ISO 25178-2:2012 includes updated terms, definitions, and parameters for 3D evaluation [33]. "Sa", a 3D parameter, offers more comprehensive data by measuring entire areas, rather than just linear profiles. Sa values are also influenced by magnification, with higher magnification yielding lower roughness values [30]. Although the values obtained for Sa exceeded the clinically acceptable limit of Ra = 0.2 μm [2], we could not directly correlate 3D–2D parameters, as they are not equivalent.

In the realm of laboratory processing, ceramics have been categorized as difficult-to-machine materials due to their high hardness and brittleness. After milling, tiny cracks may develop on the final surface [6]. Also, 5Y-ZP did not undergo transformation toughening and as a result may not be as tolerant to the surface damage introduced during the fabrication (milling, sintering), adjustment, and airborne particle abrasion of a zirconia restoration [34]. Sintering conditions have a strong impact on stability and mechanical properties, and affects surface texture. The type of sintering (traditional or fast) affects the properties. Novel speed sintering protocols have been developed to meet the demand for time and cost-effective CAD/CAM restorations [44]. Wertz et al. reported that the milling process may increase the monoclinic phase after machining, but it disappears after sintering. Moreover, glazing and sandblasting processes have minimal influence on the crystallographic structure phases [45]. However, an increase in roughness (Sa, Sz) was observed after sandblasting [46]. Kim et al. reported that translucent zirconia requires 50 μm alumina sandblasting to prevent surface damage [47]. In some cases, differences in surface roughness may not be detected using only average roughness parameters, Sa, or Ra. When this occurs, it is essential to focus on other parameters such as Sz, which allows us to assess the unevenness. In a previous study conducted by Fernández et al., the Sz parameter was evaluated in milled Cr-Co frameworks, yielding a value of 29 μm, which is comparable to the initial Sz value observed in our study for the ZF group (33 μm) [35].

This study has the typical limitations of in vitro studies. Mechanical and biological factors, such as occlusion and the oral environment, were not replicated, which limits the direct extrapolation of the data to the clinical situation. Furthermore, bacterial adhesion was not evaluated, which could have provided additional insights regarding the relationship between surface roughness and bacterial adhesion. Additionally, comparing different roughness measurement equipment was not feasible due to a lack of reported details in previous studies, highlighting the need to consider these details in future investigations.

While, traditionally, metal–ceramic prostheses have been the primary choice for CAISPs, demonstrating high clinical performance and long-term survival rates, it is important to consider the potential impact of alternative materials like zirconia and HPP, which offer biocompatibility and optimal mechanical properties. Moreover, HPP has the ability to absorb occlusal forces [48], making it interesting to evaluate its damping effects on masticatory function in order to prevent the overloading of implants and temporomandibular disorders. Ultimately, the extensive literature on surface roughness has revealed correlations with other parameters such as flexural strength [7,10], antagonist wear [49], translucency [50], etc., which could be explored in future research.

Further comparative clinical studies are essential to validate the utilization of these new materials and determine their performance and applications in clinical practice.

5. Conclusions

Considering the limitations inherent to the present in vitro study, the following conclusions were drawn:

The thermocycling process did not show a statistically significant impact on the average areal surface roughness (Sa) of the CAD/CAM studied materials, including high-performance polymers and fifth-generation zirconia. Statistically significant differences were only found for the maximum peak–valley heigh (Sz) in the zirconia groups.

Furthermore, it is noteworthy that the surface roughness observed in BioHPP (modified PEEK) groups closely resembled that of zirconia.

Significantly, microscopic observations did not reveal the presence of microcracks in the surface texture of the B and BP groups.

Author Contributions: Conceptualization, M.G.-P. and N.M.; methodology, M.G.-P. and N.M.; software, R.C. and N.M.; validation, M.G.-P., R.A.-P. and A.C.-V.; formal analysis M.G.-P., N.M., R.C. and C.G.-P.; investigation, N.M.; resources, M.G.-P. and N.M.; data curation, N.M., R.C. and C.G.-P.; writing—original draft preparation, N.M.; writing—review and editing, M.G.-P., N.M. and R.C.; visualization, A.C.-V. and R.A.-P.; supervision, M.G.-P.; project administration, M.G.-P.; funding acquisition, M.G.-P. and N.M. All authors have read and agreed to the published version of the manuscript.

Funding: This research has been partially funded by the company Bredent GmbH & Co. KG.

Institutional Review Board Statement: Not applicable.

Informed Consent Statement: Not applicable.

Data Availability Statement: The data presented in this study are available on request from the corresponding author.

Acknowledgments: The authors would like to thank Bredent GmbH for providing the materials manufactured for this research. Additionally, we extend our thanks to Euroortodoncia Laboratory, especially A. Cervera, I. García for their assistance with the test, and the Alicona support service for their guidance on using the optical profilometer.

Conflicts of Interest: The authors declare no conflict of interest.

References

1. Valente, M.; Da Silva, G.; Bachmann, L.; Agnelli, J.; Dos Reis, A. An in Vitro Analysis of the Physical and Mechanical Behavior of a Polyetheretherketone (PEEK) Component for an Implant-Supported and Retained Removable Dental Prosthesis (I-RDP). *Int. J. Prosthodont.* **2021**, *36*, 612–619. [CrossRef]
2. Bollen, C.M.L.; Lambrechts, P.; Quirynen, M. Comparison of Surface Roughness of Oral Hard Materials to the Threshold Surface Roughness for Bacterial Plaque Retention: A Review of the Literature. *Dent. Mater.* **1997**, *13*, 258–269. [CrossRef]
3. Butera, A.; Pascadopoli, M.; Pellegrini, M.; Gallo, S.; Zampetti, P.; Scribante, A. Oral Microbiota in Patients with Peri-Implant Disease: A Narrative Review. *Appl. Sci.* **2022**, *12*, 3250. [CrossRef]
4. Batak, B.; Çakmak, G.; Johnston, W.M.; Yilmaz, B. Surface Roughness of High-Performance Polymers Used for Fixed Implant-Supported Prostheses. *J. Prosthet. Dent.* **2021**, *126*, 254.e1–254.e6. [CrossRef] [PubMed]
5. Liebermann, A.; Wimmer, T.; Schmidlin, P.R.; Scherer, H.; Löffler, P.; Roos, M.; Stawarczyk, B. Physicomechanical Characterization of Polyetheretherketone and Current Esthetic Dental CAD/CAM Polymers after Aging in Different Storage Media. *J. Prosthet. Dent.* **2016**, *115*, 321–328.e2. [CrossRef] [PubMed]
6. Patil, A.; Jebaseelan, D. 3-D Surface Morphological Characterization of CAD/CAM Milled Dental Zirconia: An In Vitro Study of the Effect of Post-Fabrication Processes. *Materials* **2022**, *15*, 4685. [CrossRef]

7. Pradíes, G.; Godoy-Ruiz, L.; Özcan, M.; Moreno-Hay, I.; Martínez-Rus, F. Analysis of Surface Roughness, Fracture Toughness, and Weibull Characteristics of Different Framework-Veneer Dental Ceramic Assemblies after Grinding, Polishing, and Glazing: Influence of Grinding, Polishing, and Glazing on Ceramics Systems. *J. Prosthodont.* 2019, *28*, e216–e221. [CrossRef]
8. Hahnel, S.; Wieser, A.; Lang, R.; Rosentritt, M. Biofilm Formation on the Surface of Modern Implant Abutment Materials. *Clin. Oral. Implant. Res.* 2015, *26*, 1297–1301. [CrossRef]
9. Vulović, S.; Popovac, A.; Radunović, M.; Petrović, S.; Todorović, M.; Milić-Lemić, A. Microbial Adhesion and Viability on Novel CAD/CAM Framework Materials for Implant-Supported Hybrid Prostheses. *Eur. J. Oral. Sci.* 2022, *131*, e12911. [CrossRef]
10. Rashid, H. The Effect of Surface Roughness on Ceramics Used in Dentistry: A Review of Literature. *Eur. J. Dent.* 2014, *8*, 571–579. [CrossRef]
11. Hafezeqoran, A.; Sabanik, P.; Koodaryan, R.; Ghalili, K.M. Effect of Sintering Speed, Aging Processes, and Different Surface Treatments on the Optical and Surface Properties of Monolithic Zirconia Restorations. *J. Prosthet. Dent.* 2022, S0022-3913(21)00690-9. [CrossRef] [PubMed]
12. Schabbach, L.M.; Dos Santos, B.C.; De Bortoli, L.S.; Fabris, D.; Fredel, M.C.; Henriques, B. Translucent Multi-Layered Zirconia: Sandblasting Effect on Optical and Mechanical Properties. *Dent. Mater.* 2023, *39*, 807–819. [CrossRef] [PubMed]
13. Erjavec, A.K.; Črešnar, K.P.; Švab, I.; Vuherer, T.; Žigon, M.; Brunčko, M. Determination of Shear Bond Strength between PEEK Composites and Veneering Composites for the Production of Dental Restorations. *Materials* 2023, *16*, 3286. [CrossRef] [PubMed]
14. Sulaiman, T.A. Materials in Digital Dentistry—A Review. *J. Esthet. Restor. Dent.* 2020, *32*, 171–181. [CrossRef] [PubMed]
15. Al-Rabab'ah, M.; Hamadneh, W.; Alsalem, I.; Khraisat, A.; Abu Karaky, A. Use of High Performance Polymers as Dental Implant Abutments and Frameworks: A Case Series Report. *J. Prosthodont.* 2019, *28*, 365–372. [CrossRef]
16. Wiesli, M.G.; Özcan, M. High-Performance Polymers and Their Potential Application as Medical and Oral Implant Materials: A Review. *Implant. Dent.* 2015, *24*, 448–457. [CrossRef]
17. Najeeb, S.; Zafar, M.S.; Khurshid, Z.; Siddiqui, F. Applications of Polyetheretherketone (PEEK) in Oral Implantology and Prosthodontics. *J. Prosthodont. Res.* 2016, *60*, 12–19. [CrossRef]
18. Jin, H.-Y.; Teng, M.-H.; Wang, Z.-J.; Li, X.; Liang, J.-Y.; Wang, W.-X.; Jiang, S.; Zhao, B.-D. Comparative Evaluation of BioHPP and Titanium as a Framework Veneered with Composite Resin for Implant-Supported Fixed Dental Prostheses. *J. Prosthet. Dent.* 2019, *122*, 383–388. [CrossRef]
19. Rahmitasari, F.; Ishida, Y.; Kurahashi, K.; Matsuda, T.; Watanabe, M.; Ichikawa, T. PEEK with Reinforced Materials and Modifications for Dental Implant Applications. *Dent. J.* 2017, *5*, 35. [CrossRef]
20. Zoidis, P.; Papathanasiou, I. Modified PEEK Resin-Bonded Fixed Dental Prosthesis as an Interim Restoration after Implant Placement. *J. Prosthet. Dent.* 2016, *116*, 637–641. [CrossRef]
21. Stawarczyk, B.; Eichberger, M.; Uhrenbacher, J.; Wimmer, T.; Edelhoff, D.; Schmidlin, P.R. Three-Unit Reinforced Polyetheretherketone Composite FDPs: Influence of Fabrication Method on Load-Bearing Capacity and Failure Types. *Dent. Mater. J.* 2015, *34*, 7–12. [CrossRef] [PubMed]
22. Guo, L.; Smeets, R.; Kluwe, L.; Hartjen, P.; Barbeck, M.; Cacaci, C.; Gosau, M.; Henningsen, A. Cytocompatibility of Titanium, Zirconia and Modified PEEK after Surface Treatment Using UV Light or Non-Thermal Plasma. *Int. J. Mol. Sci.* 2019, *20*, 5596. [CrossRef] [PubMed]
23. Paratelli, A.; Perrone, G.; Ortega, R.; Gómez-Polo, M. Polyetheretherketone in Implant Prosthodontics: A Scoping Review. *Int. J. Prosthodont.* 2020, *33*, 671–679. [CrossRef]
24. Limpuangthip, N.; Poosanthanasarn, E.; Salimee, P. Surface Roughness and Hardness of CAD/CAM Ceramic Materials after Polishing with a Multipurpose Polishing Kit: An In Vitro Study. *Eur. J. Dent.* 2022, Online ahead of print. [CrossRef]
25. Spitznagel, F.A.; Boldt, J.; Gierthmuehlen, P.C. CAD/CAM Ceramic Restorative Materials for Natural Teeth. *J. Dent. Res.* 2018, *97*, 1082–1091. [CrossRef] [PubMed]
26. Stawarczyk, B.; Keul, C.; Eichberger, M.; Figge, D.; Edelhoff, D.; Lümkemann, N. Three Generations of Zirconia: From Veneered to Monolithic. Part I. *Quintessence Int.* 2017, *48*, 369–380. [CrossRef]
27. Zhang, Y.; Lawn, B.R. Evaluating Dental Zirconia. *Dent. Mater.* 2019, *35*, 15–23. [CrossRef]
28. Tong, H.; Tanaka, C.B.; Kaizer, M.R.; Zhang, Y. Characterization of Three Commercial Y-TZP Ceramics Produced for Their High-Translucency, High-Strength and High-Surface Area. *Ceram. Int.* 2016, *42*, 1077–1085. [CrossRef]
29. Alshiddi, I.F.; Habib, S.R.; Zafar, M.S.; Bajunaid, S.; Labban, N.; Alsarhan, M. Fracture Load of CAD/CAM Fabricated Cantilever Implant-Supported Zirconia Framework: An In Vitro Study. *Molecules* 2021, *26*, 2259. [CrossRef]
30. Herreño, F. *Methodology for 3D Surface Roughness Characterization*; National University of Colombia: Bogotá, Colombia, 2017.
31. Abualsaud, R.; Abussaud, M.; Assudmi, Y.; Aljoaib, G.; Khaled, A.; Alalawi, H.; Akhtar, S.; Matin, A.; Gad, M.M. Physiomechanical and Surface Characteristics of 3D-Printed Zirconia: An In Vitro Study. *Materials* 2022, *15*, 6988. [CrossRef]
32. *ISO 25178:2012(E)*; Surface Metrology—Areal—Part 1: Specification and Verification of Surface Texture Profiles. Interna-Tional Organization for Standardization (ISO): Geneva, Switzerland, 2012.
33. *ISO 25178:2012(E)*; Surface Texture: Areal—Part 2: Terms, Definitions, and Surface Texture Parameters. International Organization for Standardization (ISO): Geneva, Switzerland, 2012.
34. Alao, A.-R.; Stoll, R.; Song, X.-F.; Miyazaki, T.; Hotta, Y.; Shibata, Y.; Yin, L. Surface Quality of Yttria-Stabilized Tetragonal Zirconia Polycrystal in CAD/CAM Milling, Sintering, Polishing and Sandblasting Processes. *J. Mech. Behav. Biomed. Mater.* 2017, *65*, 102–116. [CrossRef] [PubMed]

35. Fernández, M.; Delgado, L.; Molmeneu, M.; García, D.; Rodríguez, D. Analysis of the Misfit of Dental Implant-Supported Prostheses Made with Three Manufacturing Processes. *J. Prosthet. Dent.* **2014**, *111*, 116–123. [CrossRef]
36. Matzinger, M.; Hahnel, S.; Preis, V.; Rosentritt, M. Polishing Effects and Wear Performance of Chairside CAD/CAM Materials. *Clin. Oral. Investig.* **2019**, *23*, 725–737. [CrossRef] [PubMed]
37. Yang, H.; Ji, Y. Low-Temperature Degradation of Zirconia-Based All-Ceramic Crowns Materials: A Mini Review and Outlook. *J. Mater. Sci. Technol.* **2016**, *32*, 593–596. [CrossRef]
38. Ziębowicz, A.; Oßwald, B.; Kern, F.; Schwan, W. Effect of Simulated Mastication on Structural Stability of Prosthetic Zirconia Material after Thermocycling Aging. *Materials* **2023**, *16*, 1771. [CrossRef] [PubMed]
39. Denry, I.; Kelly, J.R. State of the Art of Zirconia for Dental Applications. *Dent. Mater.* **2008**, *24*, 299–307. [CrossRef] [PubMed]
40. Kwon, S.J.; Lawson, N.C.; McLaren, E.E.; Nejat, A.H.; Burgess, J.O. Comparison of the Mechanical Properties of Translucent Zirconia and Lithium Disilicate. *J. Prosthet. Dent.* **2018**, *120*, 132–137. [CrossRef]
41. Ban, S. Classification and Properties of Dental Zirconia as Implant Fixtures and Superstructures. *Materials* **2021**, *14*, 4879. [CrossRef]
42. Maminskas, J.; Pilipavicius, J.; Staisiunas, E.; Baranovas, G.; Alksne, M.; Daugela, P.; Juodzbalys, G. Novel Yttria-Stabilized Zirconium Oxide and Lithium Disilicate Coatings on Titanium Alloy Substrate for Implant Abutments and Biomedical Application. *Materials* **2020**, *13*, 2070. [CrossRef]
43. *ISO 4287:1999*; Geometrical Product Specifications (GPS)—Surface Texture: Profile Method—Terms, Definitions and Surface Texture Parameters. International Organization for Standardization: Geneva, Switzerland, 1999.
44. Kaizer, M.R.; Gierthmuehlen, P.C.; dos Santos, M.B.; Cava, S.S.; Zhang, Y. Speed Sintering Translucent Zirconia for Chairside One-Visit Dental Restorations: Optical, Mechanical, and Wear Characteristics. *Ceram. Int.* **2017**, *43*, 10999–11005. [CrossRef]
45. Wertz, M.; Hoelzig, H.; Kloess, G.; Hahnel, S.; Koenig, A. Influence of Manufacturing Regimes on the Phase Transformation of Dental Zirconia. *Materials* **2021**, *14*, 4980. [CrossRef] [PubMed]
46. Tzanakakis, E.-G.; Dimitriadi, M.; Tzoutzas, I.; Koidis, P.; Zinelis, S.; Eliades, G. Effect of Water Storage on Hardness and Interfacial Strength of Resin Composite Luting Agents Bonded to Surface-Treated Monolithic Zirconia. *Dent. J.* **2021**, *9*, 78. [CrossRef] [PubMed]
47. Kim, H.-K.; Kim, S.-H. Effect of Hydrothermal Aging on the Optical Properties of Precolored Dental Monolithic Zirconia Ceramics. *J. Prosthet. Dent.* **2019**, *121*, 676–682. [CrossRef] [PubMed]
48. Rosentritt, M.; Schneider-Feyrer, S.; Behr, M.; Preis, V. In Vitro Shock Absorption Tests on Implant-Supported Crowns: Influence of Crown Materials and Luting Agents. *Int. J. Oral. Maxillofac. Implant.* **2018**, *33*, 116–122. [CrossRef] [PubMed]
49. Preis, V.; Behr, M.; Handel, G.; Schneider-Feyrer, S.; Hahnel, S.; Rosentritt, M. Wear Performance of Dental Ceramics after Grinding and Polishing Treatments. *J. Mech. Behav. Biomed. Mater.* **2012**, *10*, 13–22. [CrossRef]
50. Kongkiatkamon, S.; Peampring, C. Effect of Speed Sintering on Low Temperature Degradation and Biaxial Flexural Strength of 5Y-TZP Zirconia. *Molecules* **2022**, *27*, 5272. [CrossRef]

Disclaimer/Publisher's Note: The statements, opinions and data contained in all publications are solely those of the individual author(s) and contributor(s) and not of MDPI and/or the editor(s). MDPI and/or the editor(s) disclaim responsibility for any injury to people or property resulting from any ideas, methods, instructions or products referred to in the content.

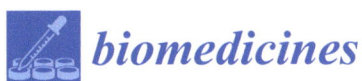 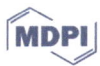

Article

The All-on-4 Concept Using Polyetheretherketone (PEEK)—Acrylic Resin Prostheses: Follow-Up Results of the Development Group at 5 Years and the Routine Group at One Year

Miguel de Araújo Nobre [1,*], Carlos Moura Guedes [2], Ricardo Almeida [2], António Silva [3] and Nuno Sereno [4]

[1] Research, Development and Education Department, MALO CLINIC, Avenida dos Combatentes, 43, Level 11, 1600-042 Lisboa, Portugal
[2] Research, Prosthodontic Department, MALO CLINIC, Avenida dos Combatentes, 43, Level 10, 1600-042 Lisboa, Portugal; cguedes@maloclinics.com (C.M.G.); ralmeida@maloclinics.com (R.A.)
[3] MALO CLINIC Ceramics, Avenida dos Combatentes, 43, Level 11, 1600-042 Lisboa, Portugal; amsilva@maloceramics.com
[4] Invibio Biomaterial Solutions & JUVORA, Global Technology Center, Hillhouse International, Thornton, Cleveleys FY5 4QD, UK; nsereno@invibio.com
* Correspondence: mnobre@maloclinics.com

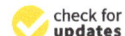

Citation: de Araújo Nobre, M.; Moura Guedes, C.; Almeida, R.; Silva, A.; Sereno, N. The All-on-4 Concept Using Polyetheretherketone (PEEK)—Acrylic Resin Prostheses: Follow-Up Results of the Development Group at 5 Years and the Routine Group at One Year. *Biomedicines* **2023**, *11*, 3013. https://doi.org/10.3390/biomedicines11113013

Academic Editors: Giuseppe Minervini and Gianmarco Abbadessa

Received: 30 September 2023
Revised: 30 October 2023
Accepted: 7 November 2023
Published: 9 November 2023

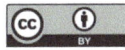

Copyright: © 2023 by the authors. Licensee MDPI, Basel, Switzerland. This article is an open access article distributed under the terms and conditions of the Creative Commons Attribution (CC BY) license (https://creativecommons.org/licenses/by/4.0/).

Abstract: Background: It is necessary to investigate the application of polymer materials in implant dentistry. The aim of this study was to examine the outcome of full-arch polyetheretherketone (PEEK)—acrylic resin implant-supported prostheses. Methods: Seventy-six patients were rehabilitated consecutively with 100 full-arch implant-supported prostheses of PEEK–acrylic resin (a development group (DG): 37 patients with 5 years of follow-up; a routine group (RG): 39 patients with 1 year of follow-up). The primary outcome measure was prosthetic survival. Secondary outcome measures were implant survival, marginal bone loss, biological complications, prosthetic complications, veneer adhesion, plaque levels, bleeding levels, and a patient subjective evaluation (including the Oral Health Impact Profile for the RG). Results: In both groups, prosthetic (DG: 93.6%; RG: 100%) and implant survival (DG: 98.9%; RG: 99.5%) were high, and marginal bone loss was low (DG: 0.54 mm; RG: 0.28 mm). The veneer adhesion rate was 28.6% of prostheses in DG (RG = 0%). Mechanical complications occurred in 49% and 11.8% of prostheses in DG and RG, respectively. Biological complications, plaque, and bleeding levels were low in both groups. The subjective patient evaluation was excellent in both groups (8.6 < DG < 8.8; 9.3 < RG < 9.5; OHIP = 1.38). Conclusions: Within the limitations of this study, PEEK can be considered a viable prosthetic alternative.

Keywords: dental implants; immediate dental implant loading; polyetheretherketone; PEEK; prostheses; implants

1. Introduction

The use of alternative materials for implant-supported rehabilitations is the object of constant development. One such alternative is polyetheretherketone (PEEK), a high-performance thermoplastic polymer whose application was extended from the aerospace and automotive industry [1] to medicine [2–4] and dentistry [5–12], either alone or reinforced with polymer composite materials [13,14]. Given its original development (Victrex plc, Lancashire, UK), the properties that make PEEK an exciting alternative include creep and wear resistance, biostability, biocompatibility, superior mechanical behavior, and compatibility with medical diagnostic imaging [15].

Its use in implant dentistry has received a significant amount of attention, from the scientific community over the last decade from implants [16] to abutments [17] to infrastructures in full-arch implant-supported rehabilitations [6–11,18–23]. Regarding the latter, the use of PEEK has been involved in some disagreement over its potential favorable or detrimental effects on bone and dental implants, with opposing conclusions from finite element analysis studies [24–29]. Concurrently, short-term clinical studies register beneficial effects for full-arch rehabilitations, particularly on marginal bone loss, where important reductions have been noted [6,9,11]. Previous studies registered positive outcomes at 1 and 3 years for PEEK—acrylic resin prosthesis—when applied to full-arch implant-supported rehabilitations, specifically the All-on-4 concept (Nobel Biocare AB, Gothenburg, Sweden) [6,9]. Nevertheless, its effects in the long term and the impact on the patient's quality of life are lacking.

A second point of debate in the use of PEEK concerns the potential difficulty of the adhesion of veneering materials (either due to PEEK's properties or the need to follow strict protocols). This renders a significant number of complications previously reported [6,9] that impact the satisfaction of both patient and clinician due to the burdensome caused by increased visits to resolve the complication. This highlights the need to establish a proper preventive protocol.

The aim of this study was to document the outcome of full-arch implant-supported fixed hybrid PEEK—acrylic resin prosthesis—applied to the All-on-4 concept at 5 years for a development group and at 1 year for a routine group with an updated protocol to prevent veneer adhesion issues.

2. Materials and Methods

This prospective cohort clinical study was performed in a private practice (Lisbon, Portugal) for a duration of 5 years. This study was approved by an independent ethical committee (Ethical Committee for Health, Lisbon, Portugal; authorization no. 008/2013). Written informed consent was obtained from all patients. Data were divided into two groups as follows: the development and routine groups. The patients were assigned consecutively to a development group and were rehabilitated between May 2015 and October 2016, and a routine group was rehabilitated between November 2017 and April 2021.

Seventy-six patients (53 females, 23 males), with an average of 58.5 years (range: 20–80 years, standard error of the mean: 1.23 years), were rehabilitated with 100 full-arch implant-supported prostheses (27 maxillary rehabilitations, 25 mandibular rehabilitations, and 24 bimaxillary rehabilitations). The development group included 37 patients (29 females, 7 males), with an average age of 59.8 years (standard error of the mean: 1.77 years), who were rehabilitated with 49 full-arch prostheses (12 maxillary rehabilitations, 13 mandibular rehabilitations, and 12 bimaxilar rehabilitations). The routine group included 39 patients (24 females, 15 males) with an average age of 57.1 years (standard error of the mean: 1.70 years), who were rehabilitated with 51 full-arch prostheses (15 maxillary rehabilitations, 12 mandibular rehabilitations, and 13 bimaxilar rehabilitations).

2.1. Inclusion and Exclusion Criteria

The patients who met the inclusion criteria were identified at the treatment planning phase. Inclusion criteria consisted of patients with full-arch rehabilitations (single arch or bimaxillary rehabilitations) performed using the All-on-4 concept (Nobel Biocare AB, Gothenburg, Sweden), in need of definitive prosthetic rehabilitation, and who provided written informed consent to participate. Exclusion criteria included patients unable to provide written informed consent, with insufficient bone volume, or inactive radiotherapy or chemotherapy.

2.2. Surgical and Prosthetic Protocols

Implant insertion (Nobelspeedy™, Nobel Biocare AB, Gothenburg, Sweden) followed standard procedures [30] except for the use of under-preparation, which was employed to guarantee a final torque of over 32 N/cm before the final implant seating. The two most anterior implants were inserted following the direction determined by the anatomy of the jaw. Two posterior implants were inserted (one implant on each quadrant) anterior to the mental foramina (in the mandible) and the anterior wall of the maxillary sinus (in the maxilla) with distal tilting between 30 and 45 degrees relative to the occlusal plane *ad modum* All-on-4 concept (Nobel Biocare AB).

Concerning the immediate prosthetic protocol, a high-density acrylic resin (PalaXpress Ultra; Heraeus Kulzer GmbH, Hanau, Germany) prostheses with titanium cylinders (Nobel Biocare AB, Gothenburg, Sweden), and a minimum of 10 teeth were manufactured at the dental laboratory and inserted on the same day. Anterior occlusal contacts and canine guidance during lateral movements were preferred as the occlusal scheme.

The definitive prosthetic protocol was described in full-on previous publications [6,9]. In brief, it consisted of a full-arch hybrid prostheses of polymeric–acrylic resin implant-supported and fixed prostheses (patent WO 2019/008368) [31] with a PEEK substructure (Juvora Ltd., Lancashire, UK), reinforcing titanium sleeves, acrylic resin prosthetic teeth (anterior teeth: Premium; posterior teeth: Mondial; Heraeus Kulzer GmbH, Hanau, Germany) and pink acrylic resin gingiva (PalaXpress Ultra, Heraeus Kulzer GmbH, Hanau, Germany). In the development group, the metal bond 1 and 2 (Heraeus Kulzer GmbH, Hanau, Germany) was used as a primer (Signum Connector, Heraeus Kulzer GmbH, Hanau, Germany) in the cases identified with veneer adhesion issues; in the routine group, the Signum connector (Heraeus Kulzer GmbH, Hanau, Germany) was used on all cases. The infrastructure CAD–CAM guidelines included an "I" shaped design in the framework, with minimum cross-sectional material dimensions of 5 mm of occlusal–cervical height, 4 mm of anterior buccal–lingual width, and 6 mm of buccal–lingual width in the areas of the titanium sleeve, together with at least 1 to 2 mm of acrylic resin. The final prostheses privileged a mutually protected occlusion scheme respecting the patients' centric relations. A clinical case is represented in Figure 1.

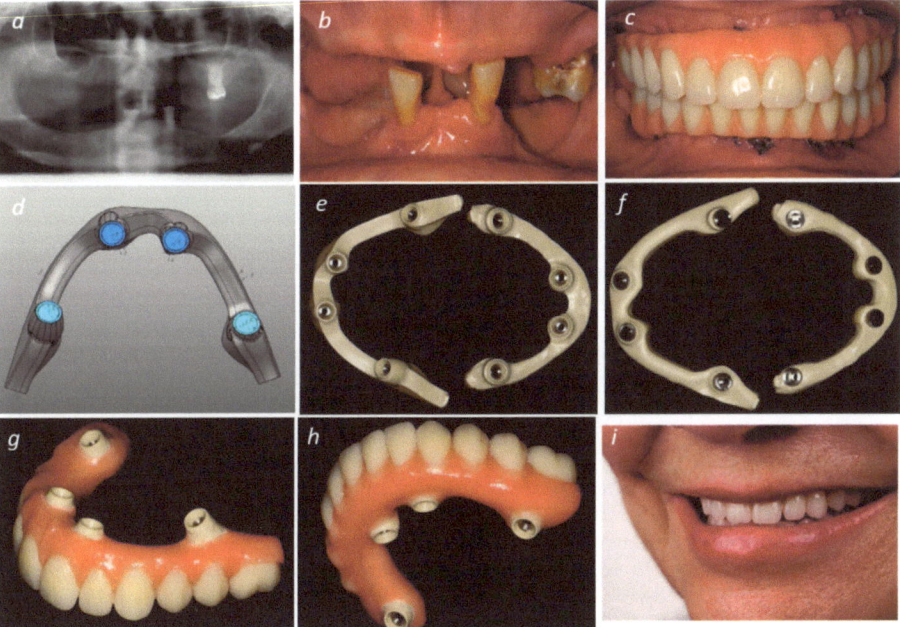

Figure 1. *Cont.*

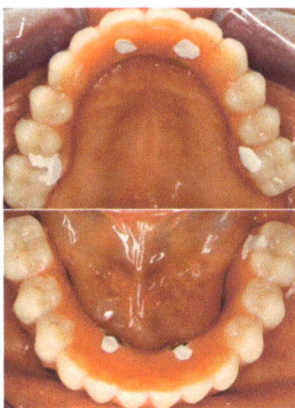
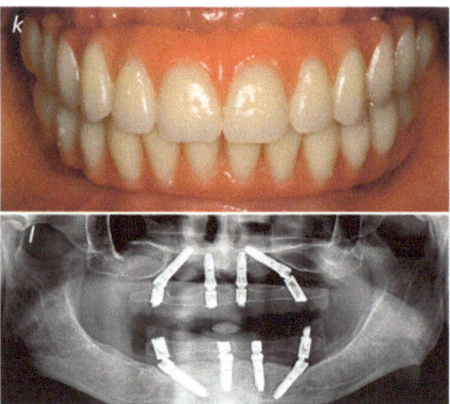

Figure 1. (**a**) Pre-treatment orthopantomography; (**b**) Pre-treatment intraoral view of both arches; (**c**) Immediate provisional prostheses after bimaxilar full-arch rehabilitation; (**d**) Infrastructure design during CAD–CAM process; (**e**) Polyetheretherketone (PEEK) infrastructures inferior view during CAD–CAM process; (**f**) PEEK infrastructures with a superior view during CAD–CAM process; (**g**) Maxillary PEEK–acrylic resin implant-supported prosthesis; (**h**) Mandibular PEEK–acrylic resin implant-supported prosthesis; (**i**) Perspective of the patient's smile after the rehabilitation process; (**j**) Intra-oral occlusal view of the maxillary and mandibular PEEK–acrylic resin implant-supported prostheses in function; (**k**) Intra-oral frontal view of the maxillary and mandibular PEEK–acrylic resin implant-supported prostheses in function; (**l**) Final post-treatment orthopantomography.

2.3. Maintenance Protocol

The connection of the definitive prosthesis was considered the baseline for clinical and radiographic evaluations, with the patients included in a maintenance protocol with clinical evaluations every 6 months and both clinical and radiographical evaluations at 1 and 5 years.

2.4. Outcome Measures

The primary outcome measure at five years was prosthetic survival (the need for replacement), including the fracture of the framework. Secondary outcome measures were implant survival, marginal bone loss, technical evaluation concerning manufacturing issues, the incidence of mechanical complications, the incidence of biological complications, modified plaque index (mPLI), modified bleeding index (mBI), and patient subjective evaluation. Implant survival was evaluated based on function and using the patient as a unit of analysis (with the first implant failure in a patient considered as a censoring event irrespective of the remaining implants maintaining their function) [6]. Marginal bone loss was evaluated through periapical radiographs employing a radiographic holder (super-bite; Hawe Neos, Bioggio, Switzerland), adjusted for the digital film's orthognathic position. The radiographs were evaluated using an outcome assessor through software for image analysis (rayMage, version 2.3, MyRay, Imola, Italy). The marginal bone level was defined as the distance between the implant's platform and the most apical bone–implant contact, while the measurement difference between the baseline (connection of the definitive prosthesis) and five-year evaluation was classified as marginal bone loss (MBL). We calibrated the measurements using the distance between implant threads and considered average values between the mesial and distal sites. The technical evaluation concerning manufacture issues was evaluated comprising the following: infrastructure manufacture issues (presence or absence), framework integrity issues (present/absent), and veneer adhesion issues (present or absent). The biological complications assessed were as follows: a probing pocket depth >4 mm, evaluated using a plastic periodontal probe calibrated to 0.25 N; abscess (presence or absence); fistulae formation (presence or absence); suppuration (presence or absence); and patient adverse soft tissue reaction (presence or absence). The mechanical complications assessed were the loosening or fracture of prosthetic screws, abutments, or prosthesis. The modified plaque index (mPLI) [32] was evaluated by inserting a periodontal plastic probe 1 mm into the peri-implant sulcus, running a circular movement all around the implant, and measuring in a scale between 0 and 3 (0, no detection of plaque; 1, plaque only recognized by running a probe across the smooth marginal surface of the implant; 2, plaque can be seen by the naked eye; and 3, abundance of soft matter). The modified bleeding index (mBI) [32] was evaluated on the same moment as mPLI and measured on a scale between 0 and 3 (0, no bleeding when a periodontal probe is passed along the mucosal margin adjacent to the implant; 1, isolated bleeding spots visible; 2, blood forms a confluent red line on mucosal margin; and 3, heavy or profuse bleeding). The patients' evaluation comprised the "in mouth comfort" defined as the following: the comfort felt by the patient with the prosthesis in function regarding an overall fulfillment of expectations, measured in a visual analog scale between 0 (poor) and 10 (excellent), and the "overall chewing feeling", defined as the patients' feeling during daily food intake routines in relation to their ability to chew any type of food and measured in a visual analog scale between 0 (poor) and 10 (excellent). Both evaluations were registered yearly. For the routine group, an additional evaluation was performed using the Oral Health Impact Profile, version 14 (OHIP-14) [33], estimating the following dimensions: functional limitations, physical pain, psychological discomfort, physical disability, psychological disability, social disability, and handicap; this was measured using a Likert scale between 0 (never occurred) and 4 (always occurs) at 6 months and 1 year of follow-up.

2.5. Statistical Analysis

Survival was estimated using life table analysis (actuarial method) and using the implant and prosthesis as a unit of analysis. Descriptive statistics (average, standard deviation) were computed for the following variables of interest: age, marginal bone loss and patient evaluation parameters, OHIP-14 dimensions, "in mouth comfort", and "overall chewing feeling". The median was computed for the variables mPLI and mBI; frequencies were computed for the technical evaluation concerning manufacturing issues, including the incidence of biological and mechanical complications. Inferential analysis was computed for the evaluation of the correlation between mPLI and mBI through the Spearman correlation coefficient. The significance level was set at 5%. Data were analyzed using the software SPSS for Windows (IBM SPSS, New York, NY, USA) version 17.

3. Results

3.1. Sample

For the development group, the median cantilever length in a prosthesis was 1 unit (average: 0.7; standard deviation: 0.6 units; range: 0–2 units). Two female patients (5.4%) with two single full-arch maxillary prostheses (4.1%) were lost to follow-up as they became inaccessible; one female patient (2.7%) with a single full-arch mandibular prosthesis (2%) deceased due to cancer after 39 months; and one female patient (2.7%) with a single full-arch mandibular prosthesis (2.0%) withdrew from the study after 48 months. A total of 33 patients (89.2%) with 45 prostheses (91.8%) were eligible for follow-up and completion at 5 years.

For the routine group, the median cantilever length in a prosthesis was 1 unit (average: 0.55; standard deviation: 0.57 units; range: 0–2 units). Two patients (5.1%) with two double full-arch prostheses (7.8%) were lost to follow-up/withdrew during the first year of follow-up: one patient deceased due to health conditions unrelated to the prosthodontic treatment, and one patient chose to be followed at another dental clinic. A total of 37 patients (94.9%) with 47 prostheses (92.2%) were evaluated at 1 year of follow-up.

3.2. Primary Outcome Measure—Prosthetic Survival

For the development group, three PEEK frameworks were fractured as follows: one mandibular framework in bimaxilar rehabilitation during the first year of follow-up in a male patient, heavy bruxer, 55 years of age requiring a new prosthesis; one mandibular framework was characterized by the complete fracture of the mandibular PEEK framework near the cylinder (position #42) during the fourth year of follow-up in a female patient 75 years of age that developed bruxing habits (and deceased due to cancer shortly after); one maxillary framework fractured on the cantilever position (position #26) in a male patient at 47 years of age (that refused its replacement as the prosthesis remained in function). This outcome rendered a 93.6% prosthetic cumulative survival rate at five years of follow-up (Table 1).

Table 1. Cumulative prosthetic survival rate for patients rehabilitated using the All-on-4 treatment concept and a hybrid polyetheretherketone (PEEK)—acrylic resin prostheses—for development and routine groups.

	Development Group				
Time	Total Number of Patients	Total Number of Prostheses	Prosthetic Failures	Lost to Follow-Up	Cumulative Survival Rate (%)
Prosthesis connection—1 year	37	49	1	2	98.0%
1 year–2 years	35	46	0	0	98.0%
2 year–3 years	35	46	0	1	98.0%
3 years–4 years	34	45	1	0	95.8%
4 years–5 years	34	44	1	2	93.6%
	Routine Group				
Time	Total Number of Patients	Total Number of Prostheses	Prosthetic Failures	Lost to Follow-Up	Cumulative Survival Rate (%)
Prosthesis connection—1 year	39	51	0	2	100%

No prosthesis failed in the routine group during the first year of follow-up, resulting in a 100% prosthesis survival rate (Table 1).

3.3. Secondary Outcome Measures

3.3.1. Implant Survival

A total of 196 implants were inserted for the rehabilitation of 49 edentulous arches in the development group. Two implant failures (implant positions #32 and #34) were registered in one female patient 75 years of age (the same patient deceased due to cancer) during the fourth year of follow-up, rendering a 98.9% implant survival rate after five years (Table 2).

Table 2. Cumulative implant survival rate for patients rehabilitated using the All-on-4 treatment concept and a hybrid polyetheretherketone (PEEK)—acrylic resin prostheses— for the development and routine groups.

	Development Group			
Time	Total Number of Implants	Implant Failures	Lost to Follow-Up	Cumulative Survival Rate (%)
Prosthesis connection—1 year	196	0	8	100.0%
1 year–2 years	188	0	0	100.0%
2 year–3 years	188	0	0	100.0%
3 years–4 years	184	2	2	98.9%
4 years–5 years	180	0	4	98.9%
	Routine Group			
Time	Total Number of Prostheses	Prosthetic Failures	Lost to Follow-Up	Cumulative Survival Rate (%)
Prosthesis connection—1 year	204	1	8	99.5%

Concerning the routine group, a total of 204 implants were inserted for the rehabilitation of 51 edentulous arches. One implant failure was registered in one female patient with mandibular rehabilitation (implant position: #32) at 7 months of follow-up, with increased marginal bone loss noted during the rehabilitation process, rendering a 99.5% implant survival rate after one year (Table 2).

3.3.2. Marginal Bone Loss

For the development group, the average (standard deviation) marginal bone loss at 5 years was 0.54 mm (0.95 mm) with the following distribution: 0.42 mm (0.95 mm) for maxillary implants; 0.65 mm (0.94 mm) for mandibular implants; 0.42 mm (0.89 mm) for bimaxillary rehabilitations; 0.78 mm (0.99 mm) for single arch maxillary rehabilitations; and 0.62 mm (1.03 mm) for single arch mandibular rehabilitations. Concerning the routine group, the average (standard deviation) marginal bone loss at one year of follow-up was 0.28 mm (0.59 mm), with 0.25 mm (0.54 mm) for maxillary implants; 0.32 (0.65 mm) for mandibular implants; 0.27 mm (0.55 mm) for bimaxillary rehabilitations; 0.22 mm (0.48 mm) for single arch maxillary rehabilitations; and 0.37 mm (0.76 mm) for single arch mandibular rehabilitations.

3.3.3. Technical Evaluation—Veneer Adhesion Issues

A total of 12 patients (32.4%) and 14 prostheses (28.6%) registered veneer adhesion issues in the development group during the 5 years of follow-up (Table 3). These were characterized by the avulsion of acrylic resin from the PEEK infrastructure. All situations were solved by leaving the cylinder areas with increased amounts of exposed PEEK to increase flexion resistance; a tungsten bur was used to increase mechanical retention on the PEEK infrastructure and the bonding primer was replaced to increase the tensile bond strength. On the routine group, no veneer adhesion issues were registered during the first year of follow-up.

Table 3. Veneer adhesion problems between acrylic resin and polyetheretherketone (PEEK) infrastructure and resolution. All situations occurred in the development group.

Patient	Gender	Follow-Up (Months)	Position (FDI)	Type Rehabilitation	Opposing Dentition	Resolution
1	Male	5	#12, #22, #25, #35	Bimaxilar	Implant-supported prosthesis	New prostheses due to fracture of PEEK infrastructure
2	Male	2	#35	Mandibular	Mucosal-retained full-arch prosthesis	To increase flexion resistance, the cylinder areas were left with increased amounts of exposed PEEK; to increase mechanical retention in the PEEK infrastructure, a tungsten bur was used; to increase the tensile bond strength, the bonding primer was replaced
3	Female	4	#46	Mandibular	Natural teeth and implant-supported prosthesis	
4	Female	10	#45	Mandibular	Mucosal-retained full-arch prosthesis	
5	Female	12	#35	Mandibular	Mucosal-retained full-arch prosthesis	
6	Female	12	#15, #22	Bimaxilar	Implant-supported prosthesis	
7	Female	16	#26	Maxillary	Natural teeth	
8	Female	30	#35	Mandibular	Implant-supported prosthesis	
9	Male	32	#12	Maxillary	Implant-supported prosthesis	
10	Female	52	#15	Maxillary	Natural teeth	
11	Male	53	#12, #13, #22, #45, #46	Bimaxilar	Implant-supported prosthesis	
12	Female	55	#13	Bimaxilar	Implant-supported prosthesis	

3.3.4. Mechanical Complications

The incidence of mechanical complications on the development group was 54.1% at the patient level (n = 20 patients) and 49% at the prostheses level (n = 24 prostheses).

In the routine group, the incidence rate of mechanical complications was 12.8% at the patient level (n = 5 patients) and 11.8% at the prostheses level (n = 6 prostheses). Table 4 describes the type of complications and remedies implemented, with all situations resolved in both groups.

Table 4. Incidence of mechanical complications and resolutions during the 5 years of follow-up of the sample.

Patient	Gender	Opposing Dentition	Cantilever Units (Left/Right)	Follow-Up in Months	Acrylic Resin Crown Fracture (Position FDI)	Abutment Wearing (Position FDI)	Abutment Loosening (Position FDI)	Prosthetic Screw Loosening (Position FDI)	Prosthetic Screw Fracture (Position FDI)	Resolution
DG 1	Male	ISP	0/0 (maxilla); 1/1 (mandible)	5	#12, #22; #35					1; Patient fractured PEEK infrastructure
DG 2	Male	ISP	1.5/0.5	16	#32		#42			1
DG 3	Male	ISP	1.5/2	22	#41					1
DG 4	Female	NT	1/1	15		#45				2
DG 5	Female	ISP	1/0.5	16			#45	#42		3
DG 6	Female	ISP	2/2	16			#42			3
DG 7	Female	ISP	1/1 (maxilla); 0/0 (mandible)	8				#25, #35, #45		3
DG 8	Female	ISP	0/0	4				#15		3
DG 9	Male	NT	1/1	20				#16, #26		3
DG 10	Female	RP	2/2	40	#35					1
DG 11	Female	NT	0/0	43					#12, #26	2
DG 12	Female	ISP	1/0	43			#32			2
DG 13	Female	ISP	1/1	47	#12					1
DG 14	Female	NT	0/0	48	#12					1
DG 15	Male	RP	1/1	49					#35	2
DG 16	Male	ISP	0/0	55			#15			2
DG 17	Female	ISP	1/1	55				#25		3
DG 18	Female	ISP	1/1	59	#11					1
DG 19	Female	ISP	1/1	59	#31					1
DG 20	Female	NT	0/0	60	#31,#41					1
RG 1	Female	RP	2/1	6				#42		3
RG 2	Female	ISP	0/0	6			#12, #22			2
RG 3	Female	ISP	1/1 (maxilla); 2/2 (mandible)	12; 6			#12, #13 #31, #32, #41			1
RG 4	Female	FPNT	1/1	12				#25		3
RG 5	Female	NT	1/1	12			#15, #25		#22	1; 2

DG: development group; RG: routine group; ISP: implant support prosthesis; NT: natural teeth; RP: removable prosthesis; FPNT: fixed prosthesis over natural teeth. Resolutions: 1—mending the prostheses and adjusting occlusion; 2—replacing the abutment/prosthetic screw and adjusting occlusion; 3—torque-controlled retightening and adjusting occlusion.

3.3.5. Biological Complications

The incidence rate of biological complications during the 5 years of follow-up for the development group was 10.8% at the patient level (n = 4 patients) and 2.6% at the implant level (n = 5 implants) consisting of a peri-implant pathology. Table 5 describes the type of complications and remedies implemented, with all situations resolved apart from two implants in two patients. No biological complications were registered for the routine group during the follow-up of 1 year.

Table 5. Incidence of biological complications (peri-implant pathology) and resolutions during the 5 years of follow-up (all from the development group).

Patient	Gender	Implant Position (FDI)	Presence of Risk Indicators	Time of Follow-Up	Resolution
1	Male	#12	Smoker; History of Periodontitis	48 months	Resolved non-surgically
2	Female	#26	Smoker; History of Periodontitis	52 months	Resolved non-surgically
3	Female	#45	History of Periodontitis	55 months	Not resolved
4	Male	#35	History of Periodontitis	58 months	Not resolved

3.3.6. Plaque and Bleeding Scores

Considering the development group, the median value for the mPLI was 2 (plaque visible by the naked eye) at five years of follow-up; while the mBI median value obtained at five years of follow-up was 1 (one isolated bleeding spot visible when tested). The correlation between plaque and bleeding levels was weak (positive) and non-significant (R = 0.240, p = 0.210; Spearman).

Regarding the routine group, the median for the mPLI was 1 (plaque was only recognized by running a probe across the smooth marginal surface of the peri-implant sulcus) at both six months and one year of follow-up. The median for the mBI was 1 (one isolated bleeding spot visible when tested) at both 6 months and one year. The correlation between mPLI and mBI was characterized by a strong positive linear relationship at both 6 months and 1 year (six months: R = 0.609, $p < 0.001$; one year: R = 0.672, $p < 0.001$; Spearman correlation coefficient).

3.3.7. Patient Subjective Evaluation and OHIP-14 Assessment

In the development group at 5 years, "in mouth comfort" registered a mean value of 8.8, while "overall chewing feeling" registered a mean value of 8.6 and both indexes were evaluated on a scale of 0 to 10 (0, poor; 10, excellent).

In the routine group, the registered mean value for "in mouth comfort" was 9.5 and 9.3 at 6 months and 1-year, respectively, whereas "overall chewing feeling" registered a mean value of 9.3 at 6 months and 9.4 at one year. In addition, concerning the patients' quality of life evaluation in the OHIP-14 dimensions, the mean total sum OHIP-14-dimension scores were 0.73 and 1.38 at 6 months and 1 year, respectively (Table 6). The distribution was skewed, with scores of 0 reported by 63% of the patients at 6 months and 60% of the patients at 1 year of follow-up (Figures 2 and 3).

Table 6. OHIP-14 scores and patient's subjective evaluation of the routine group.

OHIP-14 Evaluation Parameters	6 Months Mean (Standard Error of Mean)	1 Year Mean (Standard Error of Mean)
Functional limitation Have you had trouble pronouncing any words? Have you felt that your sense of taste has worsened?	0.23 (0.06)	0.20 (0.04)
Physical pain Have you had painful aching in your mouth? Have you found it uncomfortable to eat any foods?	0.20 (0.06)	0.35 (0.08)
Psychological discomfort Have you been self-conscious? Have you felt tense?	0.18 (0.05)	0.38 (0.09)
Physical disability Has your diet been unsatisfactory? Have you had to interrupt meals?	0.03 (0.02)	0.08 (0.04)
Psychological disability Have you found it difficult to relax? Have you been a bit embarrassed?	0.05 (0.03)	0.18 (0.06)
Social disability Have you been a bit irritable with other people? Have you had difficulty doing your usual jobs?	0.05 (0.04)	0.13 (0.05)
Handicap Have you been unable to function? Have you felt life in general was less satisfying?	0.00 (0.00)	0.08 (0.04)
Total sum	0.73 (0.00)	1.38 (0.00)

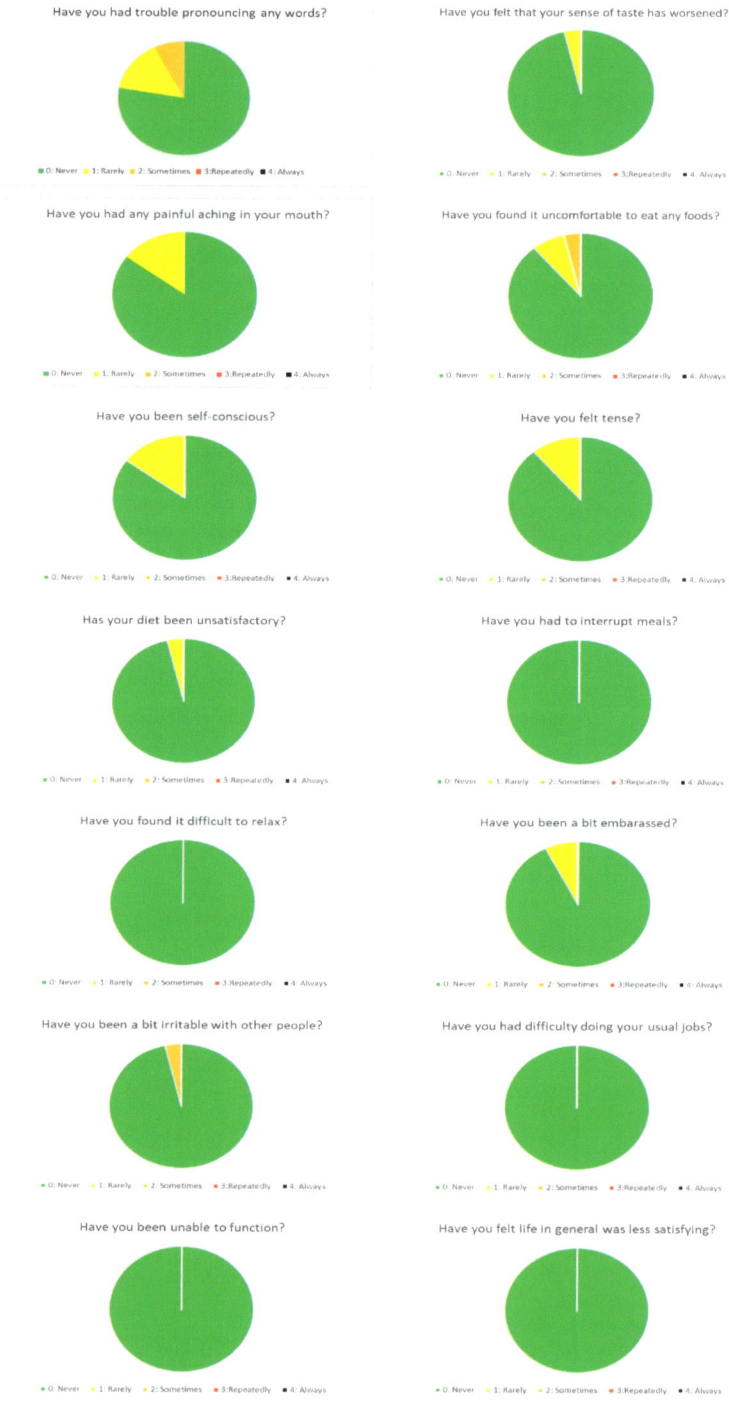

Figure 2. OHIP-14 dimensions at 6 months of follow-up.

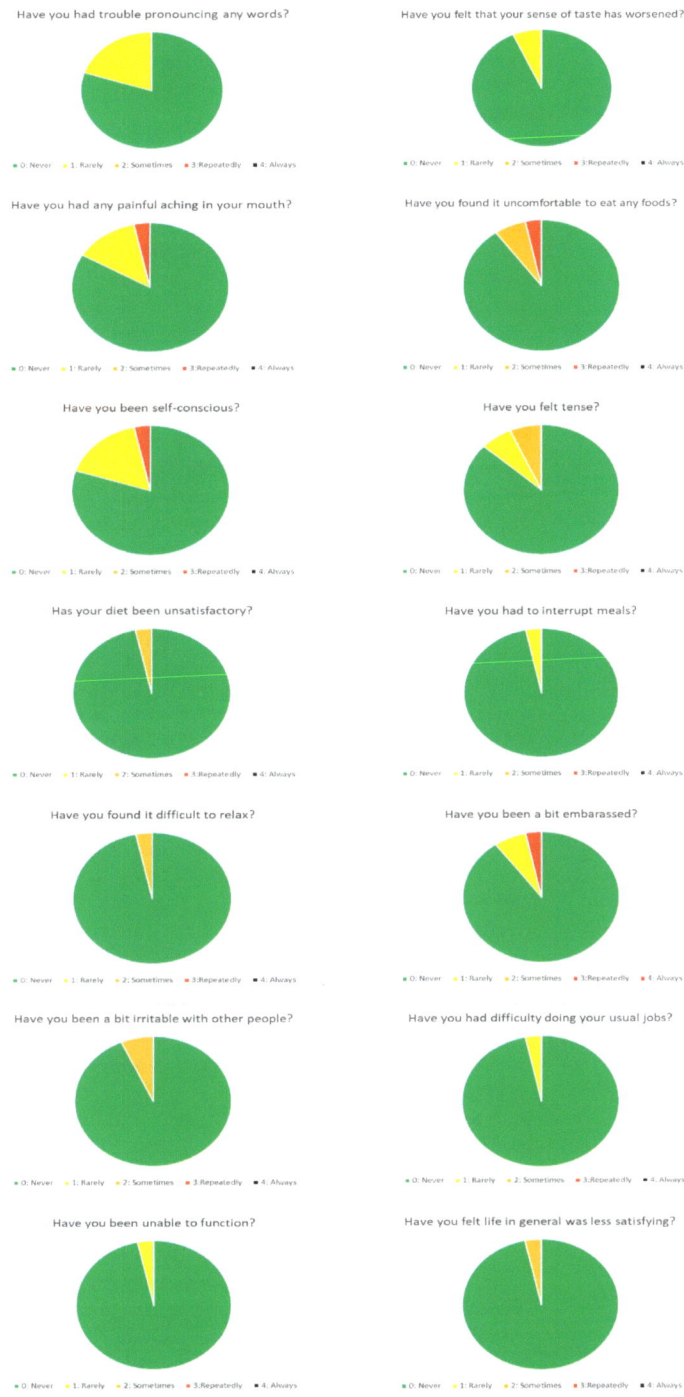

Figure 3. OHIP-14 dimensions at 1 year of follow-up.

4. Discussion

The current study reported on the outcome of a full-arch prosthodontic solution consisting of a fixed hybrid implant-supported PEEK–PMMA prosthesis produced through CAD–CAM workflow at 1 and 5 years for two different groups (routine and development, respectively).

The 100% prosthesis survival at one year registered for the routine group and the 93.6% prosthesis survival at five years for the development group are suitable taking into consideration the complexity of full-arch implant-supported rehabilitation and the broad inclusion criteria applied to this study. The PEEK infrastructure fractures corresponded to patients that were heavy bruxers and/or whose structures had >1 cantilever unit, which is a pattern that was also noted for the high incidence of mechanical complications. Bruxism and cantilever units represent two factors that significantly increase the probability of mechanical complications, with a previous study evaluating different implant distributions registering odds ratios >60 times for bruxism and >4.5 times for cantilevers [34]. Nevertheless, it is important to underline the previously mentioned limits established in CAD–CAM guidelines for full-arch PEEK infrastructures together with the limitation to one cantilever unit (≤10 mm) as these were created to compensate for material flexion [6]. Furthermore, the change in the bonding primer for the routine group was beneficial to the protocol considering the excellent results obtained (absence of veneer adhesion issues) together with the successful resolution on the development group's incident cases. The bonding primer of choice was characterized by a higher tensile bond strength enabling firmer chemical retention [35,36]. In addition, actions were taken to improve mechanical retention, including an increased amount of exposed PEEK to the cylinder areas, a PEEK rough finish [37–39], insertion of a horizontal thread in the infrastructure without smooth and round finish, and the insertion of vertical threads in the cantilever area, enabling PEEK's flexion capacity to be maintained under control. PEEK is a completely different material compared to titanium regarding its mechanical characteristics, so one should approach the prosthetic design accordingly to these features. In circumstances where the space is reduced and the infrastructure does not possess an appropriate height, the shock-absorbing property of PEEK, which is an advantage for dissipating occlusal forces, makes the infrastructure too flexible. In this situation, a titanium infrastructure designed in traditional fashion could be functional. However, in the case of a PEEK infrastructure (37 times more flexible than zirconia) [38], there is too much bending of the cantilevers and pontic areas, causing mechanical complications such as prosthetic screw loosening or fractures and fissures in the pink acrylic areas [40]. Extending the PEEK framework to the gingival tissue and creating areas in the lingual aspect that remain uncovered with acrylic resin reinforces the infrastructure and prevents or minimizes complications.

Implant survival was high (99.5% at 1-year for the routine group; 98.9% at 5 years for the development group) and compared favorably with previous publications on the outcome of full-arch rehabilitations. Recent publications on full-arch implant supported rehabilitations [41–43], including two studies on the All-on-4 concept (Nobel Biocare AB) with a long-term outcome [42,43] registered for cumulative survival rates between 98.6% and 99.6% at 1 year and between 97.7% and 98.8% at the 5 years evaluation. A recent systematic review and meta-analysis evaluating the outcome of full-arch rehabilitations supported by tilted and axially placed implants reported an implant survival proportion at 5 years of 98.2% (95% confidence intervals: 97.93%, 98.43%) [41].

The marginal bone loss registered in both groups was low with 0.28 mm (routine group at 1 year) and 0.54 mm (development group at 5 years). These results compare favorably with a recent systematic review and meta-analysis, which was lower than the overall or individual average of all included studies at 1 year or 5 years [39]. In addition, the routine group marginal bone loss at 1 year was lower (−0.09 mm) compared to the development group at the same time frame [6]. The incidence of biological complications was also low during the follow-up of this study (absence in the routine group; 2.6% of the implants in the development group), which is in line with the results from a systematic review (data extracted from study) [41]. All four patients with biological complications presented history of periodontitis or smoking habits, representing risk indicators for the incidence of biological complications [44,45]. The good results registered for these outcome measures (implant survival, marginal bone loss and biological complications) can be potentially attributable to PEEK's properties, specifically its shock absorption characteristics [9,10,46–48]. Recent finite element analysis studies reported conflicting results when evaluating PEEK infrastructures used in full-arch implant-supported rehabilitations and the *ad modum* All-on-4 concept: Tribst et al. [24], Ersöz et al. [26], Yu et al. [27] and Dayan et al. [28] reported that PEEK frameworks transferred more stress to the bone in both compression and tensile stress compared to other metallic frameworks (including titanium) in what could be perceived as placing the rehabilitations at an increased risk of biological complications. Shash et al. [25] and Haroun et al. [29] registered that PEEK material reduced the stresses and strains on bone tissue compared to titanium, and therefore, could prevent complications. In light of these results, with high implant survival and low marginal bone loss, the present study is in agreement with Shash et al. [25] and Haroun et al. [29], a result that is parallel with other clinical investigations [11,20,49]. A clinical study comparing PEEK and titanium frameworks in full-arch implant-supported fixed prosthesis with an average follow-up of 26.5 months registered a significantly lower marginal bone loss for PEEK (0.70 mm) compared to titanium (0.96 mm) [11]. A systematic review investigating the clinical performance of polymer frameworks in dental prostheses registered in their qualitative analysis lower plaque and gingival indices, probing depth, and marginal bone loss, with higher survival rates for implant-supported and fixed prostheses and overdentures fabricated with PEEK than for metal frameworks [20]. Despite the increased number of finite element analysis studies recently published on the subject [24–29], it should be noted that they do not mimic the true clinical scenario. This is due to the restrictions of these experiments and an array of possible scenarios including different types of implants; modeling only a portion of bone considered as isotropic material despite its anisotropic behavior; assuming in most cases complete osseointegration; considering compressive or oblique forces acting on the implant; or neglecting muscle forces and the bone remodeling process, thus attesting the absence of a standardized approach for finite element analysis modeling in dentistry [50].

Concerning plaque and bleeding scores, both groups were characterized by the presence of plaque around the implants, with increased plaque levels at 5 years for the development group (visible plaque) compared to a median lower score at 1 year for the routine group (plaque only visible after running the periodontal probe across the mucosal margin). On the other hand, bleeding levels were stable with the median representing mild inflammation for the routine group at 1 year and the development group at 5 years. The correlation between plaque and bleeding scores has been pointed out by previous publications, representing the causality between plaque accumulation and peri-implant breakdown [51,52]. The present study points in the same direction, with a positive correlation between plaque and bleeding scores in both groups, despite the non-significant correlation for the development group. This result should nevertheless be analyzed in the context of the risk for biological complications (which remained at a low level), in what can be inferred as the presence of stable biomechanical conditions that allow to mitigate or delay the deleterious effects of plaque accumulation in the process of peri-implant pathology [10,44]. Nevertheless, it is important to stress the importance of frequent maintenance appointments for soft tissue evaluation, prophylaxis and hygienic measures education [10].

The patients' subjective evaluation was characterized by a high satisfaction rate for the "in mouth comfort" and "overall chewing feeling" evaluation parameters, with over 90% for the routine group at 1 year and over 85% for the development group at 5 years. Both results were substantially higher (5% to 14%) than the satisfaction rate registered for the fixed mandibular full-arch implant-supported fixed prostheses of metal–acrylic resin regarding an improvement in the chewing ability and the fulfillment of expectations [53]. Moreover, an excellent impact on the patient's quality of life was registered by the low

OHIP-14 index value at both 6 months and 1 year for the routine group. The significance of this result can be described as a potential gain in quality-adjusted life years, a measure of impact which represents population health by considering the duration and quality of life. A study with 9445 subjects estimated the quality-adjusted life-expectancy loss for dental-related events including missing teeth [54]. The authors attested the substantial burden of dental conditions on quality of life, estimating an impact of approximately between ¼ to 1/3 of major causes of health burden such as diabetes, heart disease, obesity and smoking [54]. The present study, with 60% of the participants registering no impact (a score of 0), and only an average of 1.38 for the sample's quality of life, creates conditions for a large gain in years of life lived with quality by restoring the patients' function, aesthetics, and self-esteem. This confirms the results of a recent randomized controlled trial evaluating the treatment outcomes (functional and subjective through OHIP-20) of full-arch fixed hybrid rehabilitations of PEEK with milled crowns of a nano-filled composite, concluding that the treatment significantly improved the masticatory performance, bite force, occlusal pattern, quality of life, and satisfaction [18].

The study limitations include the lack of a non-polymeric control group, the short follow-up of the routine group and the fact that this was a single-center study. The strengths of this study include the low rate of dropouts (11% and 5% for the development and routine groups, respectively) which relates to an increased internal validity and the prospective study design. However, the outcomes should be interpreted with caution as even in low dropout rates, the patients missing control appointments had an increased probability of a deleterious outcome, therefore implying an overestimation of the results. Future studies should aim to assess the outcome at midterm and during the longer term for the routine group to evaluate the clinical and patient-centered impacts of the protocol modifications.

5. Conclusions

Within the limitations and considering the results of the present study, it can be concluded that when using PEEK as a framework in fixed prosthetic implant-supported prostheses for full-arch rehabilitations *ad modum*, the All-on-4 concept is an acceptable treatment approach. A high prosthetic/implant survival was registered, together with low biological complication rates, low marginal bone loss, and an excellent impact on the patient's subjective evaluation/quality of life. It further constitutes a shock-absorbing alternative that provides conditions for a beneficial and stable long-term outcome. The protocol modification resulted in an absence of veneer adhesion issues. The high incidence of mechanical complications implies strict respect for the CAD–CAM design and the number of cantilever units.

6. Patents

An international patent resulting from the work reported in this manuscript was issued on 10 January 2019: Silva, A.; Legatheaux, J.; de Araújo Nobre, M.; Guedes, C.M.; Almeida, R.; Maló, P.; Sereno, N. Dental prosthesis. International patent no. WO 2019/008368 A1.

Author Contributions: Conceptualization, M.d.A.N., C.M.G., R.A., A.S. and N.S.; methodology, M.d.A.N. and N.S.; software, A.S.; validation, M.d.A.N.; formal analysis, M.d.A.N.; investigation, M.d.A.N.; data curation, M.d.A.N.; writing—original draft preparation, M.d.A.N.; writing—review and editing, M.d.A.N., C.M.G., R.A., A.S. and N.S.; visualization, M.d.A.N., C.M.G., R.A., A.S. and N.S. All authors have read and agreed to the published version of the manuscript.

Funding: This study was supported by Juvora, grant no. 1/2013. Carlos Moura Guedes, Miguel de Araújo Nobre, and António Silva received previous educational fees from Juvora. Nuno Sereno collaborates scientifically with Juvora (an Invibio company). Ricardo Almeida declares no conflict of interest.

Institutional Review Board Statement: The study was conducted in accordance with the Declaration of Helsinki and approved by the Ethics Committee for Health (008/2013).

Informed Consent Statement: Informed consent was obtained from all subjects involved in the study. Written informed consent has been obtained from the patients to publish this paper.

Data Availability Statement: Data are available from the authors upon reasonable request.

Acknowledgments: The authors acknowledge André Pereira, Filipa Gonçalves and TLPD João Saldanha Lopes for the clinical and laboratory support; SISMA for the production support; and Sandro Catarino for the support in data management.

Conflicts of Interest: Carlos Moura Guedes, Miguel de Araújo Nobre, and António Silva received previous educational fees from Juvora. Nuno Sereno collaborates scientifically with Juvora (an Invibio company). Ricardo Almeida declares no conflict of interest. The funders had no role in the design of the study; in the collection, analyses, or interpretation of data; in the writing of the manuscript; or in the decision to publish the results.

References

1. Yurchenko, M.; Huang, J.; Robisson, A.; McKinley, G.; Hammond, P. Synthesis, mechanical properties and chemical/solvent resistance of cross-linked poly(aryl-ether-ether-ketones) at high temperatures. *Polymer* **2010**, *51*, 1914–1920. [CrossRef]
2. Toth, J.M.; Wang, M.; Estes, B.T.; Scifert, J.L.; Seim, H.B.; Turner, A.S. Polyetheretherketone as a biomaterial for spinal applications. *Biomaterials* **2006**, *27*, 324–334. [CrossRef]
3. Kurtz, S.M.; Devine, J.N. PEEK biomaterials in trauma, orthopedic, and spinal implants. *Biomaterials* **2007**, *28*, 4845–4869. [CrossRef] [PubMed]
4. El Halabi, F.; Rodriguez, J.F.; Rebolledo, L.; Hurtós, E.; Doblaré, M. Mechanical characterization and numerical simulation of polyether–ether–ketone (PEEK) cranial implants. *J. Mech. Behav. Biomed. Mater.* **2011**, *4*, 1819–1832. [CrossRef]
5. Hahnel, S.; Scherl, C.; Rosentritt, M. Interim rehabilitation of occlusal vertical dimension using a double-crown-retained removable dental prosthesis with polyetheretherketone framework. *J. Prosthet. Dent.* **2018**, *119*, 315–318. [CrossRef]
6. Maló, P.; de Araújo Nobre, M.; Moura Guedes, C.; Almeida, R.; Silva, A.; Sereno, N. Short-term report of an ongoing prospective cohort study evaluating the outcome of full-arch implant-supported fixed hybrid polyetheretherketone-acrylic resin prostheses and the All-on-Four concept. *Clin. Implant. Dent. Relat. Res.* **2018**, *20*, 692–702. [CrossRef] [PubMed]
7. Zoidis, P. The all-on-4 modified polyetheretherketone treatment approach: A clinical report. *J. Prosthet. Dent.* **2018**, *119*, 516–521. [CrossRef] [PubMed]
8. Cabello-Domínguez, G.; Pérez-López, J.; Veiga-López, B.; González, D.; Revilla-León, M. Maxillary zirconia and mandibular composite resin-lithium disilicate-modified PEEK fixed implant-supported restorations for a completely edentulous patient with an atrophic maxilla and mandible: A clinical report. *J. Prosthet. Dent.* **2020**, *124*, 403–410. [CrossRef]
9. De Araújo Nobre, M.; Moura Guedes, C.; Almeida, R.; Silva, A.; Sereno, N. Hybrid Polyetheretherketone (PEEK)-Acrylic Resin Prostheses and the All-on-4 Concept: A Full-Arch Implant-Supported Fixed Solution with 3 Years of Follow-Up. *J. Clin. Med.* **2020**, *9*, 2187. [CrossRef]
10. Mourad, K.E.; Altonbary, G.Y.; Emera, R.M.K.; Hegazy, S.A.F. Polyetheretherketone computer-aided design and computer-aided manufacturing framework for All-on-Four mandibular full-arch prosthesis: 3 Years' retrospective study of peri-implant soft tissue changes and ridge base relationship. *J. Prosthodont.* **2022**, *32*, 579–587. [CrossRef]
11. Wang, J.; Wu, P.; Liu, H.L.; Zhang, L.; Liu, L.P.; Ma, C.F.; Chen, J.H. Polyetheretherketone versus titanium CAD-CAM framework for implant-supported fixed complete dentures: A retrospective study with up to 5-year follow-up. *J. Prosthodont. Res.* **2022**, *66*, 279–287. [CrossRef]
12. Ding, L.; Lu, W.; Chen, X.; Xi, Q.; Wu, G. Complete denture fabrication with polyetherketoneketone as a framework material: A clinical report. *J. Prosthet. Dent.* **2022**, *127*, 823–826. [CrossRef]
13. Yadav, R.; Singh, M.; Shekhawat, D.; Lee, S.-Y.; Park, S.-J. The role of fillers to enhance the mechanical, thermal, and wear characteristics of polymer composite materials: A review. *Composites Part A* **2023**, *175*, 107775. [CrossRef]
14. Yadav, R.; Meena, A.; Lee, H.-H.; Lee, S.-Y.; Park, S.-J. Tribological behavior of dental resin composites: A comprehensive review. *Tribol. Int.* **2023**, *190*, 109017. [CrossRef]
15. Rivard, C.H.; Rhalmi, S.; Coillard, C. In vivo biocompatibility testing of peek polymer for a spinal implant system: A study in rabbits. *J. Biomed. Mater. Res.* **2002**, *62*, 488–498. [CrossRef]
16. Mounir, M.; Atef, M.; Abou-Elfetouh, A.; Hakam, M.M. Titanium and polyether ether ketone (PEEK) patient-specific sub-periosteal implants: Two novel approaches for rehabilitation of the severely atrophic anterior maxillary ridge. *Int. J. Oral Maxillofac. Surg.* **2018**, *47*, 658–664. [PubMed]
17. Luo, C.; Liu, Y.; Peng, B.; Chen, M.; Liu, Z.; Li, Z.; Kuang, H.; Gong, B.; Li, Z.; Sun, H. PEEK for Oral Applications: Recent Advances in Mechanical and Adhesive Properties. *Polymers* **2023**, *15*, 386. [CrossRef] [PubMed]
18. Montero, J.; Guadilla, Y.; Flores, J.; Pardal-Peláez, B.; Quispe-López, N.; Gómez-Polo, C.; Dib, A. Patient-centered treatment outcomes with full-arch PEEK rehabilitation supported on four immediate or conventionally loaded implants. A randomized clinical trial. *J. Clin. Med.* **2021**, *10*, 4589. [CrossRef] [PubMed]

19. Ayyadanveettil, P.; Thavakkara, V.; Latha, N.; Pavanan, M.; Saraswathy, A.; Kuruniyan, M.S. Randomized clinical trial of zirconia and polyetheretherketone implant abutments for single-tooth implant restorations: A 5-year evaluation. *J. Prosthet. Dent.* **2022**, *128*, 1275–1281. [CrossRef]
20. Gama, L.T.; Bezerra, A.P.; Schimmel, M.; Rodrigues Garcia, R.C.M.; de Luca Canto, G.; Gonçalves, T.M.S.V. Clinical performance of polymer frameworks in dental prostheses: A systematic review. *J. Prosthet. Dent.* **2022**, in press. [CrossRef]
21. Minervini, G.; Franco, R.; Marrapodi, M.M.; Fiorillo, L.; Cervino, G.; Cicciù, M. Prevalence of Temporomandibular Disorders (TMD) in Pregnancy: A Systematic Review with Meta-analysis. *J. Oral. Rehabil.* **2023**, *50*, 627–634. [CrossRef] [PubMed]
22. Khurshid, Z.; Nedumgottil, B.M.; Ali, R.M.M.; Bencharit, S.; Najeeb, S. Insufficient Evidence to Ascertain the Long-Term Survival of PEEK Dental Prostheses: A Systematic Review of Clinical Studies. *Polymers* **2022**, *14*, 2441. [CrossRef]
23. Di Stasio, D.; Romano, A.; Gentile, C.; Maio, C.; Lucchese, A.; Serpico, R.; Paparella, R.; Minervini, G.; Candotto, V.; Laino, L. Systemic and Topical Photodynamic Therapy (PDT) on Oral Mucosa Lesions: An Overview. *J. Biol. Regul. Homeost. Agents* **2018**, *32*, 123–126.
24. Tribst, J.P.M.; de Morais, D.C.; de Matos, J.D.M.; Lopes, G.R.S.; Dal Piva, A.M.O.; Borges, A.L.S.; Bottino, M.A.; Lanzotti, A.; Martorelli, M.; Ausiello, P. Influence of Framework Material and Posterior Implant Angulation in Full-Arch All-on-4 Implant-Supported Prosthesis Stress Concentration. *Dent. J.* **2022**, *10*, 12. [CrossRef]
25. Shash, Y.H.; El-Wakad, M.T.; Eldosoky, M.A.A.; Dohiem, M.M. Evaluation of stress and strain on mandible caused using "All-on-Four" system from PEEK in hybrid prosthesis: Finite-element analysis. *Odontology* **2022**, *111*, 618–629. [CrossRef]
26. Ersöz, T.M.B.; Mumcu, E. Biomechanical investigation of maxillary implant-supported full-arch prostheses produced with different framework materials: A finite elements study. *J. Adv. Prosthodont* **2022**, *14*, 346–359, Epub 22 December 2022. [CrossRef]
27. Yu, W.; Li, X.; Ma, X.; Xu, X. Biomechanical analysis of inclined and cantilever design with different implant framework materials in mandibular complete-arch implant restorations. *J. Prosthet. Dent.* **2022**, *127*, 783.e1–783.e10. [CrossRef]
28. Dayan, S.C.; Geckili, O. The influence of framework material on stress distribution in maxillary complete-arch fixed prostheses supported by four dental implants: A three-dimensional finite element analysis. *Comput. Methods Biomech. Biomed. Engin.* **2021**, *24*, 1606–1617. [CrossRef] [PubMed]
29. Haroun, F.; Ozan, O. Evaluation of Stresses on Implant, Bone, and Restorative Materials Caused by Different Opposing Arch Materials in Hybrid Prosthetic Restorations Using the All-on-4 Technique. *Materials* **2021**, *14*, 4308. [CrossRef] [PubMed]
30. Addel, R.; Lekholm, U.; Rockler, B.; Brånemark, P.I. A 15-year study of osseointegrated implants in the treatment of the edentulous jaw. *Int. J. Oral. Surg.* **1981**, *10*, 387–416.
31. Silva, A.; Legatheaux, J.; de Araújo Nobre, M.; Guedes, C.M.; Almeida, R.; Maló, P.; Sereno, N. Dental Prosthesis. International Patent WO 2019/008368 A1, 10 January 2019.
32. Mombelli, A.; van Oosten, M.A.C.; Schürch, E.; Lang, N.P. The microbiota associated with successful or failing osseointegrated titanium implants. *Oral. Microbiol. Immunol.* **1987**, *2*, 145–151. [CrossRef]
33. Riva, F.; Seoane, M.; Reichenheim, M.E.; Tsakos, G.; Celeste, R.K. Adult oral health-related quality of life instruments: A systematic review. *Community Dent. Oral. Epidemiol.* **2022**, *50*, 333–338. [CrossRef]
34. Maló, P.; Nobre, M.A.; Lopes, A. The rehabilitation of completely edentulous maxillae with different degrees of resorption with four or more immediately loaded implants: A 5-year retrospective study and a new classification. *Eur. J. Oral Implantol.* **2011**, *4*, 227–243.
35. Keul, C.; Liebermann, A.; Schmidlin, P.R.; Roos, M.; Sener, B.; Stawarczyk, B. Influence of PEEK surface modification on surface properties and bond strength to veneering resin composites. *J. Adhes. Dent.* **2014**, *16*, 383–392. [PubMed]
36. Stawarczyk, B.; Keul, C.; Beuer, F.; Roos, M.; Schmidlin, P.R. Tensile bond strength of veneering resins to PEEK: Impact of different adhesives. *Dent. Mater. J.* **2013**, *32*, 441–448. [CrossRef]
37. Gouveia, D.D.N.M.; Razzoog, M.E.; Sierraalta, M.; Alfaro, M.F. Effect of surface treatment and manufacturing process on the shear bond strength of veneering composite resin to polyetherketoneketone (PEKK) and polyetheretherketone (PEEK). *J. Prosthet. Dent.* **2022**, *128*, 1061–1066. [CrossRef] [PubMed]
38. Sloan, R.; Hollis, W.; Selecman, A.; Jain, V.; Versluis, A. Bond strength of lithium disilicate to polyetheretherketone. *J. Prosthet. Dent.* **2022**, *128*, 1351–1357. [CrossRef] [PubMed]
39. Taha, D.; Safwat, F.; Wahsh, M. Effect of combining different surface treatments on the surface characteristics of polyetheretherketone-based core materials and shear bond strength to a veneering composite resin. *J. Prosthet. Dent.* **2022**, *127*, 599.e1–599.e7. [CrossRef]
40. Villefort, R.F.; Diamantino, P.J.S.; Zeidler, S.L.V.V.; Borges, A.L.S.; Silva-Concílio, L.R.; Saavedra, G.D.F.A.; Tribst, J.P.M. Mechanical Response of PEKK and PEEK As Frameworks for Implant-Supported Full-Arch Fixed Dental Prosthesis: 3D Finite Element Analysis. *Eur. J. Dent.* **2022**, *16*, 115–121. [CrossRef]
41. Del Fabbro, M.; Pozzi, A.; Romeo, D.; de Araújo Nobre, M.; Agliardi, E. Outcomes of Fixed Full-Arch Rehabilitations Supported by Tilted and Axially Placed Implants: A Systematic Review and Meta-Analysis. *Int. J. Oral Maxillofac. Implant.* **2022**, *37*, 1003–1025. [CrossRef]
42. Maló, P.; de Araújo Nobre, M.; Lopes, A.; Ferro, A.; Botto, J. The All-on-4 treatment concept for the rehabilitation of the completely edentulous mandible: A longitudinal study with 10 to 18 years of follow-up. *Clin. Implant. Dent. Relat. Res.* **2019**, *21*, 565–577. [CrossRef] [PubMed]

43. Maló, P.; de Araújo Nobre, M.; Lopes, A.; Ferro, A.; Nunes, M. The All-on-4 concept for full-arch rehabilitation of the edentulous maxillae: A longitudinal study with 5-13 years of follow-up. *Clin. Implant. Dent. Relat. Res.* **2019**, *21*, 538–549. [CrossRef] [PubMed]
44. De Araújo Nobre, M.; Mano Azul, A.; Rocha, E.; Maló, P. Risk factors of peri-implant pathology. *Eur. J. Oral Sci.* **2015**, *123*, 131–139. [CrossRef]
45. Chrcanovic, B.R.; Albrektsson, T.; Wennerberg, A. Smoking and dental implants: A systematic review and meta-analysis. *J. Dent.* **2015**, *43*, 487–498. [CrossRef]
46. Conserva, E.; Meneni, M.; Bevilacqua, M.; Tealdo, T.; Ravera, G.; Pera, F.; Pera, P. The use of a masticatory robot to analyze the shock absorption capacity of different restorative materials for prosthetic implants: A preliminary report. *Int. J. Prosthodont.* **2009**, *22*, 53–55.
47. Stawarczyk, B.; Beuer, F.; Wimmer, T.; Jahn, D.; Sener, B.; Roos, M.; Schmidlin, P.R. Polyetheretherketone—A suitable material for fixed dental prostheses? *J. Biomed. Mater. Res.* **2013**, *101*, 1209–1216. [CrossRef] [PubMed]
48. Menini, M.; Conserva, E.; Tealdo, T.; Bevilacqua, M.; Pera, F.; Ravera, G.; Pera, P. The use of a masticatory robot to analyze the shock absorption capacity of different restorative materials for implant prosthesis. *J. Biol. Res.* **2011**, *84*, 118–119. [CrossRef]
49. Minervini, G.; Franco, R.; Marrapodi, M.M.; Fiorillo, L.; Cervino, G.; Cicciù, M. Economic Inequalities and Temporomandibular Disorders: A Systematic Review with Meta-analysis. *J. Oral Rehabil.* **2023**, *50*, 715–723. [CrossRef] [PubMed]
50. Falcinelli, C.; Valente, F.; Vasta, M.; Traini, T. Finite element analysis in implant dentistry: State of the art and future directions. *Dent. Mater.* **2023**, *39*, 539–556. [CrossRef] [PubMed]
51. Pontoriero, R.; Tonelli, M.P.; Carnevale, G.; Mombelli, A.; Nyman, S.R.; Lang, N.P. Experimentally induced peri-implant mucositis. A clinical study in humans. *Clin. Oral Implant. Res.* **1994**, *5*, 254–259. [CrossRef]
52. Salvi, G.E.; Aglietta, M.; Eick, S.; Sculean, A.; Lang, N.P.; Ramseier, C.A. Reversibility of experimental peri-implant mucositis compared with experimental gingivitis in humans. *Clin. Oral Implant. Res.* **2012**, *23*, 182–190. [CrossRef] [PubMed]
53. Kennedy, K.; Chacon, G.; McGlumphy, E.; Johnston, W.; Yilmaz, B.; Kennedy, P. Evaluation of patient experience and satisfaction with immediately loaded metal-acrylic resin implant-supported fixed complete prosthesis. *Int. J. Oral Maxillofac. Implant.* **2012**, *27*, 1191–1198.
54. Matsuyama, Y.; Tsakos, G.; Listl, S.; Aida, J.; Watt, R.G. Impact of Dental Diseases on Quality-Adjusted Life Expectancy in US Adults. *J. Dent. Res.* **2019**, *98*, 510–516. [CrossRef] [PubMed]

Disclaimer/Publisher's Note: The statements, opinions and data contained in all publications are solely those of the individual author(s) and contributor(s) and not of MDPI and/or the editor(s). MDPI and/or the editor(s) disclaim responsibility for any injury to people or property resulting from any ideas, methods, instructions or products referred to in the content.

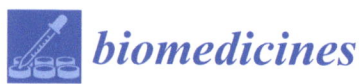 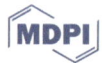

Article

Comparison of the Eggshell and the Porcine Pericardium Membranes for Guided Tissue Regeneration Applications

Horia Opris [1], Mihaela Baciut [1], Marioara Moldovan [2], Stanca Cuc [2], Ioan Petean [3], Daiana Opris [1,*], Simion Bran [1], Florin Gligor Onisor [1,*], Gabriel Armenea [1] and Grigore Baciut [1]

[1] Department of Maxillofacial Surgery and Implantology, Iuliu Hatieganu University of Medicine and Pharmacy, 400012 Cluj-Napoca, Romania; horia.opris@umfcluj.ro (H.O.); mbaciut@umfcluj.ro (M.B.); dr_brans@umfcluj.ro (S.B.); armencea.gabriel@umfcluj.ro (G.A.); gbaciut@umfcluj.ro (G.B.)

[2] Department of Polymer Composites, Institute of Chemistry Raluca Ripan, Babes-Bolyai University, 30 Fantanele Street, 400294 Cluj-Napoca, Romania; marioara.moldovan@ubbcluj.ro (M.M.); stanca.boboia@ubbcluj.ro (S.C.)

[3] Faculty of Chemistry and Chemical Engineering, Babes-Bolyai University, 11 Arany Janos Street, 400028 Cluj-Napoca, Romania; ioan.petean@ubbcluj.ro

* Correspondence: daiana.prodan@umfcluj.ro (D.O.); florin.onisor@umfcluj.ro (F.G.O.)

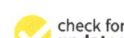

Citation: Opris, H.; Baciut, M.; Moldovan, M.; Cuc, S.; Petean, I.; Opris, D.; Bran, S.; Onisor, F.G.; Armenea, G.; Baciut, G. Comparison of the Eggshell and the Porcine Pericardium Membranes for Guided Tissue Regeneration Applications. *Biomedicines* **2023**, *11*, 2529. https://doi.org/10.3390/biomedicines11092529

Academic Editors: Giuseppe Minervini and Gianmarco Abbadessa

Received: 26 August 2023
Revised: 7 September 2023
Accepted: 12 September 2023
Published: 13 September 2023

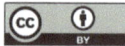

Copyright: © 2023 by the authors. Licensee MDPI, Basel, Switzerland. This article is an open access article distributed under the terms and conditions of the Creative Commons Attribution (CC BY) license (https:// creativecommons.org/licenses/by/ 4.0/).

Abstract: Guided bone regeneration is frequently used to reconstruct the alveolar bone to rehabilitate the mastication using dental implants. The purpose of this article is to research the properties of eggshell membrane (ESM) and its potential application in tissue engineering. The study focuses on the structural, mechanical, and histological characteristics of ESM extracted from *Gallus domesticus* eggs and to compare them to a commercially available porcine pericardium membrane (Jason® membrane, botiss biomaterials GmbH, Zossen, Germany). Thus, histology was performed on the ESM, and a comparison of the microstructure through scanning electron microscopy and atomic force microscopy (AFM) was conducted. Also, mechanical tensile strength was evaluated. Samples of ESM were prepared and treated with alcohol for fixation and disinfection. Histological analysis revealed that the ESM architecture is constituted out of loose collagen fibers. However, due to the random arrangement of collagen fibers within the membrane, it might not be an effective barrier and occlusive barrier. Comparative analyses were performed between the ESM and the AFM examinations and demonstrated differences in the surface topography and mechanical properties between the two membranes. The ESM exhibited rougher surfaces and weaker mechanical cohesion attributed to its glycoprotein content. The study concludes that while the ESM displays favorable biocompatibility and resorb ability, its non-uniform collagen arrangement limits its suitability as a guided bone regeneration membrane in the current non-crosslinked native form. Crosslinking techniques may enhance its properties for such applications. Further research is needed to explore modifications and processing methods that could leverage the ESM's unique properties for tissue engineering purposes.

Keywords: eggshell membrane; biocompatibility; bone regeneration; rat model

1. Introduction

Alveolar bone resorption is a process that always takes place following tooth loss due to trauma or disease [1]. Thus, reconstruction has been proposed for a long time as a treatment to compensate for lost volume [2]. Furthermore, bone block and autologous bone graft has long been the golden standard for bone rebuilding [3]. In contrast, the concept of guided bone regeneration (GBR) requires compartmentalization, which employs a barrier membrane to permit the bone to heal [4]. In addition, Urban et al. [2] found that the membrane stabilizes the graft and the surrounding tissues.

Polytetrafluoroethylene (PTFE) and titanium meshes are the most common nonabsorbable materials used for GBR [5]. However, although they have excellent space maintenance, they require a second surgery to remove and carry a greater risk of exposure and contamination [6].

The alternative, resorbable membranes, may be of natural or synthetic origin. They can also be crosslinked or non-crosslinked, a process that modifies the membrane's properties so that it absorbs water more slowly [7]. Consequently, they do not require surgical removal, but they are not suitable to maintain the space in large, particularly vertical, defects. As a matter of fact, exposure of the resorbable membranes does not always result in graft failure [8]. For instance, the bovine pericardium membranes have shown significant functional and morphological potential, which have provided the opportunity to examine cellular behavior [9].

Scanning electron microscopy (SEM) is used to evaluate the surfaces of biomaterials and bone [10]. Furthermore, it evaluates the tissue response to the graft materials and the production of the bone scaffold and osteogenic structures [11,12].

Atomic force microscopy (AFM) is used to examine the surface properties and the characteristics of materials [13]. In addition, it enables the evaluation of samples at the molecular level [14]. Moreover, by measuring forces and mapping the topography, AFM aids in evaluating the quality of graft materials, cellular adhesion, and proliferation and assists in studying the mechanical properties of regenerated bone [15].

In vivo studies on experimental animals' subcutaneous tissue give valuable information on the histology-level effects a substance might produce [16]. Especially since the ideal membrane must have a surface that does not create tissue reaction, it is easy to manage, is semipermeable, and maintains a space for proper bone healing [17].

Although there are extensive inquiries regarding the use of the eggshell membrane (ESM) in clinical trials [18] and in animal use, much research is needed to fully evaluate the proprieties and potential. The eggshell membrane is of biologic origin, composed out of natural proteins, is a semipermeable membrane for oxygen and other nutrients, and acts as a barrier membrane for the contents of the egg [19]. These qualities and the research that is already in the public domain have produced questions regarding the actual biologic use for the membrane.

The aim of this paper is to assess the histologic and microscopic structure and tensile strength of the eggshell membrane in comparison to a commercially available porcine pericardium membrane (Jason® membrane, botiss biomaterials GmbH, Zossen, Germany).

2. Materials and Methods

2.1. Production of the Membrane

Using the outer-shell membrane of *Gallus domesticus* eggshells, a collagen membrane was produced. The membrane was disinfected and fixed with a 99% alcohol solution.

The porcine pericardium membrane was procured from suppliers (Jason® membrane, botiss biomaterials GmbH, Zossen, Germany) and was used for the testing described below.

Samples from each type of membrane (ESM and Jason) were produced for each test: for biocompatibility 1×1 cm ($n = 12$), samples for tensile testing (40 mm × 5 mm), for SEM ($n = 12$) and AFM ($n = 12$).

2.2. Histology

The specimens fixed with paraformaldehyde were mounted on glass slides, dehydrated with an alcohol gradient. Paraffin-embedded 10 mm sections were washed with xylene and rehydrated before being stained with hematoxylin and eosin (Histo-Lab. Ltd., Gothenburg, Sweden).

We adopted a specific histological processing technique with the goal of precisely preserving the structure for the assessment of the eggshell membrane. To achieve this, we cut a small pocket in the liver fragments of a recently sacrificed rat using a sharp scalpel, and then we inserted a piece of membrane into the pocket. The membrane and liver fragment were immersed in a 10% formalin solution for three days to fixate them. The fragments were cleared with 1-Butanol (Histo-Lab. Ltd., Gothenburg, Sweden), dehydrated with ethyl alcohol, and then embedded in paraffin when the fixing was finished. Hematoxylin and eosin (H&E) staining was used to create sections with a 5 μm thickness. An Olympus BX41 microscope (Olympus, Tokyo, Japan) with a digital image capture camera type E-330 was used to examine histological sections. The choice for this specific technique was because it enables us to produce a clear cross-section of a relatively soft material, but it can be hard to handle and process (the eggshell membrane). Also, it allows us not to damage the structure during handling and micro slicing.

2.3. Scanning Electron Microscopy

SEM investigation was executed with an Inspect S50 SEM Microscope produced by FEI Company, Hillsboro, OR, USA. The secondary electron images were obtained at an acceleration voltage of 25 kV at low vacuum mode without metallization.

2.4. Mechanical Testing: Tensile Testing

The mechanical strength of membranes was studied using a Lloyd LR5k Plus dual-column mechanical testing machine (Ametek/Lloyd Instruments, Meerbusch, Germany), equipped with a load cell with a maximum range of 5 kN. The tested samples had a rectangular shape measuring 40 mm high and 5 mm wide. The tensile test was performed with a separation of 25 mm at an expansion speed of 25 mm/min until they failed. The membranes were evaluated wet (immediately after removal from alcoholic solution) and dry (after 15 min of absorption on suction paper).

2.5. Atomic-Force Microscopy

The eggshell membrane was dried using a filter paper until it reached the proper conditions for the AFM investigation. The porcine pericardium membrane (Jason® membrane) was extracted from the sterile envelope and a small corner was cut off for the AFM investigation. The investigation was setup with a JEOL JSPM 4210 Scanning Probe Microscope, produced by JEOL, Japan, Tokio. The probing cantilevers are of NSC 15 type produced by MicroMasch, Estonia, Talinn, with a resonant frequency of 325 kHz and a spring constant of 40 N/m. The topographic images were obtained at a scan rate of 1.5–3 Hz depending on the image size. The images were analyzed trough Jeol WIN SPM 2.0 processing soft and Ra (Surface roughness average) and Rq (root mean square roughness) roughness, measured for each image. At least three different macroscopic areas were scanned for each sample for a proper statistical average of the obtained values.

Ra represents the arithmetic average of the profile height and is described by Equation (1) and Rq root mean square of the profile height and is described by Equation (2):

$$Ra = \frac{1}{l_r} \int_0^{l_r} |z(x)| dx \tag{1}$$

and

$$Rq = \sqrt{\frac{1}{l_r} \int_0^{l_r} |z(x)^2| dx} \tag{2}$$

where l is the profile length and $\underline{z}$ is the height at x point. Both Ra and Rq are important for a various research applications [20,21].

3. Results

3.1. Histopathologic Results

Histological fixation preserved the architecture of the eggshell membrane, which does not alter in contact with bodily fluids; fixation is similar to the process of cross-linking. After histological processing, the eggshell membrane remained intact, and it could be seen on the wide surface area in direct contact with the liver parenchyma (Figures 1 and 2).

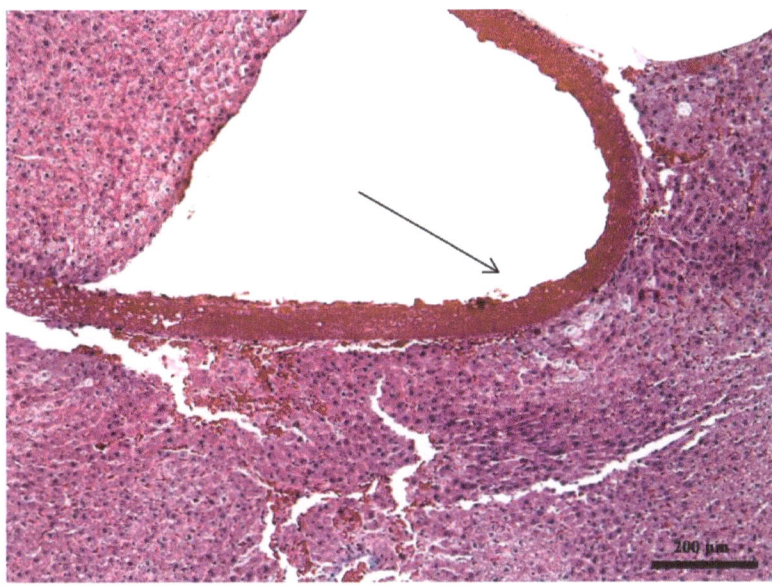

Figure 1. Intact eggshell membrane (black arrow) preserved by histological fixation, visible in direct contact with liver parenchyma (Hematoxylin eosin staining, 10×).

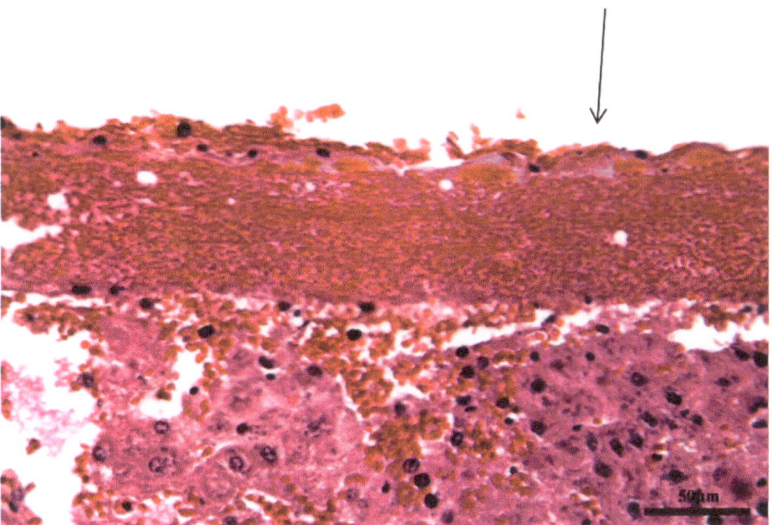

Figure 2. Eggshell membrane (black arrow) architecture remains unchanged due to histological fixation, comparable to cross-linking process; collagen fibers packed together can be seen without a rigorous union (Hematoxylin eosin staining, 40×).

The eggshell membrane is structurally made up of collagen fibers arranged closely together but without a very rigorous organization. This connective tissue can be classified as dense, non-oriented connective tissue. Because non-oriented connective tissue does not have a very rigorous arrangement of collagen fibers, it can be easily appreciated that this membrane can be considered as a protective membrane but not as a separating membrane, as desired in guided bone regeneration. In other words, this membrane has good mechanical strength, but the random arrangement of collagen fibers means that meshes with a rigorous shape and size are not defined between them but are polymorphous in shape and size. In this regard, the membrane cannot be considered an efficient separating material as desired in guided bone regeneration because cells can pass through the larger meshes between collagen fibers, whereas the separating membrane should not allow this.

3.2. SEM Analysis

The eggshell membrane general aspect of the microstructure is presented in Figure 3a. The sample was positioned at 45° to the accelerated electron beam, revealing the membrane section on the middle horizontal position within the observation field, and the membrane surface is positioned below. Both exterior and interior sides of the membrane are visible, being strongly reticulated by collagen I type fibers, while the section cohesion is assured by only a few collagen type I fibers and a lot of collagen V type small fibers that bind the glycoprotein units. The eggshell membrane has a thickness of about 50 µm as observed in Figure 3a.

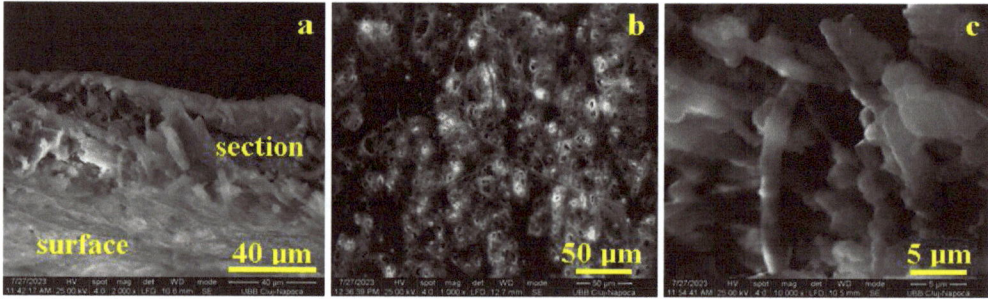

Figure 3. SEM images for the eggshell membrane: (**a**) ensemble microstructural view, (**b**) surface microstructure, and (**c**) section microstructure.

The microstructure of the eggshell membrane surface is presented in Figure 3b. The collagen I type network is clearly visible, having a lot of well interconnected fibers embedded into the glycoprotein matrix. Their average diameter is 2.5 ± 0.81 µm. The section microstructure, Figure 3c, reveals some vertical collagen type I fibers that interconnect both sides of the membrane, assuring its cohesion and consistency. Collagen type V fibers are smaller, having diameters of 0.6 ± 0.077 µm, and are predominantly horizontally oriented, assuring the texture base for the glycoprotein clusters from the membrane insight. The glycoprotein clusters are present, but it is exceedingly difficult to distinguish it from the collagen structure.

The porcine pericardium membrane is synthetically manufactured from collagen type I from porcine pericardium. Thus, it has a controlled interlaced structure based on the uniform collagen fibers. The overall microstructural aspect is presented in Figure 4a; both surface and section of the Jason membrane is visible due to the sample inclination of about 30° regarding the accelerated electron beam within SEM device. The surface is visible in the upper side of the observation field while the section is situated on the lower side of the SEM image in Figure 4a. The surface looks exceptionally smooth and is formed by a dense texture of collagen fibers. The section thickness has 100 ± 12 µm and is formed by several interlaced layers similar to the one observed in the surface. (There are about 10–12 successive collagen layers.)

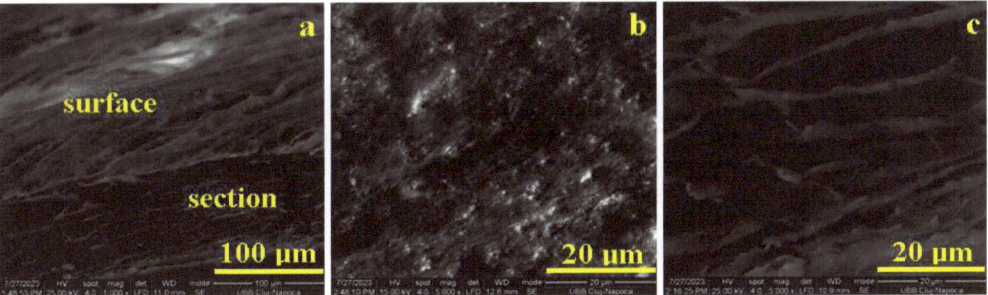

Figure 4. SEM images for Jason membrane: (**a**) ensemble microstructural view; (**b**) surface microstructure, and (**c**) section microstructure.

Surface microstructure is presented in Figure 4b. It features a dense network of collagen fibers interlaced in a compact structure. It is difficult to observe each collagen fiber due to its small diameter, but some fascicles are clearly visible. Their general direction is situated from the lower left corner to the upper right corner of Figure 4b. The section microstructure has more visible details, Figure 4c. The successive layers are also interlaced together by a dense spatial texture of fine collagen fibers. The thickness of a single layer ranges from 1.5 to 2 µm, and the free space between two successive layers is situated at 10 ± 1.3 µm. Layer cross linking occurs through local intersections under a sharp angle (about 15–30°) situation; these are more visible in the left side of Figure 4c.

3.3. Atomic Force Microscopy Analysis

The eggshell membrane is a complex biological structure based on a very well reticulated collagen matrix based on both I and V types bonded with glycoprotein. Collagen type I is found in the outermost layers of the membrane while V type is characteristic for the deeper layers of the membrane. Thus, the topography of the eggshell membrane's fine microstructure in Figure 5a reveals a dense network of collagen type I fibers with diameters of 2.5 ± 0.75 µm coated with a dense and compact glycoprotein layer that practically makes it impossible to visualize the tropocollagen units.

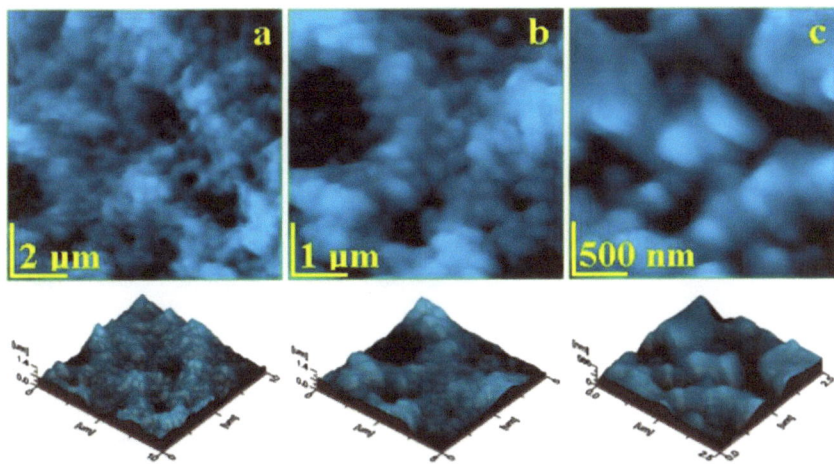

Figure 5. Eggshell membrane topographic images scanned at different images sides: (**a**) 10 µm, (**b**) 5 µm, and (**c**) 2.5 µm.

Figure 5b reveals a more detailed fine microstructure that evidences some small fibers of collagen V type in the range of 0.6–1 µm in diameter and are coated with a compact layer of rounded glycoprotein clusters of 300–400 nm. The nanostructural detail in Figure 5c reveals a single collagen V type fiber oriented from the upper left corner to the lower right corner with a diameter of 0.6 ± 0.08 µm, and glycoprotein clusters surrounds its structure.

Surface roughness, Figure 6, strongly depends on the topographic image scan side, the nanostructural aspects featuring lower roughness values (e.g., image side of 2.5 µm), while the fine microstructure has a slightly increased roughness due to the spatial orientation of the interlaced collagen fibers of type I and V. Thus, the roughness values of the fine microstructure ranges from Ra 173 to 194 nm and Rq 217 to 241 nm.

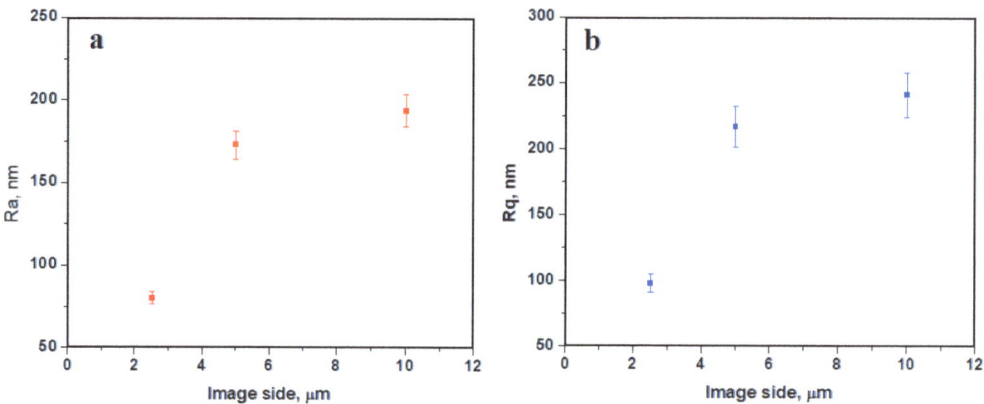

Figure 6. Roughness variation with the image side: (**a**) Ra and (**b**) Rq.

The Jason membrane is synthetically produced from collagen type I from porcine heart destined for dental application. The fine microstructure topography in Figure 7a reveals a dense texture of relative parallel fascicles of fine collagen fibers. Some of the fibers are interlaced under low angles assuring a good cohesion of the structure. It should enhance the tensile strength and avoid texture tearing under axial forces.

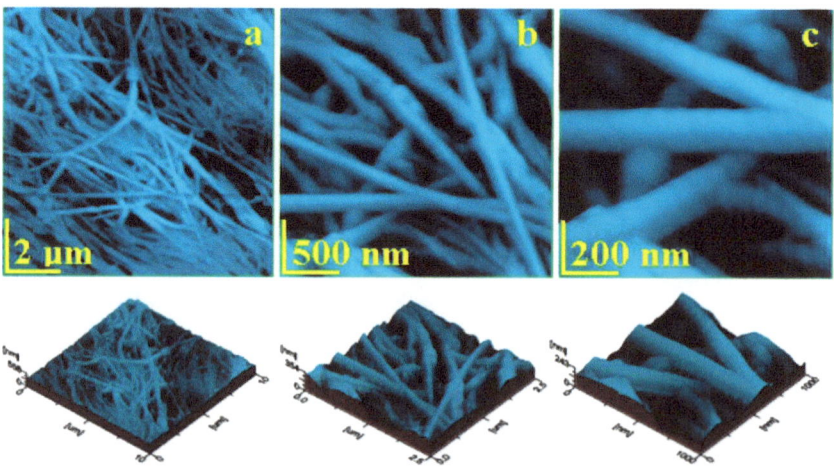

Figure 7. Jason membrane topographic images scanned at different images sides: (**a**) 10 µm, (**b**) 2.5 µm, and (**c**) 1 µm.

Figure 7b evidences a fine microstructure detail observed at a scan side of 2.5 μm, revealing the fibers interconnecting and assuring a good cohesion of the adjacent fascicles. Three concurrent fibers are situated in the lower left corner of Figure 7b and are bundled into an emergent one that passes through the right side of the structure being incorporated in the next fascicle. The nanostructural detail in Figure 7c allows us to properly observe and measure the fiber's diameter that is situated at 160 ± 15 nm. The tropocollagen units are clearly visible in the fiber's structure as rounded elements with a diameter of 67 nm.

The Jason membrane proves to be flatter than the eggshell membrane due to the synthetic interlacing and due to the lack of the glycoprotein matrix. Thus, the roughness values are less dependent on the topographic image side. However, at the nanostructural level, the roughness is slightly lower, Figure 8. The fine microstructure presents roughness ranges as follows: Ra 42.6 to 49.4 nm and Rq 54.6 to 63.5 nm.

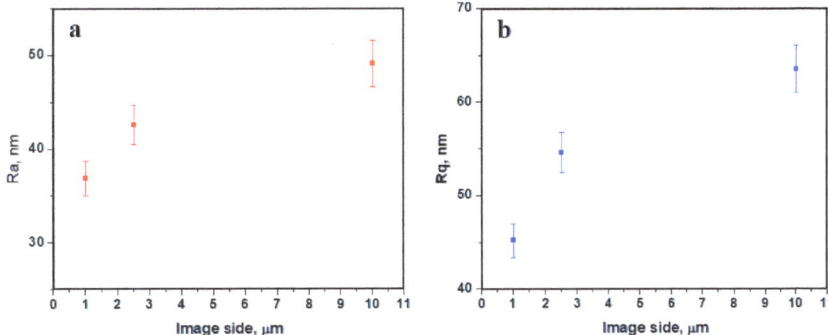

Figure 8. Roughness variation with the image side: (**a**) Ra and (**b**) Rq.

3.4. Mechanical Proprieties

The results of the mechanical testing of the membranes can be observed in Table 1, and the descriptive statistics are in Table 2. The mean of the dried membranes is 10.42 for the eggshell membrane and, for the Jason, 65.72. The same difference can be seen for the membranes observed that were immersed in SBF (simulated body fluids). This is in accordance with the histologic results and the SEM and AFM analysis. The lack of structure and the nonuniform distribution of the collagen fibers determine such a significant difference between the membranes results of the mechanical testing.

Table 1. Tensile Strength (MPa) testing on the eggshell membrane comparing to the Jason membrane.

Eggshell Membrane after 15 min of Drying	Dried Jason Membrane	Eggshell Membrane Immersed in SBF and Dried 15 min	Jason Membrane Immersed in SBF and Dried 15 min
4.93	59.65	1.20	61.91
13.74	67.01	1.20	64.22
10.09	62.25	1.27	64.32
8.35	67.01	1.25	69.63
4.36	62.25	1.25	69.87
6.37	67.01	1.23	74.44
10.75	66.08	1.22	69.73
11.70	65.78	1.24	67.00
12.46	65.65	1.23	74.18
11.82	59.91	1.21	74.14

Table 2. Descriptive statistics of the tensile strength (MPa) of the eggshell membrane and Jason membrane.

	Eggshell Membrane after 15 min of Drying	Dried Jason Membrane	Eggshell Membrane Immersed in SBF and Dried 15 min	Jason Membrane Immersed in SBF and Dried 15 min
Mean	9.46	64.26	1.23	68.94
Median	10.42	65.72	1.23	69.68
Standard Deviation	3.29	2.95	0.02	4.52
Minimum	4.36	59.65	1.20	61.91
Maximum	13.74	67.01	1.27	74.44

In Figure 9, the tensile strength curve for dry eggshell membrane after 15 min (upper left graph), dry eggshell membrane immersed in SBF (upper right graph), Jason membrane (lower left graph), and Jason membrane immersed in SBF (lower right graph) can be compared. The eggshell membrane has a higher load and break for the dried eggshell membrane. The membrane itself has significantly lower values for the load at break. The porcine pericardium origin of the collagen membrane offers a denser structure with a thicker layer which, in fact, gives it better handling capabilities and resistance at tensile testing.

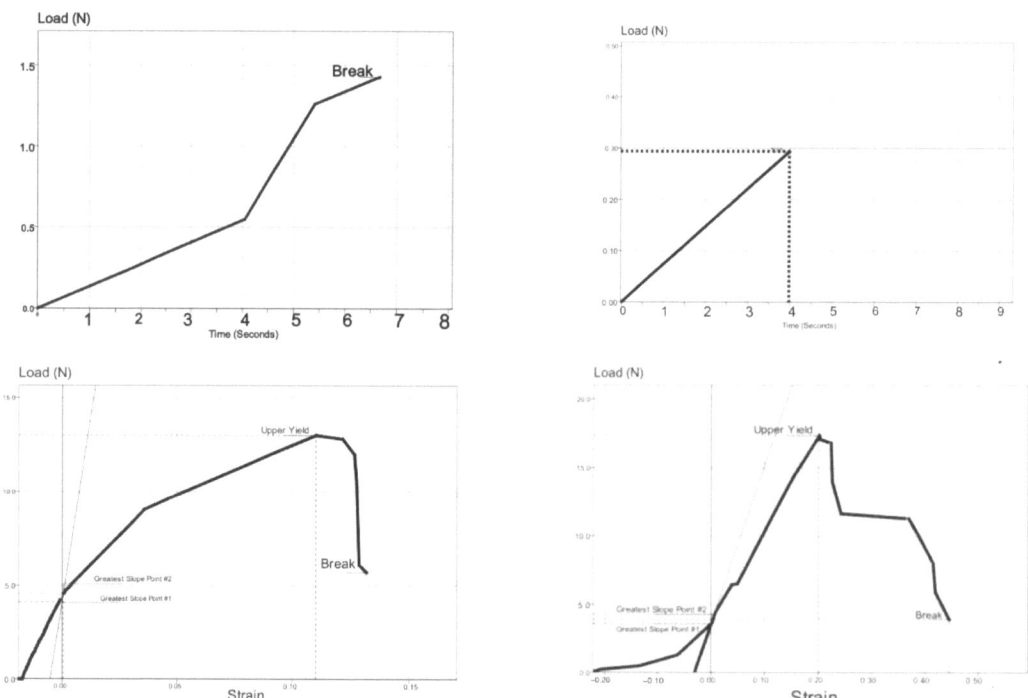

Figure 9. Tensile strength curve for dry eggshell membrane after 15 min (upper left graph), dry eggshell membrane immersed in SBF (upper right graph), Jason membrane (lower left graph), Jason membrane immersed in SBF (lower right graph).

4. Discussion

Due to the content of the membrane, it is biocompatible and resorbable. Despite this, the shell membrane cannot be an ideal separating membrane in guided bone repair because the collagen fibers are not rigorously arranged, so they do not form regular meshes of a suitable and comparable size, which could prevent cell migration through the membrane.

An early study of biocompatibility by Rothamel et al. [22] regarding the porcine pericardium membranes has revealed that they display a fibrous structure, cell proliferation, and no inflammatory reaction. Moreover, the degradation of the membranes has been shown to be around 4 to 8 weeks—for some commercial variants, even 12 weeks.

Nevertheless, the rationale behind bone regeneration techniques, not dependent on the technique itself, involves the facilitation of three-dimensional dental implant placement in a correct prosthetic position for functional loading [23]. Hence, the histologic changes that occur during alveolar bone healing can be summed up into subsequent processes: inflammatory, proliferative, and remodeling. First, it involves the blood clot formation and the inflammatory cells' migration. Secondly, it includes fibroplasia and woven bone formation. Then, the remodeling stage will reshape the alveolar bone considering the architecture and the functional loading. In conclusion, after tooth loss, it is expected that at least 50% bone loss after healing will occur, especially on the buccal side and more volume in the molar region [24]. Furthermore, the alveolar bone remodeling can be influenced by using xenograft in combination with a collagen membrane; thus, the resorption rate can be decreased. In addition, the facial aspect of the bone always resorbs in a small portion [25]. Above all, bone remodeling occurs, and usually the alveolar bone stabilizes at 9 months postoperative after GBR, to a significant degree, although it is still a better outcome than no treatment [26].

Although both resorbable and non-resorbable membranes produce the same quality of bone, when using titanium meshes, it was observed that the thickness and the stability after 1 year of loading was greater [27]. Despite all the efforts, the hard tissues resulting from GBR using resorbable membranes with xenograft material will always retract during the remodeling phase. Furthermore, Jiang et al. [28] concluded that new bone formation further than the bony envelope is not predictable.

What is a more important issue to discuss is the quality of studies found in the literature regarding the follow-up of clinical cases. In general, the median follow-up is about 60 months, not enough for what one could consider a success, and there is also a lack of prospective studies which compare different techniques and assess the long-term stability and outcome [23].

In fact, Bornert et al. [29] found that the barrier function of the pericardium porcine membrane is similar to other commercially available collagen membranes (Biogide) in regard to the resorption kinetics and resorption rate. Also, the barrier function was intact at 12 weeks, and the cell adhesion facilitated the bone formation process.

Similarly, a study on a critically sized rat calvaria defect by You et al. [30] found that the pericardium membrane, which was compared to native collagen membrane at 4 weeks, showed good biocompatibility, good barrier function, and enhanced bone regeneration. Furthermore, its surface promotes the proliferation and differentiation of the human bone mesenchymal stem cells, increased alkaline phosphatase activity, and upregulated expression of bone-specific genes.

In their in vivo tissue response study, Radenković et al. [31] compared a commercially available cross-linked porcine sugar membrane with two non-cross-linked collagen membranes. They concluded that all membranes lead to similar bone formation, but the cross-linked membrane is more stable and resorbs more slowly up to 60 days after implantation. In research recently publicized regarding an in vivo model which compares a novel membrane based on bovine dermis collagen with two commercially available alternatives, the authors found no difference between the proposed product regarding its biocompatibility [32]. Comparably, another study on calvaria's critically sized defects revealed that collagen porcine membranes promote new bone formation when compared to a negative control [33].

Strnková et al. [34] evaluated the tensile behavior of different eggshell membranes (hen, goose, and Japanese quail) and revealed that they express linear and non-linear tensile deformation. Also, the parameters increased with the loading rate, with the smallest values being measured for the quail eggs and the highest for the goose eggs. Moreover, the structure relationship of the eggshell membrane has been proven that it behaves both as Mooney–Rivlin and Hookean materials in different environmental conditions. As a result, it can stretch and restore its position, or it can have a nonlinear behavior akin to rubber [35,36].

Because of the AFM investigation, both membranes revealed significant structural and topographical differences. Nevertheless, the eggshell membrane is rougher than that of the porcine pericardium membrane due to the interpenetration of collagen types I and V bonded together with rounded glycoprotein structure while Jason membrane is synthetically textured by size-controlled collagen type I fibers of about 160 nm diameter.

Also, the microstructural aspect indicates that porcine pericardium membrane has a constant mechanical behavior under tensile strength testing due to the very well interlaced collagen fascicles. Another point is that the eggshell membrane cohesion strongly depends on the glycoprotein structure, assuring collagen network binding, whereas, in a wet state, it might exhibit significant tensile strength which might strongly decrease after glycoprotein drying because of cohesion becoming fragile.

In particular, tensile strength membranes can be influenced by a number of factors: origin of the material, processing methods, and crosslinking. Significantly, glutaraldehyde treatment of the membrane has been shown to enhance its proprieties, reduce the resorption time, and increase tensile strength [37]. Raz et al. [38], in a mechanical testing paper, examined three membranes and found comparable mechanical results as in our study: the dry state exhibited higher tensile strength values, and the denser the membrane the higher the output values.

Overall, the limitation factor for this study is the fact that it lacks a dynamic histologic and histomorphometry image of the soft and hard tissue reaction to the membrane for comparison. Also, a radiologic image could be of help to evaluate the potential of bone regeneration.

Above all, future research is needed to completely assess the membrane in an in vivo model with a bone defect. Also, investigation is needed regarding the crosslinking of the membrane, a process which might improve the mechanical and barrier functions. In addition, there could be a future perspective to research and perform an ultrastructural analysis using transmission electron microscopy.

5. Conclusions

The membrane does not determine a foreign body reaction. It can be used as an occlusive barrier but not as a separation membrane. It is a potential vehicle for other substances that may enhance its proprieties. Because it consists of collagen, it is highly biocompatible, resorbable, and biodegradable by the organism, and it does not induce a foreign body response.

Crosslinking may enhance the eggshell membranes proprieties to become a feasible, guided bone regeneration product. Further research is needed to better understand the processing needed to utilize this cheap and readily available biomaterial.

Author Contributions: Conceptualization, M.B. and G.B.; methodology, D.O.; software, G.A.; validation, F.G.O., S.B. and M.M.; formal analysis, S.C. and I.P.; investigation, I.P. and S.C.; resources, H.O.; data curation, H.O.; writing—original draft preparation, H.O. and D.O.; writing—review and editing, M.B. and D.O.; visualization, S.B.; supervision, G.B. and G.A.; project administration, F.G.O.; funding acquisition, M.B. All authors have read and agreed to the published version of the manuscript.

Funding: This work was granted by project PDI-PFE-CDI 2021, entitled Increasing the Performance of Scientific Research, Supporting Excellence in Medical Research and Innovation, PROGRES, no. 40PFE/30.12.2021 of Iuliu Hatieganu University of Medicine and Pharmacy, Cluj-Napoca, Romania which covered the APC.

Institutional Review Board Statement: The study was conducted in accordance with the Declaration of Helsinki and approved by the Institutional Ethics Committee of the University of Medicine and Pharmacy of Cluj-Napoca "Iuliu Hatieganu", Romania (number 220 from 9 June 2020).

Informed Consent Statement: Not applicable.

Data Availability Statement: Data sharing not applicable.

Conflicts of Interest: The authors declare no conflict of interest.

References

1. Omi, M.; Mishina, Y. Roles of Osteoclasts in Alveolar Bone Remodeling. *Genesis* **2022**, *60*, e23490. [CrossRef] [PubMed]
2. Urban, I.A.; Monje, A. Guided Bone Regeneration in Alveolar Bone Reconstruction. *Oral. Maxillofac. Surg. Clin. N. Am.* **2019**, *31*, 331–338. [CrossRef] [PubMed]
3. Zhao, X.; Zou, L.; Chen, Y.; Tang, Z. Staged Horizontal Bone Augmentation for Dental Implants in Aesthetic Zones: A Prospective Randomized Controlled Clinical Trial Comparing a Half-Columnar Bone Block Harvested from the Ramus versus a Rectangular Bone Block from the Symphysis. *Int. J. Oral. Maxillofac. Surg.* **2020**, *49*, 1326–1334. [CrossRef] [PubMed]
4. Arjunan, A.; Baroutaji, A.; Robinson, J.; Praveen, A.S.; Pollard, A.; Wang, C. Future Directions and Requirements for Tissue Engineering Biomaterials. *Encycl. Smart Mater.* **2022**, *1*, 195–218. [CrossRef]
5. Elgali, I.; Omar, O.; Dahlin, C.; Thomsen, P. Guided Bone Regeneration: Materials and Biological Mechanisms Revisited. *Eur. J. Oral. Sci.* **2017**, *125*, 315–337. [CrossRef]
6. Sbricoli, L.; Guazzo, R.; Annunziata, M.; Gobbato, L.; Bressan, E.; Nastri, L. Selection of Collagen Membranes for Bone Regeneration: A Literature Review. *Materials* **2020**, *13*, 786. [CrossRef]
7. Ren, Y.; Fan, L.; Alkildani, S.; Liu, L.; Emmert, S.; Najman, S.; Rimashevskiy, D.; Schnettler, R.; Jung, O.; Xiong, X.; et al. Barrier Membranes for Guided Bone Regeneration (GBR): A Focus on Recent Advances in Collagen Membranes. *Int. J. Mol. Sci.* **2022**, *23*, 14987. [CrossRef]
8. Soldatos, N.K.; Stylianou, P.; Koidou, P.; Angelov, N.; Yukna, R.; Romanos, G.E. Limitations and Options Using Resorbable versus Nonresorbable Membranes for Successful Guided Bone Regeneration. *Quintessence Int.* **2017**, *48*, 131–147. [CrossRef]
9. Bianchi, S.; Bernardi, S.; Simeone, D.; Torge, D.; Macchiarelli, G.; Marchetti, E. Proliferation and Morphological Assessment of Human Periodontal Ligament Fibroblast towards Bovine Pericardium Membranes: An In Vitro Study. *Materials* **2022**, *15*, 8284. [CrossRef]
10. Chu, C.; Deng, J.; Man, Y.; Qu, Y. Evaluation of Nanohydroxyapatite (Nano-HA) Coated Epigallocatechin-3-Gallate (EGCG) Cross-Linked Collagen Membranes. *Mater. Sci. Eng. C* **2017**, *78*, 258–264. [CrossRef]
11. Park, J.Y.; Yang, C.; Jung, I.H.; Lim, H.C.; Lee, J.S.; Jung, U.W.; Seo, Y.K.; Park, J.K.; Choi, S.H. Regeneration of Rabbit Calvarial Defects Using Cells-Implanted Nano-Hydroxyapatite Coated Silk Scaffolds. *Biomater. Res.* **2015**, *19*, 7. [CrossRef]
12. Kubosch, E.J.; Bernstein, A.; Wolf, L.; Fretwurst, T.; Nelson, K.; Schmal, H. Clinical Trial and In-Vitro Study Comparing the Efficacy of Treating Bony Lesions with Allografts versus Synthetic or Highly-Processed Xenogeneic Bone Grafts. *BMC Musculoskelet. Disord.* **2016**, *17*, 1–17. [CrossRef]
13. Ratiu, C.; Brocks, M.; Costea, T.; Moldovan, L.; Cavalu, S. PRGF-Modified Collagen Membranes for Guided Bone Regeneration: Spectroscopic, Microscopic and Nano-Mechanical Investigations. *Appl. Sci.* **2019**, *9*, 1035. [CrossRef]
14. Augustine, R.; Hasan, A.; Primavera, R.; Wilson, R.J.; Thakor, A.S.; Kevadiya, B.D. Cellular Uptake and Retention of Nanoparticles: Insights on Particle Properties and Interaction with Cellular Components. *Mater. Today Commun.* **2020**, *25*, 101692. [CrossRef]
15. Mantha, S.; Pillai, S.; Khayambashi, P.; Upadhyay, A.; Zhang, Y.; Tao, O.; Pham, H.M.; Tran, S.D. Smart Hydrogels in Tissue Engineering and Regenerative Medicine. *Materials* **2019**, *12*, 3323. [CrossRef]
16. Gabrielson, K.; Maronpot, R.; Monette, S.; Mlynarczyk, C.; Ramot, Y.; Nyska, A.; Sysa-Shah, P. In Vivo Imaging with Confirmation by Histopathology for Increased Rigor and Reproducibility in Translational Research: A Review of Examples, Options, and Resources. *ILAR J.* **2018**, *59*, 80. [CrossRef]
17. Álvarez-Ortega, O.; Ruiz-Ramírez, L.R.; Garibay-Alvarado, J.A.; Donohue-Cornejo, A.; Espinosa-Cristóbal, L.F.; Cuevas-González, J.C.; Reyes-López, S.Y. Preliminary Biocompatibility Tests of Poly-ε-Caprolactone/Silver Nanofibers in Wistar Rats. *Polymers* **2021**, *13*, 1135. [CrossRef]
18. Opris, H.; Bran, S.; Dinu, C.; Baciut, M.; Prodan, D.A.; Mester, A.; Baciut, G. Clinical Applications of Avian Eggshell-Derived Hydroxyapatite. *Bosn. J. Basic Med. Sci.* **2020**, *20*, 430–437. [CrossRef]
19. Opris, H.; Dinu, C.; Baciut, M.; Baciut, G.; Mitre, I.; Crisan, B.; Armencea, G.; Prodan, D.A.; Bran, S. The Influence of Eggshell on Bone Regeneration in Preclinical In Vivo Studies. *Biology* **2020**, *9*, 476. [CrossRef]
20. Tisler, C.E.; Moldovan, M.; Petean, I.; Buduru, S.D.; Prodan, D.; Sarosi, C.; Leucuţa, D.-C.; Chifor, R.; Badea, M.E.; Ene, R. Human Enamel Fluorination Enhancement by Photodynamic Laser Treatment. *Polymers* **2022**, *14*, 2969. [CrossRef]
21. Iosif, C.; Cuc, S.; Prodan, D.; Moldovan, M.; Petean, I.; Badea, M.E.; Sava, S.; Tonea, A.; Chifor, R. Effects of Acidic Environments on Dental Structures after Bracket Debonding. *Int. J. Mol. Sci.* **2022**, *23*, 15583. [CrossRef] [PubMed]

22. Rothamel, D.; Schwarz, F.; Fienitz, T.; Smeets, R.; Dreiseidler, T.; Ritter, L.; Happe, A.; Zöller, J. Biocompatibility and Biodegradation of a Native Porcine Pericardium Membrane: Results of in Vitro and in Vivo Examinations. *Int. J. Oral. Maxillofac. Implants* **2012**, *27*, 146–154.
23. Chatelet, M.; Afota, F.; Savoldelli, C. Review of Bone Graft and Implant Survival Rate: A Comparison between Autogenous Bone Block versus Guided Bone Regeneration. *J. Stomatol. Oral. Maxillofac. Surg.* **2022**, *123*, 222–227. [CrossRef]
24. Araújo, M.G.; Silva, C.O.; Misawa, M.; Sukekava, F. Alveolar Socket Healing: What Can We Learn? *Periodontology* **2000**, *2015*, 68. [CrossRef]
25. Couso-Queiruga, E.; Weber, H.A.; Garaicoa-Pazmino, C.; Barwacz, C.; Kalleme, M.; Galindo-Moreno, P.; Avila-Ortiz, G. Influence of Healing Time on the Outcomes of Alveolar Ridge Preservation Using a Collagenated Bovine Bone Xenograft: A Randomized Clinical Trial. *J. Clin. Periodontol.* **2023**, *50*, 132–146. [CrossRef] [PubMed]
26. Chen, H.; Gu, T.; Lai, H.; Gu, X. Evaluation of Hard Tissue 3-Dimensional Stability around Single Implants Placed with Guided Bone Regeneration in the Anterior Maxilla: A 3-Year Retrospective Study. *J. Prosthet. Dent.* **2022**, *128*, 919–927. [CrossRef]
27. Li, S.; Zhao, J.; Xie, Y.; Tian, T.; Zhang, T.; Cai, X. Hard Tissue Stability after Guided Bone Regeneration: A Comparison between Digital Titanium Mesh and Resorbable Membrane. *Int. J. Oral. Sci.* **2021**, *13*, 1–9. [CrossRef]
28. Jiang, X.; Zhang, Y.; Di, P.; Lin, Y. Hard Tissue Volume Stability of Guided Bone Regeneration during the Healing Stage in the Anterior Maxilla: A Clinical and Radiographic Study. *Clin. Implant Dent. Relat. Res.* **2018**, *20*, 68–75. [CrossRef] [PubMed]
29. Bornert, F.; Herber, V.; Sandgren, R.; Witek, L.; Coelho, P.G.; Pippenger, B.E.; Shahdad, S. Comparative Barrier Membrane Degradation over Time: Pericardium versus Dermal Membranes. *Clin. Exp. Dent. Res.* **2021**, *7*, 711–718. [CrossRef]
30. You, P.; Liu, Y.; Wang, X.; Li, B.; Wu, W.; Tang, L. Acellular Pericardium: A Naturally Hierarchical, Osteoconductive, and Osteoinductive Biomaterial for Guided Bone Regeneration. *J. Biomed. Mater. Res. A* **2021**, *109*, 132–145. [CrossRef]
31. Radenković, M.; Alkildani, S.; Stoewe, I.; Bielenstein, J.; Sundag, B.; Bellmann, O.; Jung, O.; Najman, S.; Stojanović, S.; Barbeck, M. Comparative in Vivo Analysis of the Integration Behavior and Immune Response of Collagen-Based Dental Barrier Membranes for Guided Bone Regeneration (Gbr). *Membranes* **2021**, *11*, 712. [CrossRef] [PubMed]
32. Lindner, C.; Alkildani, S.; Stojanovic, S.; Najman, S.; Jung, O.; Barbeck, M. In Vivo Biocompatibility Analysis of a Novel Barrier Membrane Based on Bovine Dermis-Derived Collagen for Guided Bone Regeneration (GBR). *Membranes* **2022**, *12*, 378. [CrossRef] [PubMed]
33. Danieletto-Zanna, C.F.; Bizelli, V.F.; Ramires, G.A.D.A.; Francatti, T.M.; De Carvalho, P.S.P.; Bassi, A.P.F. Osteopromotion Capacity of Bovine Cortical Membranes in Critical Defects of Rat Calvaria: Histological and Immunohistochemical Analysis. *Int. J. Biomater.* **2020**, *2020*, 1–9. [CrossRef] [PubMed]
34. Strnková, J.; Nedomová, Š.; Kumbár, V.; Trnka, J. Tensile Strength of the Eggshell Membranes. *Acta Univ. Agric. Silvic. Mendel. Brun.* **2016**, *64*, 159–164. [CrossRef]
35. Torres, F.G.; Troncoso, O.P.; Piaggio, F.; Hijar, A. Structure-Property Relationships of a Biopolymer Network: The Eggshell Membrane. *Acta Biomater.* **2010**, *6*, 3687–3693. [CrossRef] [PubMed]
36. Strnková, M.; Nedomová, Š.; Trnka, J.; Buchar, J.; Kumbár, V. Behaviour of Eggshell Membranes at Tensile Loading. *Bulg. Chem. Commun.* **2014**, *46*, 44–48.
37. García Páez, J.M.; Jorge-Herrero, E.; Carrera, A.; Millán, I.; Rocha, A.; Calero, P.; Cordón, A.; Salvador, J.; Sainz, N.; Méndez, J.; et al. Chemical Treatment and Tissue Selection: Factors That Influence the Mechanical Behaviour of Porcine Pericardium. *Biomaterials* **2001**, *22*, 2759–2767. [CrossRef]
38. Raz, P.; Brosh, T.; Ronen, G.; Tal, H. Tensile Properties of Three Selected Collagen Membranes. *Biomed. Res. Int.* **2019**, *2019*, 1–8. [CrossRef]

Disclaimer/Publisher's Note: The statements, opinions and data contained in all publications are solely those of the individual author(s) and contributor(s) and not of MDPI and/or the editor(s). MDPI and/or the editor(s) disclaim responsibility for any injury to people or property resulting from any ideas, methods, instructions or products referred to in the content.

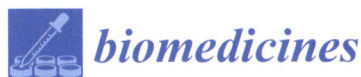

Article

The Effect of Three Desensitizing Toothpastes on Dentinal Tubules Occlusion and on Dentin Hardness

Emilia Bologa [1], Simona Stoleriu [1,*], Irina Nica [1], Ionuț Tărăboanță [1], Andrei Georgescu [1], Ruxandra Ilinca Matei [2,*] and Sorin Andrian [1]

[1] Faculty of Dental Medicine, "Grigore T. Popa" University of Medicine and Pharmacy, 16 Universitatii Str., 700115 Iași, Romania; bologa.emilia@umfiasi.ro (E.B.); nica.irina@umfiasi.ro (I.N.); ionut-taraboanta@umfiasi.ro (I.T.); andrei.georgescu@umfiasi.ro (A.G.); sorin.andrian@umfiasi.ro (S.A.)

[2] Faculty of Medicine and Pharmacy, University of Oradea, 1st December Sq., 410068 Oradea, Romania

* Correspondence: simona.stoleriu@umfiasi.ro (S.S.); dr.ruxandramatei@gmail.com (R.I.M.)

Abstract: There are two main methods used for dentin hypersensitivity (DH) treatment: dentinal tubule occlusion and blockage of nerve activity. Dentifrices are the most common vehicles for active ingredients used for DH treatment. The aim of this study was to evaluate the efficacy of three toothpastes on dentinal tubule occlusion, mineral acquisition, and dentin hardness. Forty human dentin disks were submerged in 40% citric acid for 30 s and then exposed to tooth brushing for 2 min twice a day for 14 days using three toothpastes: Dontodent Sensitive (group 1), Dr. Wolff's Biorepair (group 2), and Sensodyne Repair and Protect (group 3). In the control group (group 4), the samples were brushed with water. All of the samples were evaluated using scanning electron microscopy (SEM), energy-dispersive X-ray (EDX), and Vickers dentin hardness determination. On SEM images, the degree of dentinal tubule occlusion was assessed using a five-grade scale. The mean score values in groups 1–4 were 3.60 ± 0.69, 2.20 ± 0.91, 2.30 ± 1.16, and 5.00 ± 0.00, significantly higher in study groups when compared to the control group (Kruskal Wallis test $p < 0.05$). EDX evaluation showed significantly higher calcium and phosphorus concentrations in groups 1 and 3 when compared to control group d. The mean values of Vickers dentin hardness numbers in groups 1–4 were 243.03 ± 10.014, 327.38 ± 56.65, 260.29 ± 37.69, and 225.83 ± 29.93, respectively. No statistically significant results were obtained when comparing the hardness mean values in groups (Kruskal-Wallis statistical test, $p = 0.372 > 0.05$). All three toothpastes tested demonstrated significant occlusion of dentinal tubules. Dontodent Sensitive and Sensodyne Repair and Protect toothpastes enhanced the calcium and phosphorus content of the dentin surface. None of the toothpastes increased dentin hardness as a result of mineral acquisition.

Keywords: dentin hypersensitivity; dentin hardness; desensitizing agent; EDX; nanohydroxyapatite; SEM; zinc-nanohydroxyapatite

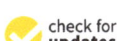

Citation: Bologa, E.; Stoleriu, S.; Nica, I.; Tărăboanță, I.; Georgescu, A.; Matei, R.I.; Andrian, S. The Effect of Three Desensitizing Toothpastes on Dentinal Tubules Occlusion and on Dentin Hardness. *Biomedicines* **2023**, *11*, 2464. https://doi.org/10.3390/biomedicines11092464

Academic Editors: Giuseppe Minervini and Gianmarco Abbadessa

Received: 30 July 2023
Revised: 26 August 2023
Accepted: 1 September 2023
Published: 5 September 2023

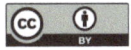

Copyright: © 2023 by the authors. Licensee MDPI, Basel, Switzerland. This article is an open access article distributed under the terms and conditions of the Creative Commons Attribution (CC BY) license (https://creativecommons.org/licenses/by/4.0/).

1. Introduction

Two conditions are mandatory for dentin hypersensitivity (DH) to occur: the dentinal tubules should be exposed into the oral cavity, and the dentinal tubules should be opened toward the pulp and toward the oral cavity [1]. Many factors are involved in DH etiology. Cervical or root dentin exposure can be a result of hard or soft tissue loss (enamel wear, gingival recession, and cementum loss) [2,3]. Dentin exposure as a result of enamel wear can frequently be determined by the association of erosive wear with abrasion, attrition, and abfraction [1,4,5]. The natural smear layer that results after dentin exposure in the absence of any acidic aggression is very stable in oral conditions and closes the dentinal tubules, preventing the occurrence of DH [6]. The exposed dentin is sensitive only if the smear layer is removed and the dentinal tubules are open [5,7]. Today, it is considered that erosion initiates the process of dentinal tubules opening, which is then amplified by abrasion, attrition, or abfraction [1,8,9]. Most frequently, root dentin exposure is caused by gingival recession and is associated with DH [10]. In gingival recession, the retraction of the gingival margin apically at the enamel-cementum junction determines coronal cementum exposure at the beginning and apical cementum exposure in more advanced cases [11]. Coronal cementum is a very thin layer (16–60 μm) that can easily be removed by tooth wear or periodontal treatment, exposing the dentin layer directly to the oral cavity [12]. Frequently, gingival recession is caused by toothbrushing, occlusal loading, periodontal disease, or periodontal treatment [13,14]; the most important risk factors are a thin periodontal biotype, the absence of attached gingiva, or a thin alveolar cortical shell [15].

There are two main methods used for DH treatment: dentinal tubule occlusion and blockage of nerve activity. Sealing of the dentin surface in occlusive therapy decreases the movement of fluid inside the tubules and reduces the DH [16]. Nerve desensitization is obtained by chemical agents that suppress or modify nerve polarization. The procedures used in DH treatment can be applied at home or in the office. In non-invasive at-home procedures, the patients apply the active ingredients by using toothpastes, mouthwashes, gels, or chewing gum. In-office therapy includes non-invasive procedures like gels, foams, vanishes, dentinal adhesive application, iontophoresis, microinvasive procedures like laser therapy, and restorative methods using composite resin or glass ionomer cements [14,17]. The products used at home are available for the treatment immediately, come at a small price, and can be self-administered. In DH associated with gingival recession, non-invasive treatment is first recommended, and then, if indicated, periodontal surgical procedures are performed.

Dentifrices are the most common vehicles for active ingredients used for DH treatment. They are preferred because of their small price, ease of use, and home application. Active ingredients such as strontium chloride, potassium nitrate, dibasic sodium citrate, formaldehyde, sodium fluoride, sodium monofluorphosphate, and stannous fluoride are included in a complex composition [18–21]. The application of fluorides seems to create a barrier by precipitating calcium fluoride crystals, which are formed especially in the inlet of the dentinal tubules. The precipitate is slowly soluble in saliva, which may explain the transitory action of this barrier [22]. Abrasive components of the dentifrices like calcium phosphate, calcium carbonate, silicate, or aluminum can determine dentin tubule obliteration by precipitation or by smear layer formation during brushing [19,20]. The multitude of products for DH treatment on the market indicates that we are far from reaching the ideal product. Choosing the method and the product for DH treatment remains the doctor's option based on their personal experience, preferences, and knowledge.

The aims of the present study were to compare the efficacy of three commercial desensitizing toothpastes on dentinal tubule occlusion by scanning electron microscopy (SEM) evaluation of dentin mineral deposition by energy-dispersive X-ray (EDX) analysis and by dentin hardness determination. The null hypothesis was that there is no difference in tubule occlusion, mineral acquisition, or dentin hardness when the selected dentifrices were used.

2. Materials and Methods

The study design is presented in Figure 1. Details of each study step are described below.

2.1. Teeth Collection and Sample Preparation

The sample size was calculated using G*Power software (version 3.1.9.7., Heinrich Heine-Universität Düsseldorf, Düsseldorf, Germany). It was used with an effect size of 0.90, an alpha value of 0.05, and a power of 95%. The results estimated a total number of 40 required samples.

Twenty extracted human permanent third molars were used for this study. In order to be included in the study, the teeth should have a complete crown and present no caries, wear, cracks, or fillings. After removing soft tissues, the teeth were stored in distilled water containing 0.2% thymol until the beginning of the study [23].

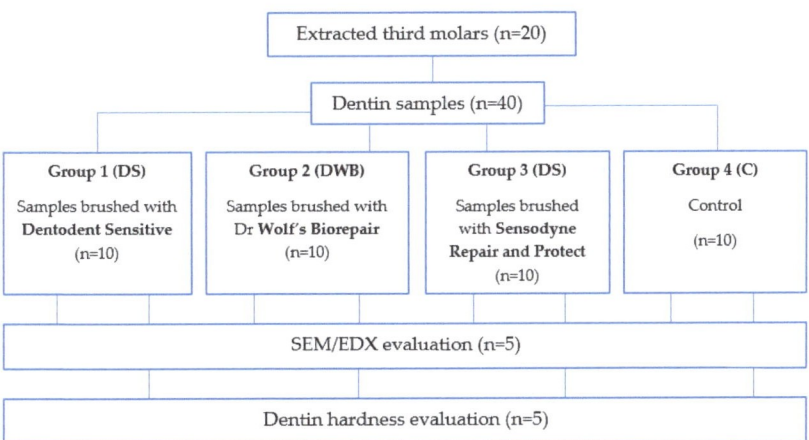

Figure 1. Study design.

For every tooth, the crown was separated from the root using a diamond disc (NTI-Kahla GmbH, Kahla, Germany) at 5000 rpm under abundant cooling water. The tooth crowns were then embedded in self-curing acrylic resin blocks (Duracryl Plus, Spofa Dental, Jičín, Czech Republic). Then, from the middle part of each crown, two dentin discs with a thickness of 1 mm were obtained by cutting the tooth perpendicular to the long axis with a diamond disc at slow speed. All the dentin sections were then polished using 600-grit silicon carbide abrasive papers for 20 s to create a uniform smear layer. To simulate the sensitive tooth model and to open the dentinal tubules, all the dentin blocks were submerged for 30 s in 40% citric acid (Cerkamed, Stalowa Wola, Poland). After that, the sections were rinsed with distilled water and introduced into an ultrasonic bath for 10 min. The resulting specimens were randomly and equally distributed into four groups. In study groups 1–3, three commercial desensitizing toothpastes were applied by brushing on dentin sample. In control group 4, the sections were brushed with water. The three toothpastes selected to be tested in the study groups were Dontodent Sensitive (DS) group 1, Dr. Wolff's Biorepair (Dr. Kurt Wolff GmbH & Co. KG, Bielefeld, Germany) group 2 (DWB), and Sensodyne Repair, and Protect (GlaxoSmithKline, Brentford, Middlesex, UK) group 3 (SRP). The brand name, manufacturer name, and chemical composition of the tested toothpastes are presented in Table 1.

Table 1. Brand name, manufacturer and chemical composition of the tested toothpastes.

Materials' Brand Name	Manufacturer	Composition
Dontodent Sensitive	DM Drogeria Markt, Karlsruhe, Germany	Hydroxyapatite, Sodium Fluoride, Tetrapotassium pyrophosphate, Aqua, Sorbitol, Propylene Glycol, Glycerin, Silica, Aroma, Cellulose Gum, Sodium C14–16 Olefin Sulfonate, Sodium Cocoyl Isethionate, Sodium Saccharin, Menthol, Eucalyptol, Limonene, CI 77891
Dr. Wolff's Biorepair	Dr. Kurt Wolff GmbH & Co. KG, Bielefeld, Germany	Zinc Hydroxyapatite, Aqua, Hydrated Silica, Glycerin, Sorbitol, Silica, Aroma, Cellulose Gum, Sodium Myristoyl Sarcosinate, Sodium Methyl Cocoyl Taurate, Tetrapotassium Pyrophosphate, Zinc Pca, Sodium Saccharin, Phenoxyethanol, Benzyl Alcohol, Propylparaben, Methylparaben, Citric Acid, Sodium Benzoate.
Sensodyne Repair and Protect	GlaxoSmithKline, Brentford, Middlesex, UK	Calcium sodium phosphosilicate, Stannous fluoride, Glycerin, PEG-8, hydrated silica, pentasodium triphosphate, sodium lauryl sulfate, flavour, titanium dioxide, polyacrylic acid, cocamidopropyl betaine, sodium saccharin

Toothpaste slurries were prepared by mixing water and toothpaste (2:1 by volume) [24]. The slurries were applied on the surface of dentin disks using a brushing machine that operates with back-and-forth movement with an amplitude of 30 mm (15 mm in each direction), a frequency of 60 cycles/minute at 1.5 Hz, and a 250 g vertical load. The application protocol was also described in a previous study [16]. The samples were brushed for 2 min twice a day for 14 days using medium-hardness bristle toothbrushes (Classic Deep Clean, Colgate-Palmolive Company, New York, NY, USA), which were changed after each brushing. After tooth brushing sessions, all the samples were rinsed under abundant deionized water and stored in artificial saliva (AFNOR NF S90–701) until the next brushing procedure. The last tooth brushing session was followed by rinsing the samples with deionized water and air drying.

2.2. Dentinal Tubules Occlusion by SEM Evaluation

Five samples from each group were morphologically evaluated using a scanning electron microscope (Vega Tescan LMH II, Tescan, Brno, Czech Republic), which operates at 30 kV and 15.5 WD. Ten photomicrographs of every sample were taken under 2000× magnification to evaluate the occlusion of the dentinal tubules. Two examiners, blinded to the protocol, independently evaluated the photomicrographs and assessed the dentinal tubules occlusion according to a scoring system with five grades: score 1 = occluded (100% of tubules occluded); score 2 = mostly occluded (50 to less than 100% of tubules occluded); score 3 = partially occluded (25 to less than 50% of tubules occluded); score 4 = mostly unoccluded (25 to less than 50% of tubules occluded); score 5 = unoccluded (0%, no tubule occlusion) [25]. In cases of disagreement on scoring, both examiners re-evaluated the specific image until they came to an agreement. For each sample, the final score of dentinal tubule occlusion was the average of the registered scores after ten images were evaluated.

2.3. Mineral Evaluation by Energy-Dispersive X-ray (EDX) Analysis

The samples evaluated using SEM were also analysed by X-ray dispersive spectroscopy. A Quantax QX2 (Bruker/Roentec, Berlin, Germany) detector was used for chemical element determination. A qualitative evaluation of the chemical elements on a selected area was performed using a P/B-ZAF database. Quantitative determination of ion concentrations (wt%) were performed in ten different areas of each dentin sample. For every sample, the ion concentrations were reported as the average value of ten determinations.

2.4. Dentin Hardness Evaluation

Five dentin samples from each group were submitted to surface hardness evaluation using a tribometer (CETR UMT-2, Bruker Corporation, Berlin, Germany). A Vickers-type indenter having a diamond cone with an angle of 120° and a tip with a radius of 200 μm was used for the microindentation test. The following parameters were used to obtain the indentations: a vertical force of 5 N, a speed of 0.005 mm/s, a preload time of 15 s, a charging time of 30 s, a holding time of 15 s, and a download time of 30 s. Surface hardness was automatically calculated by the software (Tribometer CETR UMT-2, Version 1.01 software, Bruker Corporation, Berlin, Germany) from the discharge slope curve and expressed in GPa.

2.5. Statistical Analysis

SPSS 27.0 software (SPSS Inc., Chicago, IL, USA) was used for statistical analysis. The Kolmogorov-Smirnov normality test and the non-parametric Kruskal-Wallis test were used to compare the mean scores of dentinal tubule occlusion and dentin hardness among groups. A value of 0.05 was set as a statistically significant level.

3. Results

3.1. SEM Evaluation Results

Examples of the dentin surface morphological aspects of some samples in the control and study groups are presented in Figure 2. Surface analysis of dentin samples revealed a rare area of mineral precipitation on intertubular dentin but obvious mineral deposits on tubule openings. SEM micrographs showed different degrees of dentinal tubules in groups. In group 1, the majority of the samples were evaluated with a score of 4 (70%), followed in descending order by the samples scored with 3 (20%) and the samples scored with 2 (10%). In this group, there was no sample evaluated with a score of 1 and 5. In group 2, the highest percentage of samples was scored with 2 (50%), followed by the samples scored with 1 and 3 (20%), and the samples scored with 4 (10%). No sample with a score of 5 was registered in this group. In group 3, a more homogenous distribution of scores was recorded: 20% of the samples were evaluated with scores 3 and 4, and 30% of the samples were evaluated with scores 1 and 2. There was no sample scoring 5 in this group. In group 4, all the samples were evaluated with a score of 5.

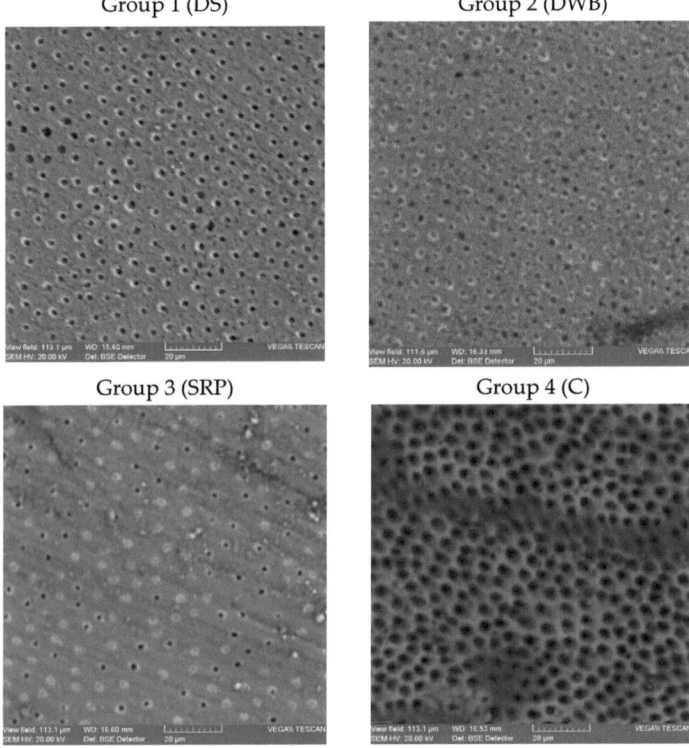

Figure 2. SEM micrographs of dentin samples in control and study groups. SEM micrographs of dentin samples in study groups (1–3) and control (4) at ×2000 magnification; DS—Dentodent Sensitive toothpaste; DWB—Dr. Wolff's Biorepair toothpaste; SRP—Sensodyne Repair and Protect toothpaste; C—control, no toothpaste.

The mean values of tubule occlusion in the study and control groups are presented in Table 2. Significantly lower mean score values were registered in the study groups when compared to the control (Table 3).

Table 2. The scores of dentinal tubule occlusion in control and study groups (mean value ± standard deviation).

	Group 1	Group 2	Group 3	Group 4
Mean score value ± SD	3.60 ± 0.69	2.20 ± 0.91	2.30 ± 1.16	5.00 ± 0.00

Table 3. Kruskal-Wallis test result of comparison of the mean values of dentinal tubule occlusion in control and study groups.

Group	Compared With	Standard Error	Significance
Group 1 (DS)	Group 2 (DWB)	5.103	0.216
	Group 3 (SRP)	5.103	0.321
	Group 4 (C)	5.103	0.048
Group 2 (DWB)	Group 3 (SRP)	5.103	1.000
	Group 4 (C)	5.103	0.000
Group 3 (SRP)	Group 4 (C)	5.103	0.000

DS—Dentodent Sensitive toothpaste; DWB—Dr. Wolff's Biorepair toothpaste; SRP—Sensodyne Repair and Protect toothpaste; C—control, no toothpaste.

3.2. Energy-Dispersive X-ray (EDX) Evaluation Results

EDX elemental analysis of the samples in groups showed the presence of carbon, oxygen, silicon, calcium, and phosphorus on the sample surface. In all groups, normalized weight percentages of oxygen were recorded, followed by calcium, carbon, and phosphorous (Table 4). A very low value of the ion weight percentage was registered in all study groups and in the control group. The fluorine ion was undetectable (mass concentration and normalized weight percent were lower than the values of absolute and relative error of detection). Carbon, silica, and oxygen ion concentrations were significantly lower in the control group when compared to all three study groups. Calcium and phosphorus ion concentrations were significantly higher in groups 1 and 3 when compared to the control group.

Table 4. Ion concentrations (wt%) in control and study groups (mean values ± standard deviation).

	Mean Value of Ion Concentration (wt%) ± Standard Deviation			
Ion	Group 1	Group 2	Group 3	Group 4
Calcium	23.657 ± 5.016 [A]	20.352 ± 7.373 [C]	24.608 ± 3.738 [A]	17.417 ± 2.381 [B]
Phosphorous	13.320 ± 3.323 [A]	11.351 ± 4.979 [C]	13.202 ± 2.910 [A]	8.983 ± 1.919 [B]
Carbon	14.135 ± 6.920 [A]	16.456 ± 9.109 [A]	11.910 ± 7.410 [A]	35.212 ± 3.712 [B]
Oxygen	46.057 ± 1.502 [A]	48.137 ± 4.631 [A]	47.581 ± 2.894 [A]	38.089 ± 2.040 [B]
Silicon	2.828 ± 0.838 [A]	3.702 ± 1.945 [A]	2.696 ± 0.980 [A]	0.296 ± 0.200 [B]

The same capital letter in rows represent no statistically significant differences among groups (ANOVA test, $p > 0.05$, post hoc LSD test, $p > 0.05$).

3.3. Dentin Hardness Test Results

The mean values of dentin surface hardness in the control and study groups are presented in Table 5. No statistically significant results were obtained when comparing the hardness values among groups (Kruskal-Wallis Chi-Square = 0.186, $p = 0.980 > 0.05$).

Table 5. Dentin hardness (GPa) in control and study groups (mean values ± standard deviation).

	Group 1	Group 2	Group 3	Group 4
Mean hardness value ± SD	243.033 ± 100.147 [A]	327.382 ± 376.653 [A]	260.299 ± 157.697 [A]	225.803 ± 89.934 [A]

The same capital letter represents no statistically significant differences among groups (Kruskal-Wallis test, $p > 0.05$).

4. Discussion

In this study, we evaluated dentinal tubule occlusion by mineral deposition on the dentin surface and the changes in dentin surface hardness after using some commercial desensitizing toothpastes. All the tested toothpastes determined significant occlusion of dentinal tubules, so the null hypothesis was rejected. An efficient toothpaste used in DH treatment should present a high capacity for dentinal tubule occlusion and a good performance during intraoral acidic attacks [26]. In a systematic review of the literature, after analyzing 35 in vitro studies, Behzadi et al. concluded that desensitizing products based on bioactive glass and n-HAP are very efficient in dentin tubule occlusion [27]. Sodium calcium phosphosilicate bioactive glass (NovaMin® technology) in Sensodyne Repair and Protect toothpaste serves as a reservoir for calcium and phosphate ions, resembling biological apatite [28,29]. In the toothpaste, calcium, phosphate, sodium, and silica dioxyde ions are included in an amorphous matrix [29]. When the product comes into contact with an aqueous environment (water or saliva), sodium ions will be released. That will cause the pH to increase, which in turn will favor a fast precipitation of calcium and phosphate ions in the form of a hydroxyapatite layer. Previous studies have demonstrated that this protective layer of amorphous calcium phosphate is formed one hour after contact with a simple buffer solution [30]. By scanning electron microscopy evaluation, it was concluded that bioglass determines apatite layer formation, which can occlude the dentinal tubules [31]. NovaMin® technology, like pure n-Hap or Zn/n-HAP, also acts by plugging formation in dentinal tubules. The bioactive glass particles attach to the dentin-exposed collagen fibers, forming a sealant layer that continuously releases calcium and phosphate ions [32]. Other studies have mentioned that an important advantage of bioactive glasses when compared to n-Hap or Zn/n-HAP is the potential to initiate cellular migration and pulp stem cell proliferation and differentiation, which will stimulate reparative dentin formation [27]. In vitro studies have shown that NovaMin® in a concentration that exceeds 3% can block at least 75% of the opened dentinal tubules after just one application and can resist frequent acidic challenges [30]. High potential for dentinal tubule occlusion of desensitizing toothpastes based on 1% n-HAP and NovaMin® technology was also reported in the study of Kulal et al. (percentage of dentin tubule occlusion of 97.62% and 81.9%, respectively) [28]. Shah et al. also found an increased capacity of dentinal tubule occlusion (95.58%) when testing SHY-NM toothpaste based on NovaMin® technology [33]. When compared to stanium fluoride, NovaMin® products can lead to protective layer formation, despite the fact that both determine dentinal tubule occlusion [32]. Mahmoodi et al.'s transversal dentin section analysis revealed occlusive deposit formation on the dentin surface and inside the dentin tubules at different depths when stanium fluoride and NovaMin® desensitizing toothpastes were used, but only the NovaMin® product determined significant tubule occlusion by this protective layer formation inside the tubules.

Decreased dentin permeability was reported in the study of Wang et al. after 24 h of immersion in saliva when a product based on NovaMin® technology was applied. After the acidic attack, a reduction in the deposits formed inside the dentinal tubules was observed, but the crystals were still present. After a prolonged period of bathing in artificial saliva, the dentin surface morphology changed, and a homogenous layer that completely sealed the dentinal tubules formed [26].

In our study, Dr. Wolff's Biorepair toothpaste (active ingredient Zn/n-HAP) determined similar dentinal tubule occlusion to Sensodyne Repair and Protect toothpaste (based on NovaMin® technology) and Dentodent Sensitive toothpaste (active ingredient n-HAP).

In a clinical study, Gopinath et al. also demonstrated that n-HAP toothpaste had the same efficiency in DH reduction as toothpaste based on NovaMin® technology [34]. The results of our study are also in agreement with the study of Poggio et al., which evaluated the capacity of desensitizing toothpastes to prevent dental erosion caused by an acidic beverage and demonstrated that Biorepair Plus-Total Protection (active ingredient Zn substituted n-HAP-MicroRepair® technology) and Sensodyne Repair and Protect (NovaMin® technology) presented high potential for dentinal tubule occlusion [35]. The same study demonstrated the remineralization capacity of both products, with the minerals being integrated into the collagen network after acidic attack.

In our study, all the tested toothpastes had the same efficacy on dentinal tubule occlusion. The same result was also reported by Arnold et al. after analyzing different desensitizing toothpastes [36]. On the contrary, other studies have concluded that n-HAP toothpaste (nanoXIM® technology) was significantly more efficient in dental tubule occlusion when compared to Sensodyne Repair & Protect toothpaste, with 66.13% of the tubules being occluded. Excellent results after seven days of using n-HAP toothpastes were also reported in Pei et al.'s study [37]. The higher efficiency of Dr. Wolff's Biorepair and Dontodent toothpastes in Pei's study when compared to the results of the present study can be explained by different experimental conditions (1% citric acid application for 20 s in Pei's study for dentin tubule occlusion). Lower concentrations and decreased time of acid action cause a reduced opening of the dentinal tubules and facilitate a more rapid and complete occlusion of the tubules when desensitizing toothpastes are applied.

Excluding calcium phosphosilicate, Sensodyne Repair and Protect toothpaste contains the active ingredient stannous fluoride. For many years, fluoride products were considered the gold standard in tooth remineralization and tooth protection against acidic attacks, but the action of fluorides in desensitizing DH is still unclear. In a review of the literature, Fiorillo L. et al. highlighted the effects of stannous fluoride compounds on dental hard tissues [38]. Previous studies demonstrated similar occlusion of dentinal tubules when using toothpastes containing 0.454% stannous fluoride and 0.76% sodium monofluorophosphate, but a greater degree of occlusion for stannous fluoride toothpaste after acidic attack [10]. Another toothpaste of the three tested products in our study, Dentodent Sensitive, has an active ingredient that is a fluoride compound (sodium fluoride). It was demonstrated that fluorides may increase the mineralization of hydroxyapatite [39] and may enhance hydroxyapatite crystal formation within the dentine tubules, which blocks dentinal fluid movement and reduces pain.

EDX analysis of the dentin surface showed increased carbon ion concentrations and decreased calcium and phosphorus ion concentrations in the control group. The dentin after desensitizing toothpaste application presented decreased carbon and increased calcium and phosphorus ion concentrations. These results confirm the hypothesis of calcium and phosphate ions being released from n-HAP and NovaMin® products. Calcium phosphate layer formation as a result of 5% and 7.5% NovaMin® product application has been reported in previous studies [40]. In this study, the increased calcium and phosphate ion concentrations on the dentin surface did not increase dentin hardness. Except the density of the mineral phase, there are other factors that can influence dentin hardness: the location, density, and direction of the dentinal tubules or the direction of the collagen fibers [41]. Other studies reported an increased dentin hardness when compared to demineralized and sound dentin after NovaMin® product application, but the research protocol was different [40].

One limitation of this study is the evaluation of dentinal tubule occlusion only by mineral deposition on the dentin surface assessment and not by the investigation of mineral penetration in tubule depth, which can allow conclusions regarding only the short-term efficacy of the products used for DH treatment. Another limitation is the use of a minimum number of dentin samples in the groups. In our study, dentin samples were obtained from the middle part of the tooth crown. There can be differences in dentinal tubule orientation and tubule diameter in this area when compared to cervical coronal or root dentin. Samples bathed in artificial saliva between toothbrushing sessions were free of acidic challenges.

Future long-term research and comparative clinical-based studies must be performed to certify the efficacy of using these products for pain relief and dentin mineralization.

5. Conclusions

Within the limitations of this in vitro study, the three tested toothpastes based on n-HAP, Zn/n-HAP, and NovaMin® technology determined the occlusion of dentinal tubules. When used twice a day for fourteen days, Dontodent Sensitive and Sensodyne Repair and Protect toothpastes increased the calcium and phosphorus ion content of the dentin surface. None of the toothpastes increased dentin surface hardness as a result of mineral (calcium and phosphate ions) acquisition. Due to their capacity for dentinal tubule blocking, the tested products can be efficiently used in immediate DH treatment.

Author Contributions: Conceptualization, E.B. and S.A.; methodology, E.B., S.S., I.N. and A.G.; software, I.T. and R.I.M.; validation, S.A. and S.S.; formal analysis, E.B. and I.N.; investigation, E.B., S.S., I.N. and I.T; resources, E.B., A.G. and I.T; writing—original draft preparation, S.S. and E.B.; writing—review and editing, S.A. and R.I.M.; visualization, I.N. and E.B.; supervision, S.A.; project administration, E.B., S.S. and S.A. All authors have read and agreed to the published version of the manuscript.

Funding: This research was co-funded by European Council- European Social Fund—Human Capital Operational Program, Project No: POCU/993/6/13/154722.

Institutional Review Board Statement: The research was conducted in accordance with the National Research Law 206/24.05.2004 and the Declaration of Helsinki, the protocol being approved by the Ethics Committee of "Grigore T. Popa" University of Medicine and Pharmacy (project no. 3390/19.01.2020).

Informed Consent Statement: The patients who agreed to donate their extracted third molars for scientific research signed the informed consent statement for biological materials.

Data Availability Statement: All the data presented in this study are available within the article.

Conflicts of Interest: The authors declare no conflict of interest.

References

1. Lussi, A. *Dental Erosion: From Diagnosis to Therapy*; Karger Medical and Scientific Publishers: Bern, Switzerland, 2006; p. 219.
2. Cunha-Cruz, J.; Wataha, J.C.; Heaton, L.J.; Rothen, M.; Sobieraj, M.; Scott, J.; Berg, J. The prevalence of dentin hypersensitivity in general dental practices in the northwest United States. *J. Am. Dent. Assoc.* **2013**, *144*, 288–296. [CrossRef]
3. Yadav, B.K.; Jain, A.; Rai, A.; Jain, M. Dentine Hypersensitivity: A Review of its Management Strategies. *J. Int. Oral Health* **2015**, *7*, 137–143.
4. Liu, X.X.; Tenenbaum, H.C.; Wilder, R.S.; Quock, R.; Hewlett, E.R.; Ren, Y.F. Pathogenesis, diagnosis and management of dentin hypersensitivity: An evidence-based overview for dental practitioners. *BMC Oral Health.* **2020**, *20*, 220. [CrossRef]
5. Gillam, D.G. *Dentine Hypersensitivity: Advances in Diagnosis, Management, and Treatment*; Springer International Publishing: Cham, Switzerland, 2015; pp. 1–190.
6. Eder, A.; Faigenblum, M. *Tooth Wear: An Authoritative Reference for Dental Professionals and Students*, 3rd ed.; Springer International Publishing: Cham, Switzerland, 2022; p. 92.
7. Borges, A.; Barcellos, D.; Gomes, C. Dentin Hypersensitivity-Etiology, Treatment Possibilities and Other Related Factors: A Literature review. *World J. Dent.* **2012**, *3*, 60–67.
8. Seligman, D.A.; Pullinger, A.G.; Solberg, W.K. The prevalence of dental attrition and its association with factors of age, gender, occlusion, and TMJ symptomatology. *J. Dent. Res.* **1988**, *67*, 1323–1333. [CrossRef]
9. Grippo, J.O.; Simring, M.; Schreiner, S. Attrition, Attrition, abrasion, corrosion and abfraction revisited: A new perspective on tooth surface lesions. *J. Am. Dent. Assoc.* **2004**, *135*, 1109–1118. [CrossRef]
10. West, N.X.; Seong, J.; Hellin, N.; Macdonald, E.L.; Jones, S.B.; Creeth, J.E. Assessment of tubule occlusion properties of an experimental stannous fluoride toothpaste: A randomised clinical in situ study. *J. Dent.* **2018**, *76*, 125–131. [CrossRef]
11. Kassab, M.M.; Cohen, R.E. The etiology and prevalence of gingival recession. *J. Am. Dent. Assoc.* **2003**, *134*, 220–225. [CrossRef]
12. Baker, P.; Spedding, C. The aetiology of gingival recession. *Dent. Update* **2002**, *29*, 59–62. [CrossRef]
13. Lussi, A.; Ganss, C. *Erosive Tooth Wear: From Diagnosis to Therapy*; Karger Medical and Scientific Publishers: Bern, Switzerland, 2014; p. 284.
14. Gillam, D.G.; Orchardson, R. Advances in the treatment of root dentin sensitivity: Mechanisms and treatment principles. *Endod. Topics* **2006**, *13*, 13–33. [CrossRef]

15. Wennstrom, J.L. Mucogingival therapy. *Ann. Periodontol.* **1996**, *1*, 671–701. [CrossRef]
16. Schmidlin, P.R.; Sahrmann, P. Current management of dentin hypersensitivity. *Clin. Oral. Investig.* **2013**, *17*, 55. [CrossRef]
17. Kazemi, R.B.; Sen, B.H.; Spångberg, L.S.W. Permeability changes of dentine treated with titanium tetrafluoride. *J. Dent.* **1999**, *27*, 531–538. [CrossRef]
18. Pashley, D.H. Dentin permeability, dentin sensitivity and treatment through tubule occlusion. *J. Endod.* **1986**, *12*, 465–474. [CrossRef]
19. Prati, C.; Chersoni, S.; Lucchese, A.; Pashley, D.H.; Mongiorgi, R. Dentin permeability after toothbrushing with different toothpastes. *Am. J. Dent.* **1999**, *12*, 190–193.
20. Prati, C.; Venturi, L.; Valdrè, G.; Mongiorgi, R. Dentin morphology and permeability after brushing with different toothpastes in presence and absence of smear layer. *J. Periodontol.* **2002**, *73*, 183–190. [CrossRef]
21. Arrais, C.A.; Micheloni, C.D.; Giannini, M.; Chan, D.C. Occluding effect of dentifrices on dentinal tubules. *J. Dent.* **2003**, *31*, 577–584. [CrossRef]
22. Orchardson, R.; Gillam, D.G. Managing dentin hypersensitivity. *J. Am. Dent. Assoc.* **2006**, *137*, 990–998. [CrossRef]
23. Öncü, E.; Karabekiroğlu, S.; Ünlü, N. Effects of different desensitizers and lasers on dentine tubules: An in-vitro analysis. *Microsc. Res. Tech.* **2017**, *80*, 737–744. [CrossRef]
24. Stoleriu, S.; Pancu, G.; Ghiorghe, A.; Sincar, D.C.; Solomon, S.; Andrian, S.; Iovan, G. Evaluation of dentinal changes following application of three different desensitizing agents. *Rev. Chim.* **2017**, *68*, 1573–1577. [CrossRef]
25. Vano, M.; Derchi, G.; Barone, A.; Pinna, R.; Usai, P.; Covani, U. Reducing dentine hypersensitivity with nano-hydroxyapatite toothpaste: A double-blind randomized controlled trial. *Clin. Oral Investig.* **2018**, *22*, 313–320. [CrossRef] [PubMed]
26. Wang, Z.; Sa, Y.; Sauro, S.; Chen, H.; Xing, W.; Ma, X.; Jiang, T.; Wang, Y. Effect of desensitising toothpastes on dentinal tubule occlusion: A dentine permeability measurement and SEM in vitro study. *J. Dent.* **2010**, *38*, 400–410. [CrossRef] [PubMed]
27. Behzadi, S.; Mohammadi, Y.; Rezaei-Soufi, L.; Farmany, A. Occlusion effects of bioactive glass and hydroxyapatite on dentinal tubules: A systematic review. *Clin. Oral Investig.* **2022**, *26*, 6061–6078. [CrossRef] [PubMed]
28. Kulal, R.; Jayanti, I.; Sambashivaiah, S.; Bilchodmath, S. An in-vitro comparison of nano hydroxyapatite, novamin and proargin desensitizing toothpastes—A SEM study. *J. Clin. Diagn. Res.* **2016**, *10*, ZC51–ZC54. [CrossRef] [PubMed]
29. Scott, R. NovaMin® Technology. *J. Clin. Dent.* **2010**, *21*, 59–60.
30. Greenspan, D.C. NovaMin® and tooth sensitivity—An overview. *J. Clin. Dent.* **2010**, *21*, 61–65.
31. Forsback, A.P.; Areva, S.; Salonen, J.I. Mineralization of dentin induced by treatment with bioactive glass S53P4 in vitro. *Acta Odontol. Scand.* **2004**, *62*, 14. [CrossRef]
32. Mahmoodi, B.; Goggin, P.; Fowler, C.; Cook, R.B. Quantitative assessment of dentine mineralization and tubule occlusion by NovaMin and stannous fluoride using serial block face scanning electron microscopy. *J. Biomed. Mater. Res. B Appl. Biomater.* **2021**, *109*, 717–722. [CrossRef]
33. Shah, S.; Shivakumar, A.T.; Khot, O.; Patil, C.; Hosmani, N. Efficacy of NovaMin- and Pro-Argin-Containing Desensitizing Dentifrices on Occlusion of Dentinal Tubules. *Dent. Hypotheses* **2017**, *8*, 104–109. [CrossRef]
34. Gopinath, N.M.; John, J.; Nagappan, N.; Prabhu, S.; Kumar, E.S. Evaluation of Dentifrice Containing Nano-hydroxyapatite for Dentinal Hypersensitivity: A Randomized Controlled Trial. *J. Int. Oral Health* **2015**, *7*, 118–122.
35. Poggio, C.; Lombardini, M.; Vigorelli, P.; Colombo, M.; Chiesa, M. The role of different toothpastes on preventing dentin erosion: An SEM and AFM study. *Scanning* **2014**, *36*, 301–310. [CrossRef]
36. Arnold, W.H.; Prange, M.; Naumova, E.A. Effectiveness of various toothpastes on dentine tubule occlusion. *J. Dent.* **2015**, *43*, 440–449. [CrossRef]
37. Pei, D.; Meng, Y.; Li, Y.; Liu, J.; Lu, Y. Influence of nano-hydroxyapatite containing desensitizing toothpastes on the sealing ability of dentinal tubules and bonding performance of self-etch adhesives. *J. Mech. Behav. Biomed. Mater.* **2019**, *91*, 38–44. [CrossRef]
38. Fiorillo, L.; Cervino, G.; Herford, A.S.; Laino, L.; Cicciù, M. Stannous Fluoride Effects on Enamel: A Systematic Review. *Biomimetics* **2020**, *5*, 41. [CrossRef]
39. Naumova, E.A.; Gaengler, P.; Zimmer, S.; Arnold, W.H. Influence of individual saliva secretion on fluoride bioavailability. *Open Dent. J.* **2010**, *4*, 185–190. [CrossRef]
40. Burwell, A.; Jennings, D.; Greenspan, D.C. NovaMin and dentin hypersensitivity--in vitro evidence of efficacy. *J. Clin. Dent.* **2010**, *21*, 66–71.
41. Cohen, S.R.; Apter, N.; Jesse, S.; Kalinin, S.; Barlam, D.; Peretz, A.I.; Ziskind, D.; Wagner, H.D. AFM investigation of mechanical properties of dentin. *Isr. J. Chem.* **2008**, *48*, 65–72. [CrossRef]

Disclaimer/Publisher's Note: The statements, opinions and data contained in all publications are solely those of the individual author(s) and contributor(s) and not of MDPI and/or the editor(s). MDPI and/or the editor(s) disclaim responsibility for any injury to people or property resulting from any ideas, methods, instructions or products referred to in the content.

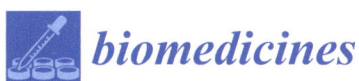 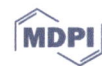

Systematic Review

Should Cone-Beam Computed Tomography Be Performed Prior to Orthodontic Miniscrew Placement in the Infrazygomatic Crest Area?—A Systematic Review

Marcin Stasiak [1,*] and Paulina Adamska [2,*]

1. Division of Orthodontics, Faculty of Medicine, Medical University of Gdańsk, Aleja Zwycięstwa 42c, 80-210 Gdańsk, Poland
2. University Dental Center, Medical University of Gdańsk, Dębowa 1a Street, 80-204 Gdańsk, Poland
* Correspondence: marcin.stasiak@gumed.edu.pl (M.S.); paulina.adamska@gumed.edu.pl (P.A.)

Abstract: There is no unequivocal scientific consensus for the temporary anchorage device (TAD) positioning in the infrazygomatic crest area (IZC). The two principal aims of this systematic review were to assess bone availability in the IZC and to establish both the target site and the need for cone-beam computed tomography (CBCT) prior to miniscrew placement. The study was performed following PRISMA guidelines (PROSPERO: CRD42023411650). The inclusion criteria were: at least 10 patients, three-dimensional radiological examination, and IZC assessment for the TAD placement. ROBINS-I tool and Newcastle-Ottawa Scale were used for quality evaluation. No funding was obtained. The study was based on the information coming from: PubMed, Google Scholar, Web of Science Core Collection, MDPI, Wiley, and Cochrane Libraries. The last search was carried out on 1 August 2023. Fourteen studies were identified for analysis. A narrative synthesis was performed to synthesize the findings of the different studies. Unfortunately, it is not possible to establish the generally recommended target site for IZC TAD placement. The reasons for this are the following: heterogeneity of available studies, inconsistent results, and significant risk of bias. The high variability of bone measurements and the lack of reliable predictors of bone availability justify the use of CBCT for TAD trajectory planning. There is a need for more high-quality studies aiming three-dimensional bone analysis of the IZC.

Keywords: CBCT; cone-beam computed tomography; temporary anchorage devices; miniscrew; infrazygomatic crest; IZC; maxilla; maxillary sinus; orthodontics; orthodontics anchorage procedures

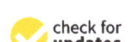

Citation: Stasiak, M.; Adamska, P. Should Cone-Beam Computed Tomography Be Performed Prior to Orthodontic Miniscrew Placement in the Infrazygomatic Crest Area?—A Systematic Review. *Biomedicines* **2023**, *11*, 2389. https://doi.org/10.3390/biomedicines11092389

Academic Editors: Giuseppe Minervini and Gianmarco Abbadessa

Received: 4 August 2023
Revised: 20 August 2023
Accepted: 24 August 2023
Published: 26 August 2023

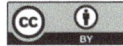

Copyright: © 2023 by the authors. Licensee MDPI, Basel, Switzerland. This article is an open access article distributed under the terms and conditions of the Creative Commons Attribution (CC BY) license (https://creativecommons.org/licenses/by/4.0/).

1. Introduction

Skeletal anchorage has expanded orthodontic treatment possibilities and is an integral part of modern orthodontic practice [1]. Temporary anchorage devices (TADs) can be placed within the maxilla in several locations such as the alveolar process [2,3], tuberosity [4], palate [5–9], and infrazygomatic crest area (IZC) [10,11]. Extra-alveolar miniscrews offer benefits such as reduced risk of root damage and the lack of interference with the mesiodistal tooth movement [11–13]. The IZC and external oblique ridge (the so-called buccal shelf) are the most frequently used extra-alveolar sites [11,14]. The TADs placed into the IZC region have been successfully used for total arch maxillary distalization with clockwise rotation of the occlusal plane [15]. Moreover, miniscrews in the IZC region seems to be more cost-effective than the palate distalizers, which offers a similar amount of tooth movement [13,15,16].

The IZC is a cortical bony eminence which is located on both sides of the zygomatic bone to the alveolar process at the level of the first molar or between first molar and second premolar (Figure 1). The IZC TADs are usually placed according to the clinical protocol, which allows to place miniscrews in the upright position in the lateral part of the posterior alveolar process between the first and second maxillary molars and to omit slipping on the bone surface [11]. However, some authors preferred to place IZC TADs in the "key ridge" above the first permanent molar [10]. Moreover, miniscrews could be placed with multiple angle adjustment technique in order to obtain more vertical orientation [17].

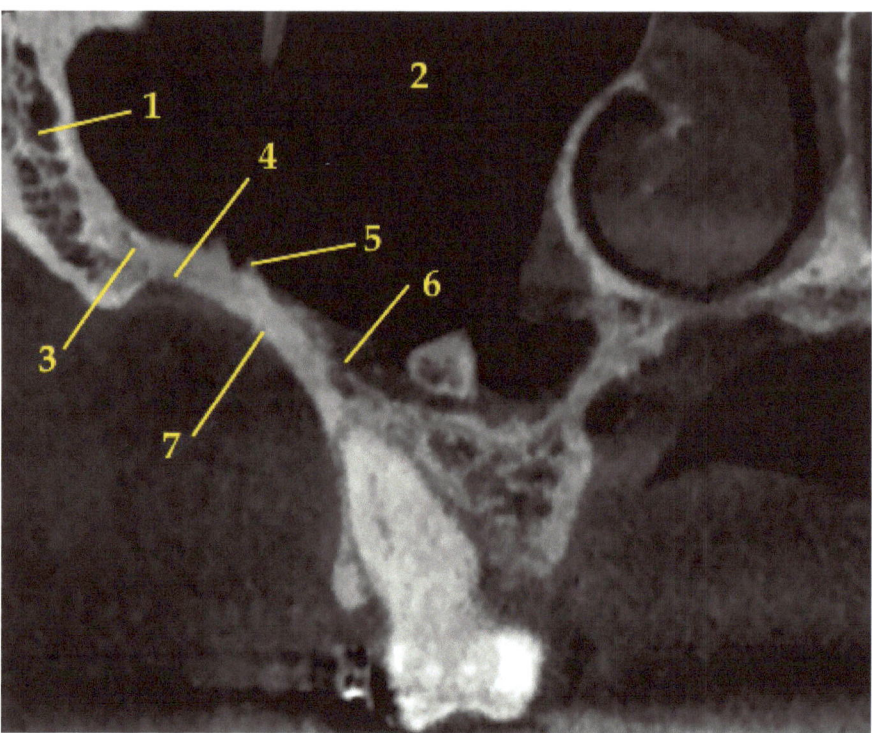

Figure 1. The anatomy of infrazygomatic crest area (1—zygomatic bone; 2—maxillary sinus; 3—zygomatico-maxillary suture; 4—zygomatic process of maxilla; 5—posterior superior alveolar artery; 6—posterior superior alveolar vein; 7—infrazygomatic crest).

The head of the miniscrew should be positioned at least 5 mm superior to the level of the soft tissue in order to facilitate oral hygiene and control soft tissue irritation [11]. It seems that the TAD should not only be placed in attached gingiva and mucogingival junction areas, but also in the zone of opportunity, which ranges to 2 mm of the mucosa apical to the mucogingival junction. It is possible to obtain greater amount of bone here with improved interradicular distance and healing response of the mucosa, which is similar to that for the attached gingiva [18–20].

On the other hand, there is a high likelihood of sinus perforation after miniscrew placement in the IZC region [21,22]. If the TAD penetrates more than 1 mm into the sinus, there is significantly higher incidence of sinus membrane thickening [21]. Concomitantly, the success rate of miniscrews placed into the IZC region is controversial and amounts from 78.2% to 96.7% [10,11,21,22].

Three-dimensional radiological examination provides detailed information about alveolar bone morphology [23]. Due to the lack of generally recommended target site and ambiguous success rate of IZC miniscrews, it was decided to perform this systematic review on papers evaluating IZC anatomy by means of three-dimensional radiological examination. The chosen research questions were as follows: What is the bone availability in the IZC area? What is the recommended target site? Should cone-beam computed tomography (CBCT) be performed prior to IZC orthodontic TAD placement for more predictable results?

2. Materials and Methods

Preferred Reporting Items for Systematic Reviews and Meta-Analyses (PRISMA) guidelines were used in this study [24]. The study protocol was registered with the Prospective Register of Systematic Reviews (PROSPERO; CRD42023411650). A narrative synthesis was performed to synthesize the findings of the different results of various studies.

2.1. Search Criteria

2.1.1. Inclusion Criteria

As a template to formulate a clinical question the PICO (P—population, I—Intervention or exposure, C—Comparison, O—Outcome) was used. Study characteristics:

P. At least 10 patients
I. Three-dimensional radiological examination
C. Not required
O. Assessment of IZC for orthodontic miniscrews placement

Only those papers written in English and study only on human were enrolled for reviewing.

2.1.2. Exclusion Criteria

Articles not meeting the PICO criteria were excluded from the systematic review. Publications that assessed the bone support after TAD placement were excluded due to two reasons—potential metal artifacts caused by the appliance and assessment driven by final placement instead of regional anatomy.

2.2. Data Collection

In order to find relevant studies, international databases including PubMed, Google Scholar, Web of Science Core Collection, MDPI, Wiley, and Cochrane Libraries were searched. We analyzed the scientific literature concerning IZC and three-dimensional radiological examination available from 2007 to the 1st of August 2023. The search terms used for the review were: [("maxilla" OR "infrazygomatic crest") AND ("mini-implant" OR "miniscrew" OR "TAD" OR "temporary anchorage device" OR "skeletal anchorage" OR "orthodontics anchorage procedures") AND ("orthodontics" OR "Tooth Movement Techniques") AND ("cone-beam CT" OR "cone beam computed tomography")] and [("infrazygomatic crest" OR "infrazygomatic crest area" OR "IZC") AND ("mini-implant" OR "mini-implants" OR "miniscrew" OR "TAD" OR "temporary anchorage device" OR "skeletal anchorage" OR "orthodontics anchorage procedures") AND ("cone-beam CT" OR "cone beam computed tomography")] and [("maxilla" OR "infrazygomatic crest") AND ("mini-implant" OR "miniscrew" OR "TAD" OR "temporary anchorage device" OR "skeletal anchorage" OR "orthodontics anchorage procedures") AND ("orthodontics" OR "Tooth Movement Techniques") AND ("CT" OR "computed tomography")] and [("infrazygomatic crest" OR "infrazygomatic crest area" OR "IZC") AND ("mini-implant" OR "mini-implants" OR "miniscrew" OR "TAD" OR "temporary anchorage device" OR "skeletal anchorage" OR "orthodontics anchorage procedures") AND ("CT" OR "computed tomography")]. References were imported into Mendeley manager. In order to identify eligible studies for the review, the papers were screened basing on titles and abstracts. Afterwards, full-text articles were assessed for eligibility.

Subsequently, data were extracted from those records retrieved for detailed text evaluation. These procedures were conducted by the first author. The second author participated in cases of disagreement. The following information was collected: first author, year of publication, study type, group characteristic (number, age, sex, ethnicity), aim of the study, assessment methods, bone measurements, and conclusions. Duplicate records, as well as letters and papers that did not contain significant information, were also excluded. Subgroup analyses were used to explore possible causes of heterogeneity among study results.

2.3. Quality Assessment

In this article the risk of bias was assessed of the included studies using the ROBINS-I tool (Risk of Bias in Non-randomized Studies of Interventions) and Newcastle-Ottawa Scale (NOS). ROBINS-I evaluates the following domains: (1) confounding; (2) selection of participants; (3) classification of interventions; (4) deviations from intended interventions; (5) missing data; (6) measurement of outcomes; and (7) selection of reported result (Table 1) [25]. Then each of the risk of bias domains was classified as: low, moderate, serious, critical, or no information. Overall risk was scored in the same gradation. NOS scale assess: (1) study selection; (2) comparability; (3) exposure (Good quality: 3 or 4 stars in sample selection category AND 1 or 2 stars in comparability category AND 2 or 3 stars in exposure category; Fair quality: 2 stars in sample selection category AND 1 or 2 stars in comparability category AND 2 or 3 stars in outcome; Poor quality: 0 or 1 star in sample selection category OR 0 stars in comparability category OR 0 or 1 stars in exposure category) [26]. These procedures were performed by both authors. In case of disagreement, a consensus reading was made.

Table 1. Criteria adopted for risk of bias assessment using ROBINS-I tool.

Domains	Criteria
Bias due to confounding	Studies are considered at **low risk** of bias if they consider the bone measurements at common sites of TAD placement in the IZC. Studies are considered at **moderate risk** of bias if they consider the presence of maxillary deciduous molars or the absence of maxillary permanent molars as confounding factors. Studies are considered at a **high risk** of bias if adjustment factors are not reported.
Bias in selection of participants into the study	Studies are considered at **low risk** of bias if the study size population was performed prospectively. Studies are considered at **moderate risk** of bias if the exposed cohort has some representation of the assessed exposure. Studies are considered at **high risk** of bias if the exposed cohort does not faithfully represent the assessed exposure.
Bias in measurement of the interventions	Studies are at **low risk** of bias if a correct measure of IZC bone is reported on CBCT or CT scans. Studies are considered at **moderate risk** of bias if the measurement of IZC bone is not performed on CBCT or CT scans. Studies are at **high risk** of bias if the way of measuring of IZC bone was not reported.
Bias due to departures from intended interventions	Studies are at **low risk** of bias if no intervention in the maxillary arch was performed, while at **moderate risk** of bias if any intervention in the opposite arch to change the reference point was performed. Studies are considered **high risk** if any intervention was performed on the maxillary arch (leveling, arch expansion, sagittal tooth movement).
Bias due to missing data	Studies are considered at **low risk** of bias if less than 10% of participants were excluded to missing data, while at **moderate risk** of bias if less than 20%. Studies with higher proportion ($\geq$20%) are considered at **high risk** of bias.
Bias in measurement of outcome	Studies are at **low risk** of bias if raters are aware of the limitations of the study or method error has been statistically evaluated. Studies are considered at **moderate risk** of bias if no reliability analysis has been performed in the intra-examiner's assessment. Studies are at **high risk** of bias if the outcome assessment is based solely on self-report, without external validation.
Bias in selection of reported results	Studies are at **low** risk of bias if all data planned by the authors in the entire sample are analyzed in accordance with a prescribed plan. Studies are considered at **moderate** risk of bias if there is no information about a prespecified plan. Studies are at **high** risk of bias if numerical result being assessed likely to have been selected on the basis of the results.
Overall risk of bias	If at least one domain was found at **high** risk of bias, the overall risk was considered **high**. If at least one domain is at some concerns, but no domains are at high risk, the overall risk was considered **moderate**. If all domains were at **low** risk of bias, the overall risk was considered **low**.

3. Results

3.1. Literature Search

In the first stage of selection, a total of 303 records were identified after duplicated references had been removed. Twenty-five studies were retrieved for full-text detailed evaluation. Next, 11 articles were excluded. Of these, two studies were excluded due to inappropriate assessment method, which did not take into consideration the recommended IZC TAD position [19,27]. Finally, 14 articles were included in the review (Figure 2 and Table 2).

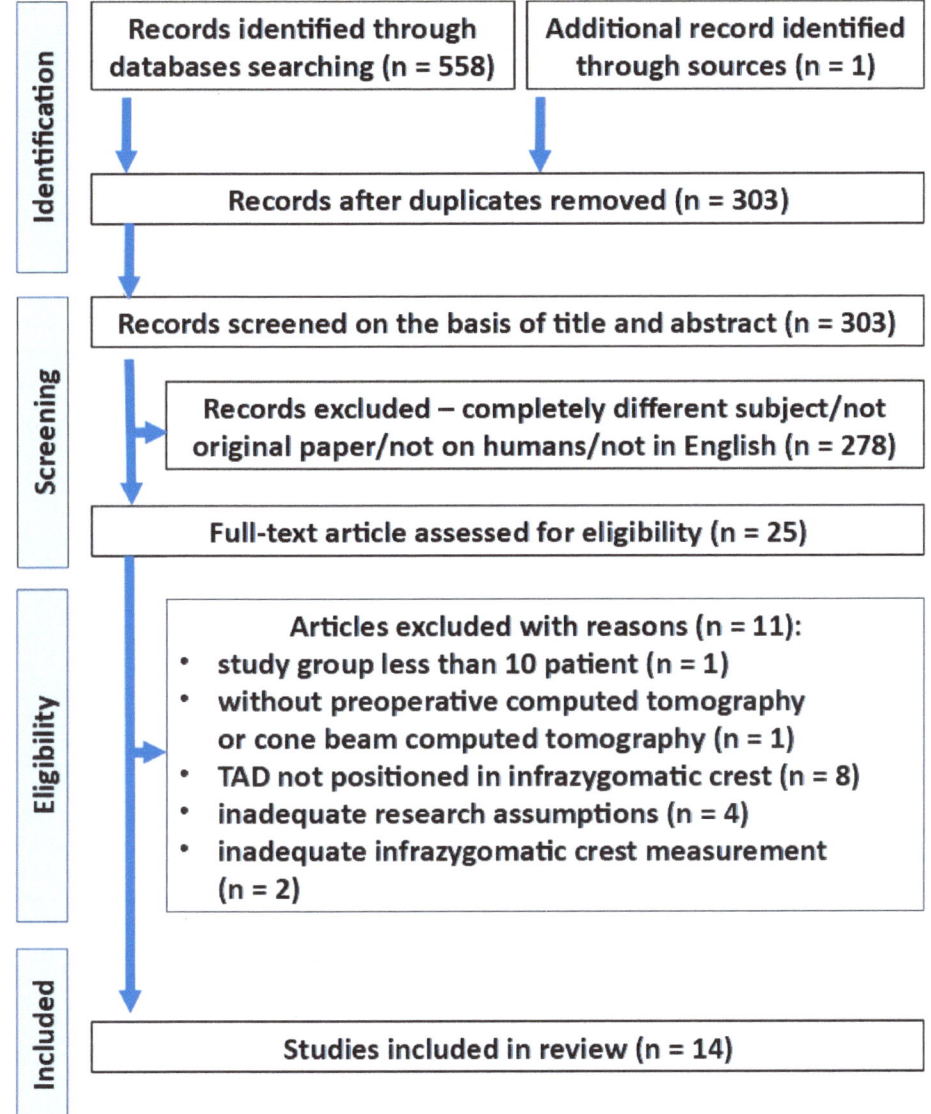

Figure 2. PRISMA flow diagram depicting the process followed for the selection of the studies.

Table 2. The studies included in the qualitative analysis and extracted data.

No	Study	Year	Study Type	Patient Characteristic				Assessment Method				Main Results—IZC Bone Measurement	Statistical Significance	Conclusions
				Country	Number	Age	Aim	Radiographical Examination	Insertion Region	Measurement Type and Method				
1	Liou [28]	2007	CSS	Taiwan	16 (M: 10, F: 6)	27.0 ± 5.2 y	The IZC depth of above the first maxillary molars, the biting depth of IZC TAD at different angles and positions to the maxillary OP; clinical implications for TAD insertion in the IZC without injuring the 6 MB root	Spiral CT	6M	Depth, eight transverse angulations: 40–70° (5° increments) to the maxillary OP; apical measurement point was the sinus point (intersection of tangent to the tooth buccal surface reference line and the floor of the maxillary sinus); 17.1 ± 3.7–12.8 ± 4.2 mm above the OP		40°: 5.2 ± 1.1 mm 45°: 5.4 ± 1.1 mm 50°: 5.6 ± 1.2 mm 55°: 6.0 ± 1.4 mm 60°: 6.3 ± 1.5 mm 65°: 7.0 ± 1.7 mm 70°: 7.7 ± 1.9 mm 75°: 8.8 ± 2.3 mm	No significant differences ($p > 0.05$) between different sides corresponding measurements	Ideal site (the adopted minimum depth of 6 mm), at an angle of 55–70° and 14–16 mm above the maxillary OP
2	Farnsworth [29]	2011	CSS	USA	52 (M: 26, F: 26)	Adolescents: 13 M: 14–16 y; 13 F: 11–13 y; Adults: 13 M; 13 F: 20–45 M and F	To examine the cortical bone thickness at common sites of TAD placement	CBCT, voxel size 0.39 mm	6M	Cortical bone thickness, one level: parallel to 6 M and 2 mm coronal to the junction of maxillary sinus and IZC cortical plates		Adolescents: 1.44 ± 0.39 mm; Adults: 1.58 ± 0.34 mm	No gender significant differences. No age significant differences	Cortical bones at commonly used TAD placement sites are thicker in adults than in adolescents except IZC
3	Liu [30]	2017	CSS	China	60 (M: 18; F: 52)	26.0 ± 7.8 y	To study the thickness and height of the alveolar bone in the IZC via the CBCT technique and to provide guidelines for choosing the appropriate TAD and the safe zone for TAD placement	CBCT, 110 kV, 0.07 mA, voxel size 0.3 mm	5-6, 6IR, 6-7	Thickness and height, five levels: 4 horizontal (5, 7, 9, 11 mm above the alveolar crest, parallel to OP), 1 vertical (parallel to the long axis of maxillary first molar)		Thickness: 5–6: 1.56 ± 0.24–1.86 ± 0.36 mm, 6IR: 2.24 ± 0.58–3.05 ± 0.58 mm, 6–7: 3.04 ± 0.55–4.07 ± 0.74 mm. Height: 5–6: 12.41 ± 5.59 mm, 6IR: 10.63 ± 4.4 mm, 6–7: 10.36 ± 3.38 mm	Significant difference in the thickness among the regions at the same plane ($p < 0.05$), no significant difference for thickness at different planes of each region ($p > 0.05$), no significant difference in height among the regions ($p > 0.05$)	6-7 should be the first choice for TAD placement in the buccal alveolar bone in the IZC for distalization of the entire maxillary dentition. Proper length of TAD is 6–8 mm for most patients. Bone tendency to get thicker apically
4	Santos [31]	2017	CSS	Brazil	40 (M:18; F:22)	22–56 y (mean 31 y)	To evaluate IZC depth in adult patients	CBCT, 120 kVp, 47 mA, voxel size 0.4 mm, FOV 20 × 25 cm	6D	Depth, two levels: 2 mm and 4 mm above FP angulation 90 ° to the cortical surface		2 mm: 2.49 mm 4 mm: 2.29 mm	No gender and side significant differences. Significantly higher depth at 2 mm level ($p = 0.019$), 2 mm no significant side differences ($p = 0.111$) and 4 mm significant side differences ($p = 0.002$)	IZC crest is significantly thinner than the length of the miniscrews. Risk of instability and sinus perforation due to insufficient bone depth

Table 2. Cont.

No	Study	Year	Study Type	Patient Characteristic				Assessment Method				Main Results—IZC Bone Measurement	Statistical Significance	Conclusions
				Country	Number	Age	Aim	Radiographical Examination	Insertion Region	Measurement Type and Method				
5	Al Amri [32]	2020	CSS	Saudi Arabia	100 (M:50, F:50)	25.4 ± 6.5 y	To assess the proximity of the maxillary sinus and nasal cavity in areas where miniscrews are usually inserted	CBCT, 120 kVp, 5 mA, voxel size 0.4 mm	6M	Depth, three transverse angulations: 45°, 55°, and 70° to the molar OP; apical measurement point was the sinus point (intersection of tangent to the tooth buccal surface reference line and the floor of the maxillary sinus)		45°: 4.94 ± 0.73 mm, 55°: 3.73 ± 0.41 mm, 70°: 3.90 ± 0.31 mm	No gender and age significant differences. IZC crest bone was significantly thicker at an insertion angle of 45° than at 55° and 70° ($p < 0.001$)	Greatest bone depth was at a 45° insertion angle. Risk of maxillary sinus perforation due to the limited available bone
6	Murugesan [33]	2020	CSS	India	36	20–30 y; average angle: 22.25 ± 4.31 y, low angle: 21.42 ± 4.52 y, high angle 21.5 ± 2.71 y	To compare the IZC crest depth in different vertical skeletal patterns (Jarabak index: S-Go and N-Me ratio and Tweed's FMA)	CBCT	6M, 7M	Depth, 70° to the molar OP; apical measurement point was the sinus point (intersection of tangent to the tooth buccal surface reference line and the floor of the maxillary sinus)		Average angle: 6M: 6.66 ± 2.80 mm, 7M: 9.20 ± 2.23 mm; Low angle: 6M: 6.09 ± 1.82 mm, 7M: 7.88 ± 1.84 mm; High angle: 6M: 3.85 ± 0.65 mm, 7M: 6.66 ± 1.63 mm	No side differences. Bone depth significant differences between insertion regions. High angle and average angle (6M,7M), high angle and low angle (6M) significant differences ($p < 0.001$, $p = 0.001$, $p = 0.001$)	IZC bone depth varied among different vertical skeletal patterns. It was least thick in high-angle group. Recommended site is 7M
7	Vargas [34]	2020	CSS	Brazil	100 (M: 42; F: 58)	19.8 ± 5.5 y	To use CBCT to determine the bone thickness in the MBS and bone depth in the IZC in individuals with different vertical skeletal patterns (gonial angle: ramus line-mandibular line through the gnathion) for the ultimate placement of TAD	CBCT, voxel size 0.3 mm, FOV 18 × 20.6 cm	6M, 6D, 6-7	Depth, two transverse angulations: 65° and 70° to the OP; height localization at the apex level on the reference line tangent to buccal cortical bone		6M 65°: 3.5 (1.3–11.8) mm, 6M 70°: 3.6 (1.3–14.1) mm, 6D 65°: 2.8 (1.0–8.3) mm, 6D 70°: 3.0 (1.1–8.7) mm, 6-7 65°: 2.4 (1.0–7.0) mm, 6-7 70°: 2.5 (1.0–7.2) mm	Significant correlation between IZC bone depth with the gonial angle: 6-7 65° $p = 0.013$, 6-7 70° $p < 0.001$, no significant correlation in other sites ($p > 0.05$)	There was no correlation between the gonial angle and bone depth in the IZC. The best site to install IZC TAD is 6M

Table 2. Cont.

No	Study	Year	Study Type	Patient Characteristic			Assessment Method			Main Results—IZC Bone Measurement	Statistical Significance	Conclusions
				Country	Number	Age	Radiographical Examination	Insertion Region	Measurement Type and Method			
									Aim			
8	Du [35]	2021	CSS	China	35 (M: 16; F: 20)	23.1 y (20–28 y)	To measure the bone depth and thickness of different insertion paths for safe placement of IZC TADs between the 6–7 by 3-dimensional reconstruction and to explore their clinical significance	CBCT, 5 mA, 120 kV, FOV 14.0 × 8.5 cm, voxel size 0.2 mm	6–7	Depth and thickness, three levels: 13 mm, 15 mm and 17 mm above posterior OP, three transverse angulations (50°, 60°, 70°), three sagittal angulations (0°, 15°, 30°)	Depth: 13 mm50°: 8.00 ± 4.64 mm, 13 mm60°: 7.16 ± 2.61 mm, 13 mm70°: 7.33 ± 2.44 mm, 15 mm50°: 5.72 ± 2.92 mm, 15 mm60°: 5.52 ± 2.38 mm, 15 mm70°: 5.73 ± 2.28 mm, 17 mm50°: 4.04 ± 2.32 mm, 17 mm60°: 4.02 ± 2.12 mm, 17 mm70°: 4.24 ± 2.08 mm, 0° distal tipping angle	No significant differences between different sides and gender ($p > 0.05$). Significant differences in bone depth between different insertion heights ($p < 0.001$). Significant differences in bone thickness between different insertion heights and transverse angulations ($p < 0.001$). Significant negative correlation between IZC bone depth and bone thickness ($p < 0.001$)	Bone depth and bone thickness may affect the safe insertion of a TAD. TADs preferred insertion path: 15 mm above the posterior OP, transversal angulation of 60–70°, and sagittal angulation of 30°. Alternative path: 13 mm above posterior OP, transversal angulation of 70°, sagittal angulation of 30°. TAD should not be inserted 17 mm above posterior OP, or with transversal angulation of 50°. A TAD with 9–11 mm in length and 1.6–2.3 mm in diameter may be proper in IZC region

Table 2. Cont.

No	Study	Year	Study Type	Patient Characteristic			Assessment Method			Main Results—IZC Bone Measurement	Statistical Significance	Conclusions
				Country	Number	Age	Radiographical Examination	Insertion Region	Measurement Type and Method			
9	Matias [12]	2021	CSS	Brazil	45 (M: 20; F: 25)	22.2 ± 7.4 y (brachyfacial) 19.24 ± 5.92 y (mesofacial) 17.79 ± 3.63 y (dolichofacial)	To identify optimal areas for the insertion of TADs into the IZC and MBS, using CBCT imaging in patients with different vertical skeletal patterns (Ricketts VERT)	CBCT, 120 kV, 8 mA, FOV 13 × 16 cm, voxel size 0.30 mm	6D	Depth, three levels: 11 mm, 13 mm and 15 mm above the cusp tip; 70° to the maxillary OP	Brachyfacial: 11 mm: 9.33 ± 2.27 mm, 13 mm: 7.51 ± 2.16 mm, 15 mm: 5.94 ± 2.15 mm. Mesofacial: 11 mm: 8.82 ± 1.83 mm, 13 mm: 7.16 ± 1.93 mm, 15 mm: 5.59 ± 1.88 mm. Dolichofacial: 11 mm: 8.87 ± 1.91 mm, 13 mm: 7.11 ± 1.95 mm, 15 mm: 5.39 ± 1.86 mm	No side significant differences. There was no statistically significant difference in the IZC bone depth among the groups ($p > 0.05$)	The IZC bone depth was similar among the brachyfacial, mesofacial and dolichofacial groups. Bone decreased as the insertion height increased
10	Arango [36]	2022	CSS	Colombia	128 (M: 59; F: 69)	9–50 y (9–13 y, 14–23 y, 24–50 y)	To compare the dimensions of the ZP, IZC, and MBS by sex and age	CBCT, 120 kV, 5 mA, voxel size 0.3 mm	5–6, 6IR, 6D	Depth, three transverse angulations: 55°, 65°, and 70° to the OP, apical measurement point was the sinus point (intersection of tangent to the tooth buccal surface reference line and the floor of the maxillary sinus)	IZC bone thickness: 5–6 at 55°: 3.06 (0.31–7.95) mm, 5–6 at 65°: 3.31 (0.31–8.84) mm, 5–6 at 70°: 3.53 (0.31–11.22) mm, 6IR at 55°: 2.62 (0.65–8.43) mm, 6IR at 65°: 3.16 (0.68–9.7) mm, 6IR at 70°: 3.78 (0.84–11.7) mm, 6D at 55°: 2.95 (0.48–8.95) mm, 6D at 65°: 3.35 (0.51–10.61) mm, 6D at 70°: 4.14 (0.51–11.4) mm	No gender significant differences. Significant differences were observed among age groups for IZC bone depth in 5–6 and 6IR ($p < 0.001$). No significant differences in 6D	IZC bone depth is bigger in younger subjects than in adults. 5–6 is the recommended site in the younger group and 6D in the older group

Table 2. Cont.

No	Study	Year	Study Type	Patient Characteristic			Assessment Method			Main Results—IZC Bone Measurement	Statistical Significance	Conclusions
				Country	Number	Age	Aim	Radiographical Examination	Insertion Region	Measurement Type and Method			
11	Lima [37]	2022	CSS	Brazil	86 (both sexes)	18–40 y	To evaluate the differences in bone thicknesses in the IZC among patients with different vertical skeletal patterns (Jarabak index: S-Go and N-Me ratio) to determine a safe zone for TAD insertion	CBCT, voxel size 0.4 mm	5–6, 6M, 6D, 6–7, 7M, 7D	Thickness; four levels: 5 mm, 7 mm, 9 mm, and 11 mm apically from a line passing through the mesial and distal alveolar bone crest	The required 3 mm minimum thickness: (1) hyperdivergent patients: 6–7 11 mm, 7M 9 mm and 11 mm, and 7D 11 mm; (2) neutral and hypodivergent patients: 6–7 11 mm and 7M 11 mm	All of the thicknesses measured at 5, 7, 9, and 11 mm presented statistically different means ($p < 0.05$) except left 5–6 in the hyperdivergent group	Safe zones for TADs—11 mm from the maxillary alveolar crest between the 6–7 and 7M for all of the facial types, thickness increase in distal and apical direction
12	Song [38]	2022	CSS	China	32 (M:16, F:16)	Adolescents: 14.4 ± 1.4 y Adults: 25.1 ± 5.5 y	To determine the optimal areas for IZC miniscrews	CBCT, 85 kV, 5 mA	6M, 6IR, 6D, 6–7, 7M, 7IR, 7D	Depth and cortical bone depth; thirteen levels: 0–12 mm (1 mm increments) from alveolar bone crest, ten transverse angulations: 0–90° (10° increments) to the OP	The most frequent shapes of IZC were the external concave shape, vertical shape, and external diagonal shape. Highest depth: 6D: 5.7 ± 5.2, 7D: 5.4 ± 4.7, Lowest depth: 6M: 3.8 ± 4.3	Cortical bone depth was significantly higher among females ($p < 0.001$). Depth was significantly higher among males ($p = 0.01$). Measurements were significantly higher among adults than adolescents ($p < 0.001$). Measurements were significantly influenced by insertion sites, heights, and angles	6D is the most ideal site. The optimal insertion heights and angles were 12 mm to 18 mm from the OP (3–9 mm from alveolar crest), and 40–70° for IZC miniscrews. Recommended insertion angle should be larger at lower insertion heights
13	Tavares [39]	2022	CSS	Brazil	58 (M:23, F:35)	29.5 ± 9.85 y (18–62 y)	To evaluate bone availability in the IZC crest in subjects with different vertical (SN-GoGn Angle) and sagittal (ANB) skeletal patterns	CBCT, 120 kV, 200 mA, FOV 32 × 32 cm, voxel size 0.6 mm	6D	Depth; three levels: 4 mm, 5 mm, and 6 mm from CEJ; three transverse angulations: 60°, 70°, and 80° to the molar OP	Bone depth was greater near the CEJ (8.7 ± 3.1 mm) and lower in the apical area (5.8 ± 2.7 mm)	Class 2—bone depth was significantly lower ($p = 0.007$) at 6 mm from CEJ at 80° when compared to 60° at 4 mm; Mesofacial subjects—bone depth was significantly lower at 80° at 6 mm from CEJ when compared to 60° at 4 mm	The best bone availability at the distance 4 mm from CEJ at an insertion angle of 60° for all individuals

Table 2. Cont.

No	Study	Year	Study Type	Patient Characteristic			Assessment Method			Main Results—IZC Bone Measurement	Statistical Significance	Conclusions
				Country	Number	Age	Radiographical Examination	Insertion Region	Measurement Type and Method			
14	Gibas-Stanek [40]	2023	CSS	Poland	100 (M:50, F:50)	28.81 ± 12.86 y (12–65 y)	CBCT, 5 mA, 120 kV, FOV 13.0 × 15.0 cm, voxel size 0.38 mm	6M, 6D, 6-7 (left side)	Depth, three levels: 12 mm, 14 mm and 16 mm above OP; 70° to the maxillary OP	6M 12 mm: 2.5 ± 2.55 mm 6M 14 mm: 2.54 ± 2.42 mm 6M 16 mm: 2.42 ± 2.16 mm 6D 12 mm: 3.71 ± 2.76 mm 6D 14 mm: 3.11 ± 2.35 mm 6D 16 mm: 2.59 ± 2.08 mm 6-7 12 mm: 6.03 ± 2.64 mm 6-7 14 mm: 4.74 ± 2.17 mm 6-7 16 mm: 3.46 ± 1.93 mm	Site significant differences 12 mm and 14 mm above OP ($p < 0.001$), 6D and 6-7 height significant differences ($p < 0.001$). 6-7 14 mm and 16 mm gender significant differences ($p = 0.012$ and $p = 0.003$). 6M and 6D significant negative correlation with age ($p < 0.001$).	6-7 12 mm above the OP is the most ideal site. 6M 16 mm above the OP presented the lowest bone depth

CBCT—cone-beam computed tomography; CEJ—cemento-enamel junction; CSS—cross-sectional study; CT—computed tomography; F—female; FOV—field of view; FP—Frankfurt plane; IZC—infrazygomatic crest; M—male; MBS—mandibular buccal shelf; OP—occlusal plane; TAD—temporary anchorage device = miniscrew; ZP—zygomatic process; 5–6—region between maxillary second premolar and first molar; 6D—distobuccal root of maxillary first molar; 6IR—middle of the maxillary first molar; 6M—mesiobuccal root of maxillary first molar; 6-7—region between maxillary first and second molars; 7D—distobuccal root of maxillary second molar; 7IR—middle of the buccal furcation of the maxillary second molar; 7M—mesiobuccal root of maxillary second molar.

3.2. Study Characteristic

All of the studies were retrospective and cross-sectional. There were five studies from Brazil, three from China, and single studies from Taiwan, USA, Saudi Arabia, India, Colombia, and Poland. The biggest study group consisted of 128 patients [36]. Only one and concomitantly the oldest paper [28] used spiral computed tomography (CT) for IZC anatomy evaluation. The rest of the studies (n = 13) performed the measurements by means of CBCT. Seven papers evaluated the IZC bone availability in relation to sex [29,31,32,35,36,38,40] and five investigated age differences [29,32,36,38,40]. Five studies analyzed the IZC anatomy in relation to different vertical skeletal patterns [12,33,34,37,39] and one in relation to different sagittal skeletal patterns [39]. One study evaluated the bone availability in relation to regional anatomy—modified palatal height index [40].

There were different measurement methods for IZC bone availability. Most popular assessment sites were mesiobuccal and distobuccal roots of maxillary first molar (n = 8), and region between maxillary first and second molars (n = 6). Other assessment sites were regions between maxillary second premolar and first molar, middle of the upper first molar, and mesiobuccal root of maxillary second molar (n = 3), distobuccal root of maxillary second molar (n = 2), and middle of the upper second molar (n = 1). Eleven studies evaluated the overall bone depth, three the bone thickness, and one the bone height in the IZC region. Single studies evaluated the buccal cortical bone depth and the buccal cortical bone thickness. Seven papers investigated different insertion regions. Eight studies investigated different insertion heights and seven compared different transversal angulations. Only one of the studies examined different sagittal angulations.

High variability of the results was found within individual studies as well as between different studies. Individual sample differences were high, as indicated the standard deviation which was often around 50% or more of the mean.

There was no consensus about best insertion region among studies, which evaluated the bone depth in different sagittal insertion sites [33,34,36,38,40]. Two studies recommended distobuccal root of first molar [36,38], one study mesiobuccal root of first molar [34], one mesiobuccal root of second molar [33], and one region between maxillary first and second molars [40]. Concomitantly, Arango et al. [36] recommended to place TADs in the region between second premolar and first molar in younger patients.

Moreover, there was no agreement among studies, which evaluated transversal angulations influence on the bone depth availability [28,32,34–36,38,39]. Only four studies performed statistical evaluation of the obtained results. On the one hand, Amri et al. [32] obtained significant negative correlation with the bone depth decrease when the insertion angle increase. On the other hand, Du et al. [35] found significant positive correlation in most sites. Instead, Tavares et al. [39] found no significant differences between different angulations at the same insertion level. Song et al. [38] assessed all of the possible angulations from 0 to 90° and obtained significant differences. The highest values were related to the transversal angulations from 60° to 70°. The transverse angulation was recommended to be larger at lower insertion heights and concomitantly the angle could be relatively smaller at higher insertion sites [28,38].

Paper, which assessed sagittal angulation effect on the bone depth availability, revealed that the bone depth increased with the higher sagittal inclination and this relation was not statistically significant only in one insertion path [35].

There was a tendency to bone depth decrease in the apical direction [12,35,38–40]. Concomitantly, in two studies which compared levels in proximity, not exceeding a distance of 2 mm between sites, no significant differences were found [12,39]. On the other hand, Gibas-Stanek et al. obtained significant differences in the region of distobuccal roots of maxillary first molar and region between maxillary first and second molars [40]. Du et al. [35] and Song et al. [38] also obtained statistical significance. The former compared the measurements performed in three levels within a distance of 4 mm and obtained significant negative correlation between insertion height and bone depth. The latter performed measurements at thirteen levels within distance of 12 mm. The results suggested an optimal range of insertion heights.

Both studies, which assessed bone thickness in various insertion regions, recommend to placing TADs more distally in the region between first and second maxillary molars or even in the region of mesiobuccal root of second maxillary molar [30,37]. One study investigated the relation between angulation and bone thickness [35]. The bone thickness increased significantly with higher transversal angulations. Concomitantly, no significant differences in bone thickness were found among different sagittal insertion angles.

There was a tendency to bone thickness increase in the apical direction [30,35,37]. Statistical significance was assessed and found in two studies [35,37]. Moreover, Lima et al. [37] found significant differences in the buccal alveolar bone thickness measurements, which tend to get higher from the region between upper premolars to the region between molars. In the same study were the alveolar bone heights evaluated. The lowest alveolar bone height was found between molars and the highest was found between premolars. However, no significant differences were obtained [30].

Only one of the studies evaluated both the bone depth and the bone thickness [35]. A statistically significant and negative correlation between these measurements was found in the study.

There was no agreement about recommended insertion height (Table 3) [12,28,30,31,35,37–40].

Table 3. Insertion height according to various authors.

No	Study	Recommended Insertion Height
1	Liou [28]	14–16 mm above OP
2	Santos [31]	2 mm above FP
3	Liu [30]	11 mm above AC
4	Du [35]	13–15 mm above OP
5	Matias [12]	11 mm above OP
6	Lima [37]	11 mm above AC
7	Song [38]	3–9 mm above AC
8	Tavares [39]	4 mm above CEJ
9	Gibas-Stanek [40]	12 mm above OP

AC—alveolar crest; CEJ—cemento-enamel junction; FP—Frankfurt plane; OP—occlusal plane.

No statistically significant differences were found between different genders in most of the studies which assessed that relationship [29,31,32,35,36]. Song et al. [38] obtained statistically significant differences, but these differences were concomitantly clinically insignificant. Gibas-Stanek et al. [40] obtained statistically significant differences only in two insertion heights (14 mm and 16 mm above the occlusal plane) in the region between maxillary first and second molars. These differences, which were both 1.2 mm, also seem to be clinically significant.

There was no consensus about age differences in IZC bone depth among studies, which obtained contrary results [36,38,40]. Al Amri et al. [32] found no significant age-related differences in bone depth, but the study group consisted of only adult patients, which were 18 years or older. Moreover, there was no consensus about differences in cortical bone dimensions in the IZC area between the adolescents and the adults [29,38].

Moreover, no consensus on vertical growth pattern differences was found [12,33,34]. There were reports, that this relationship may be related to specific sites. Two of the studies did not statistically evaluate differences between the results obtained in different growth pattern groups [37,39].

A significant and negative correlation between bone depth and modified palatal height index was found only in 30% of the measurement sites [40].

Only one of the included studies performed not only static but also dynamic evaluation by taking into consideration distal movement trajectory of roots during orthodontic treatment [35].

CBCT imaging provides accurate clinical guidance for orthodontic TAD insertion. Six studies discussed the use of CBCT prior to IZC miniscrew placement [12,31,32,34,36,40]. There was an agreement among these studies that CBCT is justified for extra-alveolar TADs placement planning. The reasons were individual variation in growth and development of the maxilla and maxillary sinus, high variability of bone measurements, high risk of maxillary sinus perforation and the fact, that facial type is not a good predictor of bone availability.

3.3. Risk of Bias

3.3.1. ROBINS-I

Of the fourteen included studies, one was judged to be at critical risk of bias, nine were rated as having a moderate risk of bias and four had a low risk of bias. Main concerns related to the risk of bias were due to no reliable analysis in the intra-examiner assessment and no prospective calculation of the study size. In the study of Song et al. [38], should have the eligible patients had the distance between maxillary sinus and alveolar ridge crest no less than 10 mm. It is a potential reason of incredible results due to overestimation. In the study of Arango et al. [36] was one of the measurements, IZC region bone length performed in three sagittal sites and in three different angulations, not described. Concomitantly, the study of Liu et al. [30] which was referenced in the above publication, did not present such a measurement. Therefore, that measurement was omitted in Table 2. The results of risk of bias assessment are shown in Figure 3.

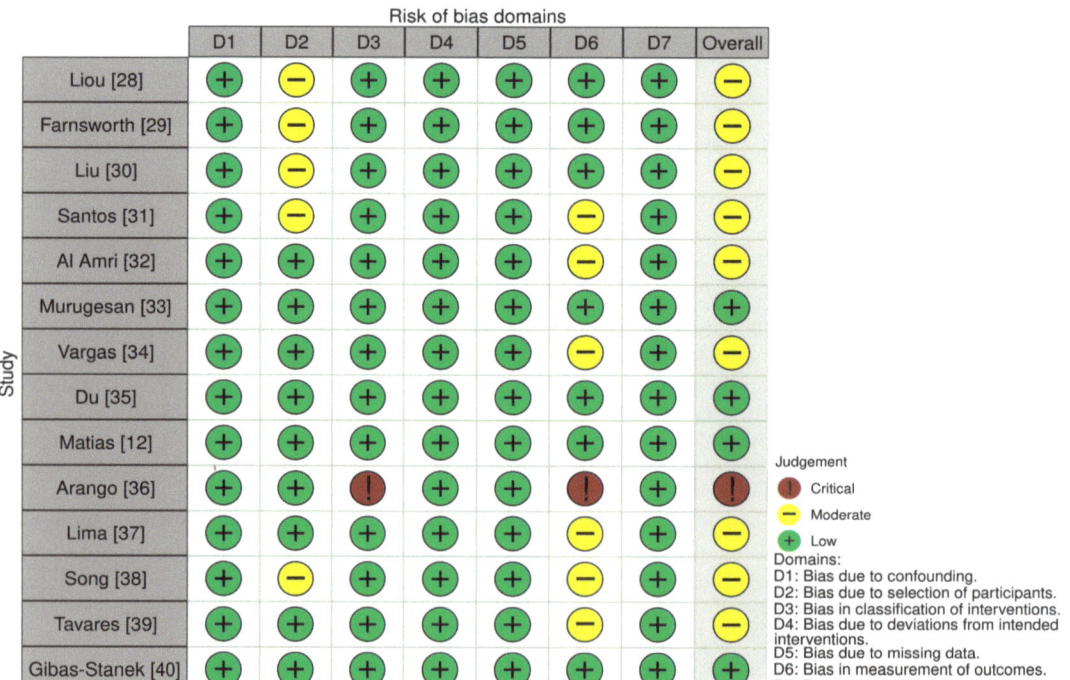

Figure 3. Risk of bias assessment using ROBINS-I tool [12,28–40].

3.3.2. Newcastle-Ottawa Scale (NOS)

It was considered that one study is of good quality and 13 are of fair quality. The risk of bias assessment using the NOS was described in Table 4.

Table 4. Risk of bias using the Newcastle-Ottawa Scale for quality assessment.

No	Study	Sample Selection				Comparability		Exposure		Total
		Adequate Case Definition	Representativeness of the Cases	Selection of Control	Definition of Control	Comparability of Cases	Controls Based on the Analysis	Ascertainment of Exposure	Non-Response Rate	
1	Liou [28]	★	-	-	-	★	-	★	★	4
2	Farnsworth [29]	★	-	-	-	★	-	★	-	3
3	Liu [30]	★	-	-	-	★	-	★	-	3
4	Santos [31]	★	-	-	-	★	-	★	-	3
5	Al Amri [32]	★	★	-	-	★	-	★	-	4
6	Murugesan [33]	★	★	-	-	★	-	★	-	4
7	Vargas [34]	★	★	-	-	★	-	★	-	4
8	Du [35]	★	★	★	★	★	★	★	★	8
9	Matias [12]	★	★	-	-	★	-	★	-	4
10	Arango [36]	★	★	-	-	★	-	★	★	5
11	Lima [37]	★	★	-	-	★	-	★	★	5
12	Song [38]	★	★	-	-	★	-	★	★	5
13	Tavares [39]	★	★	-	-	★	-	★	-	4
14	Gibas-Stanek [40]	★	★	-	-	★	-	★	-	4

Star (★) = item present.

4. Discussion

Recent development in three-dimensional X-ray diagnostics have enabled more precise measurements of alveolar bone structure [41]. Concomitantly, CBCT provides lower radiation dose than spiral CT [42]. Only four studies included in the review discussed the radiation dose during the CBCT examination [32,34,36,39]. Current guidelines state, that CBCT is not normally indicated for planning the placement of TADs in orthodontics. This examination is needed preoperatively for placement of miniscrews in cases of borderline dimensions [43]. High variability of the results was associated with different root lengths, anatomy of the maxilla and the maxillary sinus, transversal inclination of the adjacent teeth, and height of the alveolar process [30,31,33,35,37–40]. However, not only high variability of IZC bone architecture, but also no reliable predictors of bone availability were found during the review. It seems that only CBCT with adequate parameters can provide information about the bone amount, possibility of IZC miniscrew placement and preferred insertion path. It seems that insertion of the IZC TAD needs to be patient specific and one site is not adequate for all. Therefore, CBCT may be necessary to install IZC miniscrews correctly. It enables one to develop individual TAD insertion protocol for each patient to obtain desirable primary stabilization for orthodontic anchorage and to reduce complication risk. Not only insertion height and depth but also bone thickness, cortical bone amount and different transversal and sagittal angulations should be taken into consideration. When considering favorable risk-benefit ratio, it seems justified to use CBCT for IZC miniscrew placement planning. However, radiological protection is needed for this type of examination especially in young patients [44]. It is recommended to reduce the field of view to the maxilla region if there are no other indications for increasing the imaging area size. This approach is in conformity with the ALARA (as low as reasonably achievable) principle. This rule involves maintaining exposures to radiation as far below the dose limits as is practical, while being consistent for which the activity is undertaken [45].

According to the literature, decreasing the CBCT voxel size can improve the accuracy of alveolar bone measurements [44]. Examination with a 0.2-mm voxel size provides on average spatial resolution of 0.4 mm. Therefore, it can distinguish objects with a minimum 0.4-mm distance [46]. It provides clearer images, easier identification of alveolar crests, and enables closer to the gold standard (direct measurements) results [47]. Voxel size of approximately 0.4 mm can potentially be a limitation due to insufficiency accurate measurements [40]. On the other side, Farnsworth et al. [29] showed high reliability for both the 0.2 mm and 0.4 mm scans with high interclass correlations.

The positioning of the orthodontic miniscrew in the IZC area relative to the anatomical structures of the maxilla is of great importance. Only with the use of CBCT, it is possible to precisely determining the availability of the bone limited by the maxillary sinus floor location or the position of the posterior superior alveolar artery and vein. Moreover, the presence of septa in the maxillary sinus can be used as an additional bone support for the IZC TAD stability. The prevalence of sinus septa is estimated at 31.7% [48]. The posterior superior alveolar artery is located on or in the lateral wall of the maxillary sinus. The intraosseous variant is usually located at a height of 19 mm from the bone crest, and the extraosseous variant at a height of 23 mm from the bone crest. The average distance from the bottom of the maxillary sinus is about 6–9 mm. Moreover, the position of posterior superior alveolar vein should be also taken into consideration. It is in a more inferior position, which is more adjacent to the IZC insertion site than the artery. Both vessels can be damaged during the positioning of the miniscrew. This can lead to postoperative complications in the form of prolonged bleeding [49–51]. Jia et al. [21] assessed the incidence of TADs penetration into the maxillary sinus and penetration depth influence on sinus tissue. The frequency of penetration of miniscrews into the maxillary sinus was high. The incidence of membrane thickening was 88.2% in a group in which penetration exceeded 1 mm, and the mean value of thickening was 1 mm. In a group with membrane penetration of 1 mm was the membrane thickening observed at 37.5%, and the mean value of thickening was 0.2 mm. According to Chang et al. [22] perforation of the sinus reduced both the length of the bone contact and the terminal insertion torque, but did not significantly increase the failure rate of TADs.

Thick cortical bone is associated with good primary stability. Therefore, it is not recommended to place the miniscrews in thin cortical bone, which is less than 1 mm thick [52]. However, there is no consensus how does the insertion torque affect the survival rate of orthodontic TADs [22,52]. Placement failure might be associated with low as well as excessive torque values [52]. IZC are might be expected to undergo greater damage, such as crushing and heat, due to thick cortical bone during placement [29]. Pilot holes might be preferred to omit this potential damage in certain patients [29,52].

Nine studies presented requirements for adequate bone availability [28,33–40]. There was no consensus about preferred values of the bone measurements. Liou et al. [28], Arango et al. [36], Tavares et al. [39], and Gibas-Stanek et al. [40] suggested the required bone depth value of 6 mm. Concomitantly, all of the patients met this requirement in the study of Liou et al. Moreover, mean bone depths obtained the required value except one insertion path in class 2 patients in the study performed by Tavares et al. [39]. However, significant variability was noticed. Whereas Arango et al. obtained a significant bone variability with mean measurements beneath the adopted limit value. Gibas-Stanek et al. found that bone depth rarely reaches recommended value of 6 mm. Murugesan et al. [33] and Song et al. [38] required bone depth of 5 mm. In the former study was that mean bone amount not obtained only in high angle patients' group above the mesiobuccal root of first molar. The mean bone depth was adequate above the mesiobuccal root of a second molar in all skeletal patterns. In the latter study was the recommended areas, with greater bone depth than required 5 mm, presented. There is a possibility, that border value of 5–6 mm might be exaggerated and significantly limits the choice of sites for miniscrew safe insertion in the IZC region. Therefore, Vargas et al. [34] and Du et al. [35] preferred values of 4 mm and 3.8 mm, respectively. Most of the measurements in the IZC were lower than 4 mm in the former study. In the study of Du et al., the median bone depths of most paths did not reach 3.8 mm only at the 17 mm insertion height. Farnsworth et al. [29], following the study of Motoyoshi et al. [52], preferred the cortical bone depth of 1 mm. Most of the patients met this condition [29,38]. Other requirements were presented according to the bone thickness measurements. Lima et al. [37] preferred bone thickness of 3 mm, when Du et al. [35] recommended 1.3 mm. This value was calculated as a sum of 0.8 mm TAD radius and 0.5 mm safety distance from root surface. According to Lima et al. mean values of bone thickness were larger than 3 mm between first and second molar, and in the mesial second molar root area 11 mm from the alveolar crest. In the study of Du et al. [29], was the median bone thickness of each path at 13 mm height less than 1.3 mm when transversal angulation of 50° was adopted. A statistically significant and negative correlation between the bone depth and the bone thickness was found. Therefore, both measurements should be taken into consideration for insertion path analysis. The extent of the results and obtained standard deviations in sites with adequate mean bone values indicate that there is no universality of the measurements and some patients presented inadequate bone availability. There is a need for comprehensive studies considering different aspects of regional bone anatomy to establish the bone requirements. The aspects of bone quantity and quality with possible bicortical fixation that could increase the clinical success should be considered.

Dynamic evaluation presented by Du et al. [35] seems to be more adequate for orthodontic purposes than static measurements. Potential collision of the miniscrew with orthodontic tooth movement may prevent the clinician from obtaining the desired treatment results and may lead to root injuries or failure of the miniscrews. Therefore, continuous evaluation taking into consideration distal movement trajectory of roots is justified. Future studies should take this approach into consideration.

Orthodontic biomechanics should be also considered when IZC miniscrew placement planning. Tooth movement patterns during total maxillary arch distalization with different force directions were recognized [53]. None of the included studies discussed in this aspect of miniscrew placement. More distal and occlusal placement sites provide higher relation between values of horizontal and vertical force vectors when comparing with mesial and more apical placement sites. Therefore, power arms should be more frequently considered in forward and apical locations.

There was no consensus that higher transversal angulations were associated with greater bone depth. On the other hand, it seems that it is better to implant TADs closer to the occlusal plane to ensure the appropriate depth of implant insertion, and the apically increasing bone thickness provides support and distance to root surfaces despite transverse angulation of the miniscrew. This also seems to be advantageous considering the biomechanical aspects. Moreover, additional stabilization increase may be obtained due to miniscrews' sagittal angulation. However, more acute insertion angle is associated with more technically difficult placement due to slipping [28]. Precise TAD insertion may still be a challenge for manual manipulation, especially for inexperienced physicians. Du et al. [35] indicated a need for assistive device or intelligent robot to be developed. Implementation of optical scanning and 3D printing to fabricate customized appliances including guides for patients with craniofacial disorders was proved to be efficient way in the individualization of the treatment [54]. Moreover, there is a possibility to use insertion guides for more predictable results [6,55]. Surgical guides for IZC miniscrew placement can be obtained based on CBCT examinations and intraoral scans. Implementation of optical scanning and 3D printing to fabricate customized appliances including guides for patients with craniofacial disorders is proved to be efficient way in the individualization of the treatment. This approach could potentially improve the primary stability and reduce both the TAD collision risk during orthodontic tooth movement and the sinus penetration risk. Moreover, it could solve the slipping problem during insertion. The use of surgical guides for IZC miniscrew placement should be further researched.

An interesting issue is the use of artificial intelligence-supported determination of available sites for orthodontic miniscrews based on bone analysis using the CBCT [56,57]. Today, it is not common in dentistry and orthodontics. The AI system demonstrated high accuracy in bone segmentation and measurement, which is helpful in identifying available sites and designing a surgical template for palatal TADs [56]. The use of AI for IZC miniscrew placement planning should be researched in the future.

The differences of IZC TADs' success rates among previously mentioned studies might be caused by different localizations and miniscrews' dimensions. Uribe et al. [10] preferred the "key ridge" above the first permanent molar, where reduced bone depth due to high insertion position could be present. These authors favored also TADs of smaller width than the other authors did [11,21,22]. Both factors seem to affect the obtained results. There is no consensus on the ideal IZC position in terms of vertical dimension. Some authors propose positioning relative to the occlusal plane [12,35,40,58]. It may not be a reproducible place for positioning TADs in cases of pathological tooth wear or disturbed occlusal plane. Also, the height of the crown of the teeth varies. The use of the mean height of clinical crowns measured between the cusp tip and the cemento-enamel junction is not reliable due to individual variability. Another aspect is the clinical significance of the variables, which potentially could be insignificant in case of minor deviation. Moreover, adjustment of the single molar occlusal plane as the referential [33,39] seems to be even more limited due to the common compensatory transversal inclination of the molars. A repetitive location could be positioning using the mucogingival line as a landmark. As a rule, miniscrews should be located within the safe zone adjacent to the mucogingival line. This protects the oral mucosa from excessive exposure to inflammation caused by the implant irritating the mobile mucosa. Due to both diverse gingival biotypes of patients and different height of keratinized gingiva, it is difficult to define uniform standards for the positioning of TADs. Alveolar crest in the condition of healthy periodontium or cemento-enamel junction should be considered as the potentially good referential site. Establishing a reference value would allow more accurate positioning of miniscrews.

Cross-sectional studies have limited reliability in the age-related assessments. Therefore, it is justified to perform cohort studies. However, there are ethic aspects as well as radiological protection requirements, which should be taken into consideration when performing two CBCT examinations in the untreated study group.

Only in the study of Santos et al. [31] was a need for maxillary anchorage during orthodontic treatment stated as an inclusion criterion.

The available literature lacks a systematic review on the positioning TADs in the IZC area. The presented study shows limitations of existing evidence, new directions of research, and their degree of advancement on the way to implementation in everyday practice. The limitation of this article is the scarcity of literature reports on this subject. The most studies included in the systematic review was the assessment of the location of miniscrews in IZC without clear standards. The studies differ in the methods of measuring the depth and angulation of the inserted TADs, the level of insertion relative to the horizontal plane, the diversity of patients in terms of ethnic group or age of patients. Moreover, the IZC position was commonly not assessed in the absence of maxillary molars or the presence of significant congenital disorders such as cleft palate. The influence of the alveolar bone loss due to periodontal disease on the bone depth in IZC region was not investigated. Also, periodontal biotype and recessions presence were not evaluated as potential prognostic factors of the bone availability. These aspects should be researched in the future.

5. Conclusions

It is not possible to establish the generally recommended target site for the placement of the miniscrews in the IZC area. The reasons for this were the heterogeneity of available studies, inconsistent results, and significant risk of bias. The high variability of bone measurements and the lack of reliable predictors of bone availability justify the use of CBCT for TAD trajectory planning. Finally, there is a need for more high-quality studies aiming three-dimensional bone analysis of IZC area.

Author Contributions: Conceptualization, M.S.; methodology, M.S. and P.A.; software, M.S. and P.A.; validation, M.S. and P.A.; formal analysis, M.S. and P.A.; investigation, M.S. and P.A.; resources, M.S. and P.A.; data curation, M.S. and P.A.; writing—original draft preparation, M.S. and P.A.; writing—review and editing, M.S. and P.A.; visualization, M.S. and P.A.; supervision, M.S., and P.A.; project administration, M.S. and P.A. All authors have read and agreed to the published version of the manuscript.

Funding: This research received no external funding.

Institutional Review Board Statement: Not applicable.

Informed Consent Statement: Not applicable.

Data Availability Statement: The data presented in this study are available on request from the corresponding author. The data are not publicly available due to privacy restrictions.

Acknowledgments: We would like to thank Marcela Burdzy-Pogonowska for proofreading the article.

Conflicts of Interest: The authors declare no conflict of interest.

Abbreviations

AC	alveolar crest
CBCT	cone-beam computed tomography
CEJ	cemento-enamel junction
CSS	cross-sectional study
CT	computed tomography
F	female
FOV	field of view
FP	Frankfurt plane
IZC	infrazygomatic crest
M	male
MBS	mandibular buccal shelf
OP	occlusal plane
TAD	temporary anchorage device = miniscrew
ZP	zygomatic process
5–6	region between maxillary second premolar and first molar
6D	distobuccal root of first maxillary molar
6IR	middle of the buccal furcation of the maxillary first molar (equal distances to mesial and distal buccal root)
6M	mesiobuccal root of maxillary first molar
6–7	region between maxillary first and second molar
7D	distobuccal root of maxillary second molar
7IR	middle of the buccal furcation of the maxillary second molar (equal distances to mesial and distal buccal root)
7M	mesiobuccal root of second maxillary molar

References

1. Melsen, B. Mini-Implants: Where Are We? *J. Clin. Orthod.* **2005**, *39*, 539–547.
2. Park, H.S.; Jeong, S.H.; Kwon, O.W. Factors Affecting the Clinical Success of Screw Implants Used as Orthodontic Anchorage. *Am. J. Orthod. Dentofac. Orthop.* **2006**, *130*, 18–25. [CrossRef]
3. Antoszewska-Smith, J.; Sarul, M.; Łyczek, J.; Konopka, T.; Kawala, B. Effectiveness of Orthodontic Miniscrew Implants in Anchorage Reinforcement during En-Masse Retraction: A Systematic Review and Meta-Analysis. *Am. J. Orthod. Dentofac. Orthop.* **2017**, *151*, 440–455. [CrossRef] [PubMed]
4. Paredes-Gallardo, V.; Bellot-Arcís, C.; García-Sanz, V. Miniscrew Mechanics for Molar Distalization and Incisor Intrusion in a Patient with a Class II Brachyfacial Pattern and Gummy Smile. *Am. J. Orthod. Dentofac. Orthop.* **2020**, *158*, 273–285. [CrossRef] [PubMed]
5. Nienkemper, M.; Pauls, A.; Ludwig, B.; Drescher, D. Stability of Paramedian Inserted Palatal Mini-Implants at the Initial Healing Period: A Controlled Clinical Study. *Clin. Oral Implant. Res.* **2015**, *26*, 870–875. [CrossRef] [PubMed]

6. Wilmes, B.; Tarraf, N.E.; de Gabriele, R.; Dallatana, G.; Drescher, D. Procedure Using CAD/CAM-Manufactured Insertion Guides for Purely Mini-Implant-Borne Rapid Maxillary Expanders. *J. Orofac. Orthop.* **2022**, *83*, 277–284. [CrossRef] [PubMed]
7. Sa'aed, N.L.; Park, C.O.; Bayome, M.; Park, J.H.; Kim, Y.J.; Kook, Y.A. Skeletal and Dental Effects of Molar Distalization Using a Modified Palatal Anchorage Plate in Adolescents. *Angle Orthod.* **2015**, *85*, 657–664. [CrossRef] [PubMed]
8. Bud, E.S.; Bică, C.I.; Păcurar, M.; Vaida, P.; Vlasa, A.; Martha, K.; Bud, A. Observational Study Regarding Possible Side Effects of Miniscrew-Assisted Rapid Palatal Expander (MARPE) with or without the Use of Corticopuncture Therapy. *Biology* **2021**, *10*, 187. [CrossRef] [PubMed]
9. Park, J.J.; Kim, K.A.; Kim, H.R.; Hong, S.O.; Kang, Y.G. Treatment Effects of Miniscrew-Assisted Rapid Palatal Expansion in Adolescents Using Cone-Beam Computed Tomography. *Appl. Sci.* **2023**, *13*, 6309. [CrossRef]
10. Uribe, F.; Mehr, R.; Mathur, A.; Janakiraman, N.; Allareddy, V. Failure Rates of Mini-Implants Placed in the Infrazygomatic Region. *Prog. Orthod.* **2015**, *16*, 31. [CrossRef]
11. Chang, C.H.; Lin, J.S.; Eugene Roberts, W. Failure Rates for Stainless Steel versus Titanium Alloy Infrazygomatic Crest Bone Screws: A Single-Center, Randomized Double-Blind Clinical Trial. *Angle Orthod.* **2019**, *89*, 40–46. [CrossRef] [PubMed]
12. Matias, M.; Flores-Mir, C.; de Almeida, M.R.; Vieira, B.d.S.; de Freitas, K.M.S.; Nunes, D.C.; Ferreira, M.C.; Ursi, W. Miniscrew Insertion Sites of Infrazygomatic Crest and Mandibular Buccal Shelf in Different Vertical Craniofacial Patterns: A Cone-Beam Computed Tomography Study. *Korean J. Orthod.* **2021**, *51*, 387–396. [CrossRef]
13. Wilmes, B.; Drescher, D. Application and Effectiveness of the Beneslider: A Device to Move Molars Distally. *World J. Orthod.* **2010**, *11*, 331–340.
14. Seo, Y.J.; Park, J.H.; Chang, N.Y.; Chae, J.M. Non-Surgical Camouflage Treatment of a Skeletal Class III Patient with Anterior Open Bite and Asymmetry Using Orthodontic Miniscrews and Intermaxillary Elastics. *Appl. Sci.* **2023**, *13*, 4535. [CrossRef]
15. Nunes Rosa, W.G.; de Almeida-Pedrin, R.R.; Oltramari, P.V.P.; de Castro Conti, A.C.F.; Fernandes Poleti, T.M.F.; Shroff, B.; de Almeida, M.R. Total Arch Maxillary Distalization Using Infrazygomatic Crest Miniscrews in the Treatment of Class II Malocclusion: A Prospective Study. *Angle Orthod.* **2023**, *93*, 41–48. [CrossRef] [PubMed]
16. Lee, S.K.; Abbas, N.H.; Bayome, M.; Baik, U.B.; Kook, Y.A.; Hong, M.; Park, J.H. A Comparison of Treatment Effects of Total Arch Distalization Using Modified C-Palatal Plate vs Buccal Miniscrews. *Angle Orthod.* **2018**, *88*, 45–51. [CrossRef]
17. Van Giap, H.; Lee, J.Y.; Nguyen, H.; Chae, H.S.; Kim, Y.H.; Shin, J.W. Cone-Beam Computed Tomography and Digital Model Analysis of Maxillary Buccal Alveolar Bone Thickness for Vertical Temporary Skeletal Anchorage Device Placement. *Am. J. Orthod. Dentofac. Orthop.* **2022**, *161*, e429–e438. [CrossRef] [PubMed]
18. Baumgaertel, S. Hard and Soft Tissue Considerations at Miniimplant Insertion Sites. *J. Orthod.* **2014**, *41*, S3–S7. [CrossRef]
19. Baumgaertel, S.; Hans, M.G. Assessment of Infrazygomatic Bone Depth for Mini-Screw Insertion. *Clin. Oral Implant. Res.* **2009**, *20*, 638–642. [CrossRef]
20. Baumgaertel, S.; Tran, T.T. Buccal Mini-Implant Site Selection: The Mucosal Fallacy and Zones of Opportunity. *J. Clin. Orthod.* **2012**, *46*, 434–436.
21. Jia, X.; Chen, X.; Huang, X. Influence of Orthodontic Mini-Implant Penetration of the Maxillary Sinus in the Infrazygomatic Crest Region. *Am. J. Orthod. Dentofac. Orthop.* **2018**, *153*, 656–661. [CrossRef]
22. Chang, C.H.; Lin, J.H.; Roberts, W.E. Success of Infrazygomatic Crest Bone Screws: Patient Age, Insertion Angle, Sinus Penetration, and Terminal Insertion Torque. *Am. J. Orthod. Dentofac. Orthop.* **2022**, *161*, 783–790. [CrossRef]
23. Stasiak, M.; Wojtaszek-Słomińska, A.; Racka-Pilszak, B. Alveolar Bone Heights of Maxillary Central Incisors in Unilateral Cleft Lip and Palate Patients Using Cone-Beam Computed Tomography Evaluation. *J. Orofac. Orthop.* **2021**, *82*, 198–208. [CrossRef]
24. Page, M.J.; McKenzie, J.E.; Bossuyt, P.M.; Boutron, I.; Hoffmann, T.C.; Mulrow, C.D.; Shamseer, L.; Tetzlaff, J.M.; Akl, E.A.; Brennan, S.E.; et al. The PRISMA 2020 Statement: An Updated Guideline for Reporting Systematic Reviews. *BMJ* **2021**, *372*, n71. [CrossRef]
25. Sterne, J.A.; Hernán, M.A.; Reeves, B.C.; Savović, J.; Berkman, N.D.; Viswanathan, M.; Henry, D.; Altman, D.G.; Ansari, M.T.; Boutron, I.; et al. ROBINS-I: A Tool for Assessing Risk of Bias in Non-Randomised Studies of Interventions. *BMJ* **2016**, *355*, i4919. [CrossRef]
26. Wells, G.; Shea, B.; O'Connell, D.; Peterson, J.; Welch, V.; Losos, M.; Tugwell, P. The Newcastle-Ottawa Scale (NOS) for Assessing the Quality of Nonrandomised Studies in Meta-Analyses. Available online: https://www.ohri.ca/programs/clinical_epidemiology/oxford.asp?fbclid=IwAR3xy9Cb0mD2ec2WCQwn0MY7dvcXUFJRDK5YsG-YrxxNq8NqKJ8_j2EzmCc (accessed on 1 August 2023).
27. Husseini, B.; Younes, R.; Baumgaertel, S.; El Wak, T.; El Osta, N.; Bassil-Nassif, N.; Bouserhal, J. Assessment of Infrazygomatic Crest Dimensions in Different Vertical Facial Growth Types for Miniscrew Insertion: A Cone-Beam Computed Tomography Study. *Am. J. Orthod. Dentofac. Orthop.* **2022**, *162*, 917–926. [CrossRef] [PubMed]
28. Liou, E.J.W.; Chen, P.H.; Wang, Y.C.; Lin, J.C.Y. A Computed Tomographic Image Study on the Thickness of the Infrazygomatic Crest of the Maxilla and Its Clinical Implications for Miniscrew Insertion. *Am. J. Orthod. Dentofac. Orthop.* **2007**, *131*, 352–356. [CrossRef] [PubMed]
29. Farnsworth, D.; Rossouw, P.E.; Ceen, R.F.; Buschang, P.H. Cortical Bone Thickness at Common Miniscrew Implant Placement Sites. *Am. J. Orthod. Dentofac. Orthop.* **2011**, *139*, 495–503. [CrossRef]
30. Liu, H.; Wu, X.; Yang, L.; Ding, Y. Safe Zones for Miniscrews in Maxillary Dentition Distalization Assessed with Cone-Beam Computed Tomography. *Am. J. Orthod. Dentofac. Orthop.* **2017**, *151*, 500–506. [CrossRef] [PubMed]

31. Santos, A.R.; Castellucci, M.; Crusoé-Rebello, I.M.; Sobral, M.C. Assessing Bone Thickness in the Infrazygomatic Crest Area Aiming the Orthodontic Miniplates Positioning: A Tomographic Study. *Dental Press J. Orthod.* **2017**, *22*, 70–76. [CrossRef]
32. Al Amri, M.S.; Sabban, H.M.; Alsaggaf, D.H.; Alsulaimani, F.F.; Al-Turki, G.A.; Al-Zahrani, M.S.; Zawawi, K.H. Anatomical Consideration for Optimal Position of Orthodontic Miniscrews in the Maxilla: A CBCT Appraisal. *Ann. Saudi Med.* **2020**, *40*, 330–337. [CrossRef]
33. Murugesan, A.; Jain, R.K. A 3D Comparison of Dimension of Infrazygomatic Crest Region in Different Vertical Skeletal Patterns: A Retrospective Study. *Int. Orthod.* **2020**, *18*, 770–775. [CrossRef] [PubMed]
34. Vargas, E.O.A.; Lopes de Lima, R.; Nojima, L.I. Mandibular Buccal Shelf and Infrazygomatic Crest Thicknesses in Patients with Different Vertical Facial Heights. *Am. J. Orthod. Dentofac. Orthop.* **2020**, *158*, 349–356. [CrossRef] [PubMed]
35. Du, B.; Zhu, J.; Li, L.; Fan, T.; Tan, J.; Li, J. Bone Depth and Thickness of Different Infrazygomatic Crest Miniscrew Insertion Paths between the First and Second Maxillary Molars for Distal Tooth Movement: A 3-Dimensional Assessment. *Am. J. Orthod. Dentofac. Orthop.* **2021**, *160*, 113–123. [CrossRef] [PubMed]
36. Arango, E.; Plaza-Ruíz, S.P.; Barrero, I.; Villegas, C. Age Differences in Relation to Bone Thickness and Length of the Zygomatic Process of the Maxilla, Infrazygomatic Crest, and Buccal Shelf Area. *Am. J. Orthod. Dentofac. Orthop.* **2022**, *161*, 510–518.e1. [CrossRef] [PubMed]
37. Lima, A.; Domingos, R.G.; Cunha Ribeiro, A.N.; Rino Neto, J.; de Paiva, J.B. Safe Sites for Orthodontic Miniscrew Insertion in the Infrazygomatic Crest Area in Different Facial Types: A Tomographic Study. *Am. J. Orthod. Dentofac. Orthop.* **2022**, *161*, 37–45. [CrossRef]
38. Song, Q.; Jiang, F.; Zhou, M.; Li, T.; Zhang, S.; Liu, L.; Pu, L.; Lai, W.; Long, H. Optimal Sites and Angles for the Insertion of Orthodontic Mini-Implants at Infrazygomatic Crest: A Cone Beam Computed Tomography (CBCT)-Based Study. *Am. J. Transl. Res.* **2022**, *14*, 8893–8902.
39. Tavares, A.; Montanha-Andrade, K.; Cury, P.R.; Crusoé-Rebello, I.; Neves, F.S. Tomographic Assessment of Infrazygomatic Crest Bone Depth for Extra-Alveolar Miniscrew Insertion in Subjects with Different Vertical and Sagittal Skeletal Patterns. *Orthod. Craniofacial Res.* **2022**, *25*, 49–54. [CrossRef]
40. Gibas-Stanek, M.; Ślusarska, J.; Urzędowski, M.; Żablicki, S.; Pihut, M. Quantitative Evaluation of the Infrazygomatic Crest Thickness in Polish Subjects: A Cone-Beam Computed Tomography Study. *Appl. Sci.* **2023**, *13*, 8744. [CrossRef]
41. Stasiak, M.; Wojtaszek-Słomińska, A.; Racka-Pilszak, B. Current Methods for Secondary Alveolar Bone Grafting Assessment in Cleft Lip and Palate Patients—A Systematic Review. *J. Craniomaxillofac. Surg.* **2019**, *47*, 578–585. [CrossRef]
42. Chau, A.C.M.; Fung, K. Comparison of Radiation Dose for Implant Imaging Using Conventional Spiral Tomography, Computed Tomography, and Cone-Beam Computed Tomography. *Oral Surg. Oral Med. Oral Pathol. Oral Radiol. Endod.* **2009**, *107*, 559–565. [CrossRef] [PubMed]
43. European Comission Radiation Protection N° 172-Cone Beam CT For Dental and Maxillofacial Radiology (Evidence-Based Guidelines). Available online: https://sedentexct.eu/files/radiation_protection_172.pdf (accessed on 1 August 2023).
44. Stasiak, M.; Wojtaszek-Słomińska, A.; Racka-Pilszak, B. A Novel Method for Alveolar Bone Grafting Assessment in Cleft Lip and Palate Patients: Cone-Beam Computed Tomography Evaluation. *Clin. Oral Investig.* **2021**, *25*, 1967–1975. [CrossRef]
45. United States Nuclear Regulatory Commission NRC Regulations Title 10, Code of Federal Regulations. Available online: https://www.nrc.gov/reading-rm/basic-ref/glossary/alara.html (accessed on 1 August 2023).
46. Ballrick, J.W.; Palomo, J.M.; Ruch, E.; Amberman, B.D.; Hans, M.G. Image Distortion and Spatial Resolution of a Commercially Available Cone-Beam Computed Tomography Machine. *Am. J. Orthod. Dentofac. Orthop.* **2008**, *134*, 573–582. [CrossRef]
47. Sun, Z.; Smith, T.; Kortam, S.; Kim, D.-G.; Tee, B.C.; Fields, H. Effect of Bone Thickness on Alveolar Bone-Height Measurements from Cone-Beam Computed Tomography Images. *Am. J. Orthod. Dentofac. Orthop.* **2011**, *139*, 117–127. [CrossRef] [PubMed]
48. Ulm, C.W.; Solar, P.; Krennmair, G.; Matejka, M.; Watzek, G. Incidence and Suggested Surgical Management of Septa in Sinus-Lift Procedures. *Int. J. Oral Maxillofac. Implant.* **1995**, *10*, 462–465.
49. la Encina, A.C.; Martínez-Rodríguez, N.; Ortega-Aranegui, R.; Cortes-Bretón Brinkmann, J.; Martínez-González, J.M.; Barona-Dorado, C. Anatomical Variations and Accessory Structures in the Maxilla in Relation to Implantological Procedures: An Observational Retrospective Study of 212 Cases Using Cone-Bean Computed Tomography. *Int. J. Implant Dent.* **2022**, *8*, 59. [CrossRef]
50. Tofangchiha, M.; Hematzadeh, S.; Vali, M.E.; Ghonche, M.R.A.; Mirzadeh, M.; Reda, R.; Testarelli, L. Anatomical Localization of Posterior Superior Alveolar Artery: A Retrospective Study by Cone-Beam Computed Tomography. *Dent. Med. Probl.* **2022**, *59*, 407–412. [CrossRef]
51. Rathod, R.; Singh, M.P.; Nahar, P.; Mathur, H.; Daga, D. Assessment of Pathway and Location of Posterior Superior Alveolar Artery: A Cone-Beam Computed Tomography Study. *Cureus* **2022**, *14*, e22028. [CrossRef]
52. Motoyoshi, M.; Matsuoka, M.; Shimizu, N. Application of Orthodontic Mini-Implants in Adolescents. *Int. J. Oral Maxillofac. Surg.* **2007**, *36*, 695–699. [CrossRef]
53. Kawamura, J.; Park, J.H.; Kojima, Y.; Tamaya, N.; Kook, Y.A.; Kyung, H.M.; Chae, J.M. Biomechanical Analysis for Total Distalization of the Maxillary Dentition: A Finite Element Study. *Am. J. Orthod. Dentofac. Orthop.* **2021**, *160*, 259–265. [CrossRef] [PubMed]
54. Thurzo, A.; Urbanová, W.; Neuschlová, I.; Paouris, D.; Čverha, M. Use of Optical Scanning and 3D Printing to Fabricate Customized Appliances for Patients with Craniofacial Disorders. *Semin. Orthod.* **2022**, *28*, 92–99. [CrossRef]

55. Pozzan, L.; Migliorati, M.; Dinelli, L.; Riatti, R.; Torelli, L.; Di Lenarda, R.; Contardo, L. Accuracy of the Digital Workflow for Guided Insertion of Orthodontic Palatal TADs: A Step-by-step 3D Analysis. *Prog. Orthod.* **2022**, *23*, 27. [CrossRef]
56. Tao, T.; Zou, K.; Jiang, R.; He, K.; He, X.; Zhang, M.; Wu, Z.; Shen, X.; Yuan, X.; Lai, W.; et al. Artificial Intelligence-Assisted Determination of Available Sites for Palatal Orthodontic Mini Implants Based on Palatal Thickness through CBCT. *Orthod. Craniofac. Res.* **2023**, *26*, 491–499. [CrossRef]
57. Urban, R.; Haluzová, S.; Strunga, M.; Surovková, J.; Lifková, M.; Tomášik, J.; Thurzo, A. AI-Assisted CBCT Data Management in Modern Dental Practice: Benefits, Limitations and Innovations. *Electronics* **2023**, *12*, 1710. [CrossRef]
58. Liou, E.J.W.; Pai, B.C.J.; Lin, J.C.Y. Do Miniscrews Remain Stationary under Orthodontic Forces? *Am. J. Orthod. Dentofac. Orthop.* **2004**, *126*, 42–47. [CrossRef] [PubMed]

Disclaimer/Publisher's Note: The statements, opinions and data contained in all publications are solely those of the individual author(s) and contributor(s) and not of MDPI and/or the editor(s). MDPI and/or the editor(s) disclaim responsibility for any injury to people or property resulting from any ideas, methods, instructions or products referred to in the content.

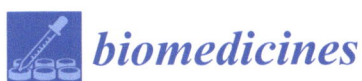

Article

Changes in Molar Tipping and Surrounding Alveolar Bone with Different Designs of Skeletal Maxillary Expanders

Javier Echarri-Nicolás [1], María José González-Olmo [2,*], Pablo Echarri-Labiondo [3] and Martín Romero [2]

1. Doctoral Program in Health Sciences, International PhD School, Rey Juan Carlos University (URJC), 28922 Alcorcón, Spain; j.echarri.2020@alumnos.urjc.es
2. Department of Orthodontics, Rey Juan Carlos University, 28922 Alcorcón, Spain; martin.romero@urjc.es
3. Athenea Dental Institute, San Jorge University, 50830 Zaragoza, Spain; echarri@centroladent.com
* Correspondence: mariajose.gonzalez@urjc.es

Abstract: This study compared the buccolingual angulation (BLA) of the upper and lower first permanent molars before and after using the different methods of microimplant-assisted expansion in adults and its influence on bone insertion loss. Methods: Cone-beam computed tomography scans taken before and after the expansion in 36 patients (29.9 ± 9.4 years) were used to assess dental and periodontal changes and compare changes between the groups. Results: This research shows a statistically significant increase in the BLA of the upper first molars. An increase of the BLA of the lower molars is also observed in MARPE. Regarding the comparison between cases treated with MARPE (4.42° ± 10.25°; 3.67° ± 9.56°) and BAME (−0.51° ± 4.61°; 2.34° ± 4.51°), it was observed that upper molar torque increased significantly less in cases treated with BAME. In cases with CWRU < 96° at T0, a slight bone insertion gain was observed at T1, whereas if CWRU ≥ 96°, a slight bone insertion loss was observed. Regarding the labial cortical bone loss, a slight gain of CBW was observed in all cases. This labial cortical enlargement (T0–T1) is greater in cases where the CWRU < 96° at T0. Conclusions: Patients treated with MARPE show torque increase in the teeth selected to support the expansion appliance compared to cases treated with BAME. In cases where the BLA at T0 < 96°, an increase in thickness and cortical insertion is observed in the upper molars after treatment with disjunction appliances assisted with microscrews.

Keywords: rapid maxillary expansion; maxillary skeletal expander; cone-beam computed tomography (CBCT); miniscrew-assisted rapid palatal expansion (MARPE); bone-anchored maxillary expander (BAME)

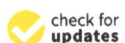

Citation: Echarri-Nicolás, J.; González-Olmo, M.J.; Echarri-Labiondo, P.; Romero, M. Changes in Molar Tipping and Surrounding Alveolar Bone with Different Designs of Skeletal Maxillary Expanders. *Biomedicines* 2023, 11, 2380. https://doi.org/10.3390/biomedicines11092380

Academic Editors: Giuseppe Minervini and Gianmarco Abbadessa

Received: 1 August 2023
Revised: 22 August 2023
Accepted: 23 August 2023
Published: 25 August 2023

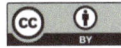

Copyright: © 2023 by the authors. Licensee MDPI, Basel, Switzerland. This article is an open access article distributed under the terms and conditions of the Creative Commons Attribution (CC BY) license (https://creativecommons.org/licenses/by/4.0/).

1. Introduction

Non-surgical rapid palatal expansion (RPE) in adults can provoke purely orthodontic expansion, i.e., undesired dentoalveolar effects [1] This limitation is due to the mid-palatal suture ossification, which makes the orthopedic separation of hemimaxillary portions impossible with the use of tooth-borne separators [2]. An expansion with increased torque and descent of the palatine cusps occurs in the upper posterior teeth [2]. In addition, adverse effects have been found, such as gingival inflammation, labial gingival recession, labial fenestration, and root resorption, due to their contact with the labial cortical bone [3].

The use of this technique is contraindicated in adults with maxillary compression, correct or positive molar torque, periodontal disease, generalized recessions, or absence of posterior teeth. If treatment is required, a surgical approach with surgical assisted rapid palatal expansion (SARPE) should be chosen. In SARPE, a surgical separation of the already ossified midpalatal suture is performed. In this way, we can increase the skeletal transverse dimension with an intraoral expansion device [4].

The microimplant-assisted rapid palatal expansion (MARPE) technique described by Moon [5] is characterized by a reduction of the excessive load exerted by conventional appliances to the labial periodontal ligament of the teeth, which is used as anchorage. The technique consists of a tooth-bone-borne device that uses retention in the form of two or four bicortical microscrews placed in the posterior area of the palate. The bone-anchorage maxillary expansion (BAME) appliance has been described as consisting of two or four bicortical microimplants without dental support [6].

The main side effect of MARPE is the buccolingual angulation (BLA) of the posterior teeth [7]. Increased molar torque has also been related to bone dehiscence [8]. Few studies have studied the change of BLA of the molars after treatment with MARPE or BAME using CBCTs [7,9–12].

Complications with microscrew-assisted separators occur in patients who have already completed the midpalatal suture ossification when the orthopedic forces are applied near the maxillary, frontal maxillary, and frontal zygomatic-maxillary buttresses. These buttresses distribute the applied force. There are reports of cases with fractures in the frontonasal suture or ocular area. In addition, there have also been cases with device impaction or microscrews fracture that can be solved only by a surgical intervention [13–15].

The BLA of the upper and lower molars forms the curve of Wilson (COW), which has a convex shape in the upper posterior teeth and a concave shape in the lower posterior teeth [16]. According to Hayes [16], the correct BLA of both the canines and the upper and lower molars is assumed to be essential to ensuring the functional balance of the patient and the stability of orthodontic treatment. The objective of having correct molar occlusion are twofold: (i.) the centering and uprighting of the teeth in their alveolus and (ii.) ensuring their correct intercuspation. These factors are important for achieving the proper functioning of dentition, dental stability, temporomandibular joint health, and periodontal viability [17].

The correct relationship of COW has been studied in treatments performed with fixed appliances [18–21] and with aligners [22], but it has not been studied in treatments performed with MARPE or BAME.

The literature also describes how cortical bone insertion (CBI) affects the molars in MARPE or BAME treatments [7,23–25], but no relation has been found with the increased torque of the affected teeth.

This article has two main objectives. The first is to analyze and compare the change of the BLA of the upper and the lower first permanent molars before and after using the different methods of microimplant-assisted expansion (MARPE and BAME). The second is to evaluate whether the initial buccolingual inclination of the upper first molars affects periodontal health after MARPE treatment.

This article has great clinical significance for orthodontists since it provides rigorous information on which expansion therapy has the most dental effect on the maxillary and mandibular molars, and it is important to evaluate the inclination of the upper molars before treatment for the control of periodontal health.

2. Materials and Methods

2.1. Design and Participants

Patients' data were involved retrospectively. Those patients under treatment with MARPE or BAME in a private dental office (Athenea Dental Institute, Barcelona, Spain) from September 2021 to March 2023 were involved.

The inclusion criteria of the study were adult patients with maxillary compression without counter-indications for surgery and who were to undergo microimplant-assisted maxillary expansion treatment. The exclusion criteria from the study were patients with craniofacial malformations, patients with fissured palates, patients who did not accept orthodontic treatment, and patients who refused to participate in the study or refused to sign the informed consent. Demographics and sample images were used, and the information was anonymized. The sample size was calculated using Jamovi 2.3.18. As there were no previous studies comparing dental changes using BAME and MARPE, sample size calculations were based on the results of a pilot study performed with ten patients.

The calculated means ± standard deviations (SDs) of the maxillary width change of BAME and MARPE were 1.96 mm ± 0.22 and 2.31 mm ± 0.35, respectively. Based on comparison of means using the two-tailed test, it was calculated that accepting an alpha risk of 0.05 and a beta risk of 0.2 in a bilateral contrast, 16 subjects per group are required to detect a difference equal to or greater than 0.35 mm. Finally, we were able to include 36 subjects, which increased the robustness of the data. The MARPE technique was used in 18 subjects, and the BAME technique was used in 18 subjects. See Figures 1 and 2.

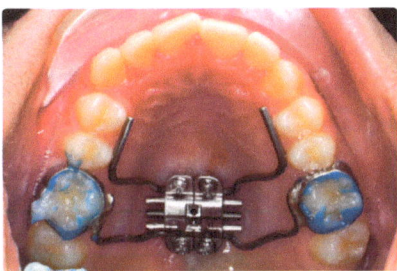 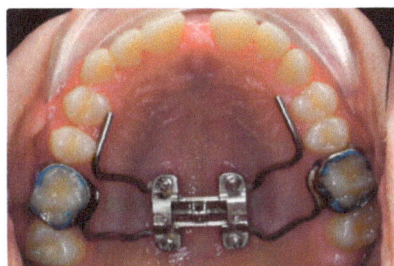

Figure 1. Pre- and post-expansion MARPE device design.

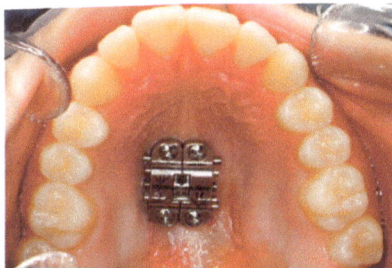 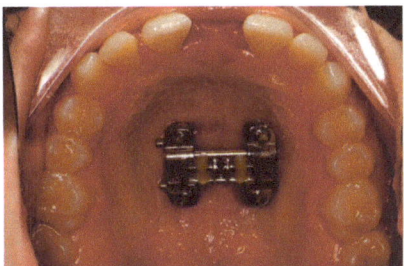

Figure 2. Pre- and post-expansion BAME device design.

2.2. Digital Procedure and Measurements in the CBCT

Palalign Round Head Type (Osteonic Co., Ltd., Seoul, Republic of Korea), an Ti6Al4V alloy, with diameter of 1.8 mm diameter and 10, 12, 14, or 16 mm long (depending on the case) microimplants are used to ensure bicorticality. It has been described that this bicorticality is mandatory to ensure the increase the stability and decrease mini-implant deformation and fracture [25]. All appliances were designed digitally, and all the microscrews were placed with digital guidance to reduce clinical placement error [26]. A Power MARPE Type 1 (Osteonic Co., Ltd., Seoul, Republic of Korea) expansion screw was used with an activation rate of four turns per day until the interincisal diastema appeared and then, two turns per day until a 1.5 mm overcorrection per side is achieved. All treatments were performed by the same orthodontist. The study was conducted according to the guidelines of the Declaration of Helsinki. The protocol was reviewed and approved by the Ethics Committee of the Rey Juan Carlos University with internal number (1504202110721).

2.2.1. CBCT Data Acquisition

The patient was subjected to a CT-type radiographic recording (NewTom Giano HR (QR, Verona, Italy) with 300 μm voxel size and a 16 × 18 cm fov before and after MARPE or BAME treatment, and the following indicators were calculated on that 3D X-ray before (T0) and after treatment (T1). All treatments were performed by the same orthodontist.

2.2.2. CBCT Measurement

For the CBCT BLA measurements, the transverse analysis of Case Western Reserve University (CWRU) was followed [27]. Maxillary first molar BLA was measured in the coronal view as the angle between the major axis of the palatal root and the mesiopalatal cusp and the line tangent to the nasal floor. The BLA of the lower molars was the angle between the mesial cusp and the mesial root and the tangent line at the lower edge of the mandibular corpus [28]. The indicators are shown in Table 1 and Figure 3.

Table 1. Description of indicators (BLA: buccolingual angulation, CBI: cortical bone insertion, and CBW: cortical bone width).

Measurements	Description
Bucolingual angulation of the first right upper molar (BLA 16)	Angle between the line passing through the palatal cusp and the root apex of the palatal root of the right upper first molar and the tangent line to the floor of the nostrils.
Bucolingual angulation of the first left upper molar (BLA 26)	Angle between the line passing through the palatal cusp and the root apex of the palatal root of the left upper first molar and the line tangent to the floor of the nostrils.
Bucolingual angulation of the first left lower molar (BLA 36)	Angle between the line passing through the central fossa and the root apex of the lingual root of the first right lower molar and the line tangent to the lower edge of the mandibular corpus.
Bucolingual angulation of the first right lower molar (BLA 46)	Angle between the line passing through the central fossa and the root apex of the lingual root of the first lower left molar and the line tangent to the lower edge of the mandibular body.
Cortical bone insertion (CBI)	Labial cortical bone insertion with respect to the cementoenamel junction of the upper first molars
Cortical bone width (CBW)	Labial cortical bone thickness. The distance from the furca of the upper first molars to the most external point of the labial cortical bone was taken.

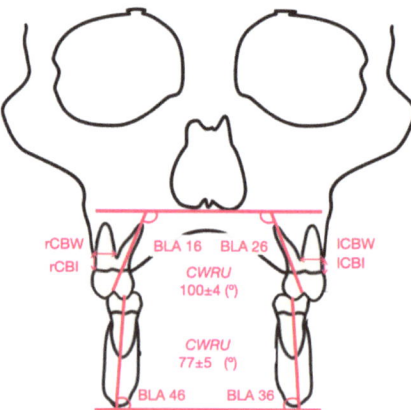

Figure 3. Indicators of BLA, CBI, and CBW. Angulation standard in the maxillary and mandibular molars according to CWRU.

Cortical bone insertion (CBI) and cortical bone width (CBW) of the right and left upper first molars were also measured (Figure 3).

An example of how the measurements were carried out can be found in the Supplementary Material.

2.3. Statistical Analysis

All statistical analyses were performed using the Statistical Package for the Social Sciences version 28.0 for Windows (IBM, Armonk, NY, USA). The Kolmogorov–Smirnov test was used to evaluate the assumption of normality, which was confirmed. A descriptive analysis was carried out to expose the details of the sample, such as age, sex, appliance type, maturation stage of the suture, and type of suture opening achieved after treatment. An intraclass correlation coefficient (ICC) was used to determine the intra-observer reliability of the measurements through reliability analysis in SPSS. The intraclass correlation coefficient (ICC) was calculated considering poor (ICC < 0.40), fair to good ($0.40 \leq ICC \leq 0.75$), and excellent (ICC > 0.75). Three measurements were also carried out for each indicator and for each investigation time, and the measurement error was calculated. Subsequently, a paired sample *t*-test was performed to evaluate the T0–T1 change of dental measurements obtained with MARPE and BAME, and a student *t*-test to compare changes in skeletal measurements between MARPE and BAME. In addition, Cohen's d was used for the effect of the sample in the analysis of the differences of the means with the *t*-test. A measurement with low effect was considered as d ≈ 0.2, medium d ≈ 0.5, and high d ≈ 0.8 [29]. An ANOVA one-factor analysis was performed to evaluate the loss of CBI and CBW after treatment with both therapies. Then, a univariate analysis was done to evaluate the loss of CBI and CBW and their relationship with the CWRU at T0. Statistical significance was established at $p < 0.05$.

3. Results

This study presents an ICC > 0.9 in the evaluations performed (Table 2).

Table 2. Intraclass Correlation Coefficient (ICC) and Measurement Error (ME).

	ICC	ME
BLA 16	0.972	0.26° ± 0.56
BLA 26	0.912	0.19° ± 0.42
BLA 36	0.998	0.37° ± 0.67
BLA 46	0.986	0.25° ± 0.55

3.1. General Descriptive Analysis

The sample size was 36 subjects, and 41.7% of the subjects were male and 58.3% were female. The mean age of the subjects was 27.42 ± 8.53, with an age range of 18 to 49. The MARPE technique was used in 18 subjects (50%), and the BAME technique was used in 18 subjects (50%). Regarding the relationship between device type and sex, MARPE was used in 60% of the male subjects, whilst BAME was used in the remaining 40%, and MARPE was used in 42.9% of the female subjects, whilst BAME in the remaining 57.1%. No differences in gender distribution were found (X(1) = 1.029; $p = 0.310$).

3.2. Evaluation of Variables Baseline

To evaluate the similarity between groups at T0, age was compared (MARPE: 29.9 ± 9.4 and BAME: 24.8 ± 6.8; t = 1.83, $p = 0.076$) finding no significant differences. The clinical variables (See Table 3) are right cortical bone insertion (MARPE: 2.9 ± 1.3 y BAME: 2.9 ± 1.7; t = 0.01, $p = 0.496$) and left (MARPE: 3.1 ± 0.9 y BAME: 2.8 ± 1.2; t = 0.667, $p = 0.255$), right cortical bone width (MARPE: 6.66 ± 1.6 BAME: 7.1 ± 0.8; t = 1.044, $p = 0.153$) and left (MARPE: 6.8 ± 1.0 y BAME: 7.1 ± 0.9; t = 0.947, $p = 0.175$), buccal lingual angulation in right upper molar (MARPE: 99.5 ± 7.3 y BAME: 101.4 ± 6.4; t = 0.829, $p = 0.413$), and buccal lingual angulation in left upper molar (MARPE: 97.4 ± 7.8 y BAME: 102.8 ± 10.1; t = 0.1.782, p = 0.08). No differences were found between either groups.

Table 3. Descriptive and comparative analysis of changes in BLA for MARPE T1–T0 and descriptive and comparative analysis of changes in BLA for BAME T1–T0.

	MARPE T0 M (SD)	MARPE T1 M (SD)	MARPE T1–T0 M (SD)	p Value T1–T0
BLA 16 (°)	99.52 (7.35)	103.94 (8.02)	4.42 (10.25)	0.085
BLA 26 (°)	97.47 (7.89)	101.14 (7.69)	3.67 (9.56)	0.122
BLA 36 (°)	76.01 (5.50)	77.26 (5.95)	1.02 (4.21)	0.222
BLA 46 (°)	76.46 (8.13)	77.58 (6.93)	1.12 (6.04)	0.440
	BAME T0	BAME T1	BAME T1–T0	p value T1–T0
BLA 16 (°)	101.44 (5.88)	100.93 (8.82)	− 0.51 (4.61)	0.644
BLA 26 (°)	102.88 (10.16)	105.22 (8.75)	2.34 (4.51)	0.042 *
BLA 36 (°)	77.06(5.81)	75.96 (6.41))	− 1.10 (6.71)	0.496
BLA 46 (°)	77.57(7.61)	78.36 (6.51)	0.79 (4.17)	0.434

* = p< 0.05.

3.3. Changes in T1–T0 Bucolingual Angulation of First Molar

The angulations of the upper and lower right molars as well as the left first molars were calculated according to the expansion therapy used. Torque increases of 4.42 ± 10.25° and 3.67 ± 9.56° in the right and left upper first molars, respectively, were observed in the cases treated with MARPE. Torque increases of − 0.51 ± 4.61° and 2.34 ± 4.51° in the right and left upper first molars, respectively, were observed in the cases treated with BAME. Compared with the used therapies (Table 4), MARPE produced a greater bucolingual inclination compared to BAME, although these differences were not statistically significant.

Table 4. Comparative analysis of T1–T0 for MARPE and BAME appliances.

	MARPE T1–T0	BAME T1–T0	p Value	Cohen's d
BLA 16 (°)	4.42 (10.25)	− 0.51 (4.61)	0.071	0.620
BLA 26 (°)	3.67 (9.56)	2.34 (4.51)	0.594	0.177
BLA 36 (°)	1.02 (4.21)	− 1.10 (6.71)	0.274	0.378
BLA 46 (°)	1.12 (6.04)	0.79 (4.17)	0.847	0.063

In relation to BLA 36 and BLA 46, there was an increase in BLA for the cases treated with MARPE (BLA 36: 1.02 ± 4.21°; BLA 46: 1.12 ± 6.04°), but for BAME, this increase was lower than MARPE for only one of the lower molars (BLA 46: 0.79 ± 4.17°), whereas for BLA 36, there was an inclination loss (−1.1 ± 6.71°) (see Table 4).

3.4. The Loss of CBI and CBW and Their Relationship with the CWRU at T0

In cases where the CWRU was less than 96° at the beginning of the treatment, a slight bone insertion gain (0.24 ± 0.61 mm) was observed, whereas if the CWRU was 96–104° (−0.08 ± 1.05 mm) or higher than 104° (−0.29 ± 1.06 mm), a slight bone insertion loss was observed. These differences were not significant (F = 0.874, p = 0.427), as seen in Figure 4.

Regarding labial cortical bone loss, a slight loss was observed in all the groups, but the least loss was observed in the CWRU = 96–104° group (−0.01 ± 0.69 mm). There was a greater loss for the CWRU > 104° group (−0.24 ± 0.61 mm) and a median loss for the CWRU < 96° group (−0.13 ± 0.53 mm).

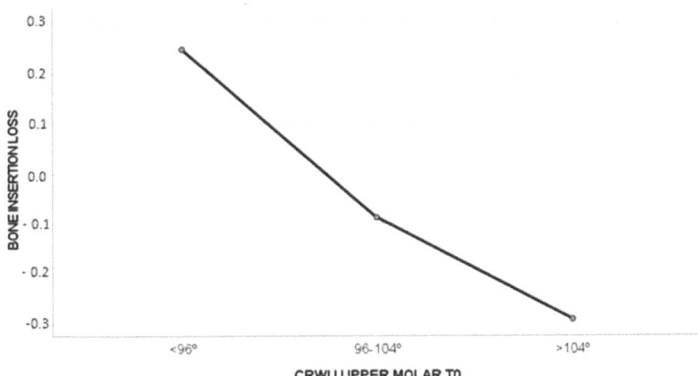

Figure 4. Amount of CBI loss (mm) compared to CWRU T0.

This loss of labial cortical bone was less in cases where the posterior molar torque was correct at T0, but these differences were not significant ($F = 0.440$, $p = 0.648$), as seen in Figure 5.

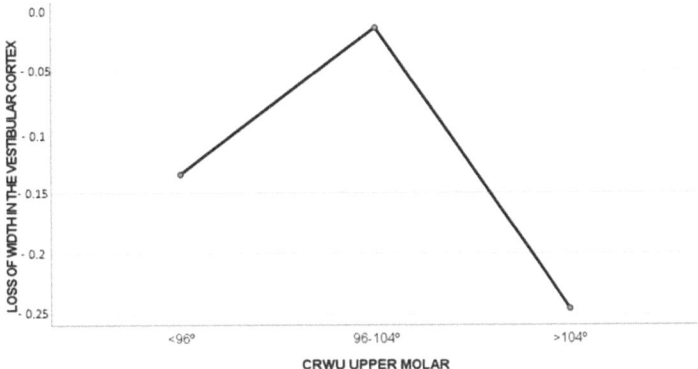

Figure 5. Amount of CBW loss (mm) compared to CWRU T0.

4. Discussion

The two main objectives of this research were to study (i.) the BLA changes in the first upper and lower molars and (ii.) the loss of CBI and CBW in patients with maxillary compression treated with MARPE and BAME. For this study, different measurements were taken in the CBCT, and they were taken before (T0) and after (T1) maxillary expansion therapy. Several studies, such as those by Shewinvanakitkul [27], Evangelinakis [30], Shewinvanakitkul et al. [31], Karamitsou [32], Miyamoto [33], Copeland [34], Streit [35], and Palomo et al. [36], have described the CWRU method for measuring the BLA in canines and the upper and lower molars, and these studies have established some standards. Those standards were (i) $100 \pm 4°$ of BLA in upper first molars and (ii) $77 \pm 4°$ of BLA in lower first molars.

The labial molar angulation after MARPE therapy is commonly found in the literature [8,37–39], but it has not been compared with the labial angulation of the lower molars or in treatments performed with MARPE and BAME techniques.

In the article by Jia et al. [38], dental changes were compared in 30 patients treated with MARPE and 30 patients treated with conventional bone-borne maxillary expansion. CBCTs were taken before expansion and 1 week after expansion, and the change of the labiolingual inclination of the upper right and left first molars was studied, which resulted in the obtainment of the angle between the lines passing through the palatal orifice of the chamber and the apex of the palatal root and the original horizontal line. Torque increases of 3.82 ± 4.07° and 2.72 ± 3.44° were shown in the right and the left upper first molars, respectively. The results obtained in our research for the cases treated with MARPE do not coincide with the results obtained in the article by Jia et al. [38], and this disparity may be because our research was conducted in adults.

De Oliveira et al. [39] compared skeletal and dental changes in 17 patients treated with MARPE and 15 patients treated with SARPE. Three-dimensional radiographic records were also taken just before and after the expansion. In the group of patients treated with MARPE, the increase in BLA of the upper right and left first molars was 2.87 ± 1.94° and in the SARPE group, it was 3.39 ± 2.41°.

Gunyuz Toklu et al. [37] compared periodontal, dentoalveolar, and skeletal changes in cases treated with tooth-borne and tooth-bone-borne expansion appliances in 26 patients. CBCTs were taken before treatment (T1) and at the end of 3 months of retention (T2). It measured the changes in the molar mesiobuccal bone thickness (M1 MBBT) and molar dental inclination (M1 D1) of the upper right and left first molar between T1 and T2. The results of the MARPE group for M1 MBBT were 0.89 ± 0.72 mm and 0.98 ± 0.61 mm and for M1D1 were −2.43 ± 5.54° and −2.89 ± 4.90° for right and left upper first molar, respectively, between T1 and T2. The results obtained in our research for the cases treated with MARPE do not coincide with the results in the article of Gunyuz Toklu et al. [37], and this disparity may be because our second measurement in the CBCT was immediately after expansion.

This research shows an increase in the BLA of the upper first molars. A variation in the BLA of the lower molars was also observed. Regarding the comparison between the cases treated with MARPE and BAME, it was observed that the molar torque increased significantly less in cases treated with BAME. This increase may be due to the dental anchorage at the level of upper first molars of the design in MARPE appliances. These results contradict the conclusions drawn by Khosravi et al. [40] in their systematic review of tooth tipping in treatments carried out using MARPE and BAME devices. The article by Khosravi et al. [40] compared four studies that examined rapid maxillary expansion between bone-borne and tooth-borne appliance following surgical assisted maxillary expansion. Similar dental tippings were reported for both bone-borne and tooth-borne appliances with no significant difference between the two devices.

Whether the initial BLA in the upper first molars at T0 affected the loss of CBI and CBW was also considered. It was observed that when the BLA (100 ± 4° according to CWRU) at T0 was correct, there is increased bone insertion. In cases where the buccolingual angulation did not fall within the CWRU standard, slight bone insertion loss was observed. The gains were slight, but there were differences. Regarding the CBW loss, CBW gain was observed. If the T0 BLA was negative and MARPE or BAME therapies were performed, the labial cortical bone gained some width. These differences were not statistically significant. The results of this research coincide with those previously observed in the study by Baysal et al. [41] regarding CBI loss, but our findings do not support the conclusions drawn in a previous study [41] that also showed CBW loss.

The contribution of this study should be evaluated after taking into account its limitations. The data presented in this research should be interpreted with caution due to the limited sample size. The observation period of the results was also short, and a measurement after the removal of the device may prove useful to corroborate the stability of the results. As for the periodontal measurements, an investigation in which they will be performed using a periodontal probe instead of measurements taken from CBCTs would also be beneficial.

Other variables, such as root resorption of the first molars, were not taken into account. These variables have been assessed in the literature [42], demonstrating root resorption even in teeth not anchored to the appliance; however, this resorption was lower in cases treated with skeletal-supported appliances [43].

The results of this study have a number of important implications for the future practice of orthodontists. On the one hand, the microimplant-assisted expander will bring about a series of dentoalveolar changes in the upper molars. The choice between MARPE and BAME will play an important role in the amount of torque increase as well as the CBI and CBW loss in the upper molars.

5. Conclusions

- Patients treated with MARPE show torque increases in the teeth selected to support the expansion appliance compared to cases treated with BAME.
- In cases where the upper molar torque was correct at the beginning of the treatment, a slight bone insertion gain was observed.
- In cases where the upper molar torque was negative or positive, a slight bone insertion loss was observed.
- Regarding the labial cortical bone loss, a slight gain of CBW was observed in all cases. This increase in labial cortical is higher in cases where posterior molar torque was negative before treatment.

Supplementary Materials: The following supporting information can be downloaded at: https://www.mdpi.com/article/10.3390/biomedicines11092380/s1, Figure S1: Example of measurements taken.

Author Contributions: J.E.-N. contributed to acquisition, drafted the manuscript, and critically revised the manuscript. M.J.G.-O. contributed to conception and design and analysis and interpretation, drafted the manuscript, and critically revised the manuscript. P.E.-L. contributed to acquisition, drafted the manuscript, and critically revised the manuscript. M.R. contributed to conception and design and critically revised the manuscript. All authors have read and agreed to the published version of the manuscript.

Funding: This research received no external funding.

Institutional Review Board Statement: The study was conducted according to the guidelines of the Declaration of Helsinki and was approved by the Ethics Committee of Rey Juan Carlos University (protocol code 1504202110721).

Informed Consent Statement: Informed consent was obtained from all subjects involved in the study.

Data Availability Statement: The data that support the findings of this study are available on request from the corresponding author. The data are not publicly available due to privacy and ethical restrictions.

Acknowledgments: Thank you to all that participated in this research.

Conflicts of Interest: The authors declare no conflict of interest.

References

1. Bucci, R.; Montanaro, D.; Rongo, R.; Valletta, R.; Michelotti, A.; D'Antò, V. Effects of maxillary expansion on the upper airways: Evidence from systematic reviews and meta-analyses. *J. Oral. Rehabil.* **2019**, *46*, 377–387. [CrossRef] [PubMed]
2. Suzuki, H.; Moon, W.; Previdente, L.H.; Suzuki, S.S.; Garcez, A.S.; Consolaro, A. Miniscrew-assisted rapid palatal expander (MARPE): The quest for pure orthopedic movement. *Dent. Press. J. Orthod.* **2016**, *21*, 17–23. [CrossRef] [PubMed]
3. Wilmes, B.; Tarraf, N.; Drescher, D. Treatment of maxillary transversal deficiency by using a mini-implant-borne rapid maxillary expander and aligners in combination. *Am. J. Orthod. Dentofac. Orthop.* **2021**, *160*, 147–154. [CrossRef] [PubMed]
4. Lee, K.J.; Park, Y.C.; Park, J.Y.; Hwang, W.S. Miniscrew-assisted nonsurgical palatal expansion before orthognathic surgery for a patient with severe mandibular prognathism. *Am. J. Orthod. Dentofac. Orthop.* **2010**, *137*, 830–839. [CrossRef]
5. Moon, W. An interview with Won Moon. By André Wilson Machado, Barry Briss, Greg J Huang, Richard Kulbersh and Sergei Godeiro Fernandes Rabelo Caldas. *Dent. Press. J. Orthod.* **2013**, *18*, 12–28.
6. Winsauer, H.; Vlachojannis, J.; Winsauer, C.; Ludwig, B.; Walter, A. A bone-borne appliance for rapid maxillary expansion. *J. Clin. Orthod.* **2013**, *47*, 375–381.
7. Garib, D.G.; Henriques, J.F.; Janson, G.; de Freitas, M.R.; Fernandes, A.Y. Periodontal effects of rapid maxillary expansion with tooth-tissue-borne and tooth-borne expanders: A computed tomography evaluation. *Am. J. Orthod. Dentofac. Orthop.* **2006**, *129*, 749–758. [CrossRef]

8. Kim, H.; Park, S.H.; Park, J.H.; Lee, K.J. Nonsurgical maxillary expansion in a 60-year-old patient with gingival recession and crowding. *Korean J. Orthod.* **2021**, *51*, 217–227. [CrossRef]
9. Kapetanović, A.; Theodorou, C.I.; Bergé, S.; Schols, J.G.J.H.; Xi, T. Efficacy of miniscrew-assisted rapid palatal expansion (MARPE) in late adolescents and adults: A systematic review and meta-analysis. *Eur. J. Orthod.* **2021**, *43*, 313–323. [CrossRef]
10. Lagravère, M.O.; Gamble, J.; Major, P.W.; Heo, G. Transverse dental changes after tooth-borne and bone-borne maxillary expansion. *Int. Orthod.* **2013**, *11*, 21–34. [CrossRef]
11. Park, J.J.; Park, Y.C.; Lee, K.J.; Cha, J.Y.; Tahk, J.H.; Choi, Y.J. Skeletal and dentoalveolar changes after miniscrew-assisted rapid palatal expansion in young adults: A cone-beam computed tomography study. *Korean J. Orthod.* **2017**, *47*, 77–86. [CrossRef] [PubMed]
12. Lim, H.M.; Park, Y.C.; Lee, K.J.; Kim, K.H.; Choi, Y.J. Stability of dental, alveolar, and skeletal changes after miniscrew-assisted rapid palatal expansion. *Korean J. Orthod.* **2017**, *47*, 313–322. [CrossRef] [PubMed]
13. Ghoneima, A.; Abdel-Fattah, E.; Hartsfield, J.; El-Bedwehi, A.; Kamel, A.; Kula, K. Effects of rapid maxillary expansion on the craial and circummaxillary sutures. *Am. J. Orthod. Dentofac. Orthop.* **2011**, *140*, 510–519. [CrossRef]
14. Cantarella, D.; Dominguez-Mompell, R.; Moschik, C.; Sfogliano, L.; Elkenawy, I.; Pan, H.C.; Mallya, S.M.; Moon, W. Zygomatico-maxillary modifications in the horizontal plane induced by micro-implant-supported skeletal expander, analyzed with CBCT images. *Prog. Orthod.* **2018**, *19*, 1–8. [CrossRef]
15. Lee, S.C.; Park, J.H.; Bayome, M.; Kim, K.B.; Araujo, E.A.; Kook, Y.A. Effect of bone-borne rapid maxillary expanders with and without surgical assistance on the craniofacial structures using finite element analysis. *Am. J. Orthod. Dentofac. Orthop.* **2014**, *145*, 638–648. [CrossRef]
16. Hayes, J. A Clinical Approach to Identify Transverse Discrepancies. In Proceedings of the Pennsylvania Association of Orthodontists, Philadelphia, PA, USA, 8 March 2003.
17. Tamburrino, R.K.; Boucher, N.S.; Vanarsdall, R.L.; Secchi, A. The transverse dimension: Diagnosis and relevance to functional occlusion. *RWISO J.* **2010**, 13–22.
18. Gioka, C.; Eliades, T. Materials-induced variation in the torque expression of preadjusted appliances. *Am. J. Orthod. Dentofac. Orthop.* **2004**, *125*, 323–328. [CrossRef] [PubMed]
19. Mestriner, M.A.; Enoki, C.; Mucha, J.N. Normal torque of the buccal surface of mandibular teeth and its relationship with bracket positioning: A study in normal occlusion. *Braz. Dent. J.* **2006**, *17*, 155–160. [CrossRef]
20. McLaughlin, R.P.; Bennett, J.C. Finishing with the preadjusted orthodontic appliance. *Semin. Orthod.* **2003**, *9*, 165–183. [CrossRef]
21. Lucchese, A.; Manuelli, M.; Albertini, P.; Ghislanzoni, L.H. Transverse and torque dental changes after passive self-ligating fixed therapy: A two-year follow-up study. *Am. J. Orthod. Dentofac. Orthop.* **2019**, *156*, 94–103. [CrossRef]
22. Goh, S.; Dreyer, C.; Weir, T. The predictability of the mandibular curve of Wilson, buccolingual crown inclination, and transverse expansion expression with Invisalign treatment. *Am. J. Orthod. Dentofac. Orthop.* **2023**, *163*, 109–116. [CrossRef] [PubMed]
23. Canan, S.; Şenışık, N.E. Comparison of the treatment effects of different rapid maxillary expansion devices on the maxilla and the mandible. Part 1: Evaluation of dentoalveolar changes. *Am. J. Orthod. Dentofac. Orthop.* **2017**, *151*, 1125–1138. [CrossRef]
24. Moon, H.W.; Kim, M.J.; Ahn, H.W.; Kim, S.J.; Kim, S.H.; Chung, K.R.; Nelson, G. Molar inclination and surrounding alveolar bone change relative to the design of bone-borne maxillary expanders: A CBCT study. *Angle Orthod.* **2020**, *90*, 13–22. [CrossRef]
25. Bazzani, M.; Cevidanes, L.H.S.; al Turkestani, N.N.; Annarumma, F.; McMullen, C.; Ruellas, A.C.O.; Massaro, C.; Rego, M.V.N.N.; Yatabe, M.S.; Kim-Berman, H.; et al. Three-dimensional comparison of bone-borne and tooth-bone-borne maxillary expansion in young adults with maxillary skeletal deficiency. *Orthod. Craniofac Res.* **2022**, *26*, 151–162. [CrossRef] [PubMed]
26. Ronsivalle, V.; Venezia, P.; Bennici, O.; D'Antò, V.; Giudice, A. Accuracy of digital workfloe for placing orthodontic miniscrews using generic and licensed open systems. A 3d imaging analysis of non-native.stl files for guided protocols. *BMC Oral Health* **2023**, *494*, 23.
27. Shewinvanakitkul, W. A New Method to Measure Buccolingual Inclination Using Cbct. Master's Thesis, Case Western Reserve University, Cleveland, OH, USA, 2009.
28. Yehya Mostafa, R.; Bous, R.M.; Hans, M.G.; Valiathan, M.; Copeland, G.E.; Palomo, J.M. Effects of Case Western Reserve University's transverse analysis on the quality of orthodontic treatment. *Am. J. Orthod. Dentofac. Orthop.* **2019**, *152*, 178–192, Erratum in: *Am. J. Orthod. Dentofac. Orthop.* **2019**, *155*, 618. [CrossRef]
29. Cohen, J. *Statistical Power Analysis for the Behavioral Sciences*, 2nd ed.; Lawrence Erlbaum Associates: Hillsdale, NJ, USA, 1988.
30. Evangelinakis, N. Changes in Buccolingual Inclination of Mandibular Canines and First Molars after Orthodontic Treatment using CBCT. Ph.D. Thesis, Case Western Reserve University, Cleveland, OH, USA, 2010.
31. Shewinvanakitkul, W.; Hans, M.G.; Narendran, S.; Martin Palomo, J. Measuring Buccolingual Inclination of Mandibular Canines and First Molars using CBCT. *Orthod. Craniofac. Res.* **2011**, *14*, 168–174. [CrossRef] [PubMed]
32. Karamitsou, E. Pretreatment Buccolingual Inclination of Maxillary Canines and First Molars. Master's Thesis, Case Western Reserve University, Cleveland, OH, USA, 2011.
33. Miyamoto, M.J. Changes in Buccolingual Inclination of Maxillary Canines and First Molars after Orthodontic Treatment Using CBCT. Ph.D. Thesis, Case Western Reserve University, Cleveland, OH, USA, 2011.
34. Copeland, G. Case Western Reserve University Transverse Analysis: Clinical Application. Ph.D. Thesis, Case Western Reserve University, Cleveland, OH, USA, 2012.

35. Streit, L. Case Western Reserve University Transverse Analysis—Developing Norms. Ph.D. Thesis, Case Western Reserve University, Cleveland, OH, USA, 2012.
36. Palomo, J.M.; Valiathan, M.; Hans, G.M. 3D Orthodontic Diagnosis and Treatment Planning. In *Cone Beam Computed Tomography in Orthodontics: Indications, Insights, and Innovations*; Kapila, S.D., Ed.; John Wiley & Sons Inc.: Ames, IA, USA; Hoboken, NJ, USA, 2014; pp. 221–246.
37. Gunyuz Toklu, M.; Germec-Cakan, D.; Tozlu, M. Periodontal, dentoalveolar, and skeletal effects of tooth-borne and tooth-bone-borne expansion appliances. *Am. J. Orthod. Dentofac. Orthop.* **2015**, *148*, 97–109. [CrossRef]
38. Jia, H.; Zhuang, L.; Zhang, N.; Bian, Y.; Li, S. Comparison of skeletal maxillary transverse deficiency treated by microimplant-assisted rapid palatal expansion and tooth-borne expansion during the post-pubertal growth spurt stage: A prospective cone beam computed tomography study. *Angle Orthod.* **2021**, *91*, 36–45. [CrossRef]
39. De Oliveira, C.B.; Ayub, P.; Ledra, I.M.; Murata, W.H.; Suzuki, S.S.; Ravelli, D.B.; Santos-Pinto, A. Microimplant assisted rapid palatal expansion vs surgically assisted rapid palatal expansion for maxillary transverse discrepancy treatment. *Am. J. Orthod. Dentofac. Orthop.* **2021**, *159*, 733–742. [CrossRef]
40. Khosravi, M.; Ugolini, A.; Miresmaeili, A.; Mirzaei, H.; Shahidi-Zandi, V.; Soheilifar, S.; Karami, M.; Mahmoudzadeh, M. Tooth-borne versus bone-borne rapid maxillary expansion for transverse maxillary deficiency: A systematic review. *Int. Orthod.* **2019**, *17*, 425–436. [CrossRef] [PubMed]
41. Baysal, A.; Uysal, T.; Veli, I.; Ozer, T.; Karadede, I.; Hekimoglu, S. Evaluation of alveolar bone loss following rapid maxillary expansion using cone-beam computed tomography. *Korean J. Orthod.* **2013**, *43*, 83–95. [CrossRef] [PubMed]
42. Leonardi, R.; Ronsivalle, V.; Barbato, E.; Lagravère, M.; Flores-Mir, C.; Lo Giudice, A. External root resorption (ERR) and rapid maxillary expansion (RME) at post-retention stage: A comparison between tooth-borne and bone-borne RME. *Prog. Orthod.* **2022**, *23*, 1–9. [CrossRef]
43. Leonardi, R.; Ronsisvalle, V.; Isola, G.; Cicciù, M.; Lagravère, M.; Flores-Mir, C.; Lo Giudice, A. External root resorption and rapid maxillary expansion in the short-term: A CBCT comparative study between tooth-borne and bone-borne appliances, using 3D imaging digital technology. *BMC Oral. Health* **2023**, *558*, 23. [CrossRef] [PubMed]

Disclaimer/Publisher's Note: The statements, opinions and data contained in all publications are solely those of the individual author(s) and contributor(s) and not of MDPI and/or the editor(s). MDPI and/or the editor(s) disclaim responsibility for any injury to people or property resulting from any ideas, methods, instructions or products referred to in the content.

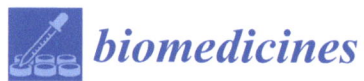 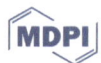

Systematic Review

Effect of Silver Diamine Fluoride on Bacterial Biofilms—A Review including In Vitro and In Vivo Studies

Hind Mubaraki [1], Navin Anand Ingle [1,*], Mohammad Abdul Baseer [1], Osamah M AlMugeiren [1], Sarah Mubaraki [1], Marco Cicciù [2] and Giuseppe Minervini [3,*]

1. Preventive Dentistry Department, College of Dentistry, Riyadh Elm University, Riyadh 13244, Saudi Arabia; o.almugeiren@riyadh.edu.sa (O.M.A.)
2. Department of Biomedical and Surgical and Biomedical Sciences, Catania University, 95123 Catania, Italy; mcicciu@unime.it
3. Multidisciplinary Department of Medical-Surgical and Dental Specialties, University of Campania, 80138 Naples, Italy
* Correspondence: navin.ingle@riyadh.edu.sa (N.A.I.); giuseppe.minervini@unicampania.it (G.M.)

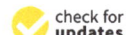

Citation: Mubaraki, H.; Ingle, N.A.; Baseer, M.A.; AlMugeiren, O.M.; Mubaraki, S.; Cicciù, M.; Minervini, G. Effect of Silver Diamine Fluoride on Bacterial Biofilms—A Review including In Vitro and In Vivo Studies. *Biomedicines* 2023, 11, 1641. https://doi.org/10.3390/biomedicines11061641

Academic Editor: Guruprakash Subbiahdoss

Received: 19 March 2023
Revised: 29 May 2023
Accepted: 31 May 2023
Published: 5 June 2023

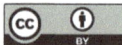

Copyright: © 2023 by the authors. Licensee MDPI, Basel, Switzerland. This article is an open access article distributed under the terms and conditions of the Creative Commons Attribution (CC BY) license (https://creativecommons.org/licenses/by/4.0/).

Abstract: Caries/carious lesions are a growing concern among the general population across the world, and different strategies are evolving to combat the bacterial invasion that resultantly leads to caries. In this systematic review, we are looking to analyse the role of silver diamine fluoride (SDF) on the growth of bacterial biofilms. The search strategy for the studies to be selected for the review was initiated by a search across multiple databases, which ultimately yielded 15 studies that were in accordance with our objectives. The reviewed articles indicate a very clear correlation between the usage of SDF and the decrease in bacterial biofilms, which are limited not just to one or two but multiple bacterial species. As shown by the events favoring SDF's odds ratio of 3.59 (with a 95% confidence interval of 2.13 to 6.05), a risk ratio of 1.63 (1.32 to 2.00), and a risk difference of 0.28 (0.16 to 0.40), there was strong evidence that SDF is a successful treatment for reducing bacterial biofilms in dental practice. This study offers substantial proof that SDF works well to reduce bacterial biofilms in dentistry practices. We advise further investigation to examine the potential of SDF as a standard therapy choice for dental caries and related conditions given the obvious relationship between the use of SDF and the reduction in bacterial biofilms.

Keywords: bacteria; biofilms; caries; SDF; *Streptococcus*

1. Introduction

Oral biofilms, also known as dental plaque, are complex microbial communities that form on the surfaces of teeth and other structures in the mouth [1–4]. These biofilms are composed of a variety of microorganisms, including bacteria, fungi, and viruses, and can vary in composition depending on factors such as diet, hygiene habits, and genetics [5]. The formation of oral biofilms begins with the attachment of bacteria to the surface of the tooth, known as the pellicle layer [6]. Over time, the biofilm can become thicker and more complex, with different layers of microorganisms forming different niches based on their specific needs and environmental preferences. For example, some bacteria may prefer to live in areas with more oxygen, while others may thrive in areas with less oxygen [7]. While they are a natural part of the mouth's ecology, they can also pose a threat to oral health if left unchecked [8,9]. For example, certain types of bacteria in the biofilm can produce acids that damage tooth enamel and lead to cavities. Additionally, the build-up of plaque can lead to gum disease, which can cause tooth loss and other oral health problems [10,11].

The primary pathogens responsible for tooth decay come in various numbers and ratios and generate bacteria that make acids and bases [12–14]. Mutans streptococci (MS), one of the speculated acid-producing bacteria, was discovered to be crucial in the early stages of dental caries on both enamel and root surfaces after a comprehensive literature analysis [15–17]. This is true for several reasons, including the fact that MS is the species that is frequently isolated from a caries lesion, that it is highly acidogenic and aciduric, and that it can produce surface antigens and water-insoluble glucan, which promote bacterial adhesion to other bacteria and to the tooth's surface. To break the closed loop of the process, a measure that can prevent the microorganisms that produce acid must be taken [18,19].

SDF is a unique and versatile liquid treatment that has garnered a great deal of attention in recent years [20]. SDF is a highly effective and cost-effective treatment for a wide range of dental issues, including tooth decay, gum disease, and oral infections [21,22]. In this article, we will explore the properties of SDF and the role it plays in modern dentistry [23,24]. SDF is a clear, odorless liquid that contains two main ingredients: silver and fluoride [25]. Silver is a powerful antimicrobial agent that has been used for centuries to treat various infections, while fluoride is a mineral that is known to strengthen tooth enamel and prevent cavities. When these two ingredients are combined, they create a powerful solution that is highly effective at killing bacteria and preventing the spread of infection [26].

One of the key advantages of SDF is its ability to penetrate deep into the tooth structure, where it can kill bacteria and prevent further decay [27]. This makes it an excellent choice for treating cavities and other dental issues that are difficult to reach with traditional dental tools. SDF is also highly effective at killing the bacteria that cause gum disease, which is a major contributor to tooth loss in adults [28].

In addition to its antimicrobial properties, SDF is also highly effective at preventing the spread of infection [29]. When applied to an infected tooth or gum tissue, it quickly kills the bacteria and prevents it from spreading to other parts of the mouth. This can be particularly important for patients who are at risk of developing oral infections due to weakened immune systems or other medical conditions [30].

Another important property of SDF is its ability to strengthen tooth enamel and prevent cavities [31]. Fluoride is a mineral that is known to bond with tooth enamel, making it stronger and more resistant to decay [31]. When applied to the teeth, SDF releases fluoride ions that bond with the enamel and help to prevent the development of cavities. This makes it an excellent choice for patients who are at risk of developing tooth decay due to poor oral hygiene or other factors [32]. Moreover, unlike traditional dental treatments, which can be painful and time-consuming, SDF can be applied quickly and easily in a single visit. This makes it an excellent choice for patients who are anxious about dental procedures or who have difficulty sitting still for long periods of time [33–35].

The creation of in vitro biofilm models has simplified the investigation of mouth biofilm today [36,37]. But this approach isn't without several drawbacks [38]. An option is to use an in-situ biofilm model to study natural oral biofilms and various therapeutic approaches. Several gaps in the literature need to be addressed when examining the effect of SDF on bacterial biofilms. Firstly, there is a need for standardized protocols and methodologies to study the effect of SDF on biofilms. Varying experimental conditions, biofilm models, SDF concentrations, and application methods make it difficult to compare and synthesize findings across studies. Developing standardized protocols would enhance the reliability and reproducibility of research outcomes. Additionally, there is a lack of evidence regarding the long-term effects and durability of SDF on biofilms. Most studies focus on short-term effects, but understanding the persistence and long-term effectiveness of SDF in controlling biofilms is crucial. Furthermore, there is a need for more clinical research assessing the clinical outcomes and patient-centered effects of SDF on biofilms. Comparative studies that assess the effectiveness of SDF compared to other treatments for bacterial biofilms are also lacking. Comparative research would shed light on the relative efficacy, safety, and cost-effectiveness of SDF as a treatment option. Finally, further mechanistic understanding is needed to elucidate the underlying mechanisms of SDF's action on bacterial biofilms. Investigating the interaction between SDF and biofilm components, as well as its impact on biofilm formation, maturation, and eradication, would enhance our understanding of its mode of action. Addressing these gaps in the literature might provide a comprehensive understanding of the effect of SDF on bacterial biofilms and guide its optimal clinical use. Therefore, this investigation aimed to systematically review and meta-analyse the available literature on the effect of SDF on bacterial biofilms. Secondarily, we also wanted to provide an overview of the existing evidence regarding the efficacy of SDF in reducing bacterial biofilms in dental practice. Additionally, the study aimed to evaluate the effectiveness of SDF compared to other biomarkers used in dental practice and to identify potential limitations or biases in the available literature.

2. Materials and Methods

2.1. Eligibility Criteria

All studies were assessed for eligibility according to the following participants, intervention, comparison, and outcomes (PICO) model:

(P) Participants in this systematic review are patients with bacterial biofilms. To include all relevant studies, the Boolean operator "OR" was used to combine different keywords related to bacterial biofilms, such as "biofilm", "plaque" and "microbial colonies".

(I) The intervention consisted of Silver Diamine Fluoride (SDF). To ensure that all relevant studies on SDF were included in the review, the Boolean operator "OR" was used to combine different variations of the keyword, such as "silver diamine fluoride" or "AgF".

(C) The comparison consisted of control groups that compared SDF to other chemical compounds. To identify studies that compare SDF to other biomarkers/control groups, the Boolean operator "AND" was used to combine the intervention and comparison groups that were considered as interventions.

(O) The outcome measures the effect of SDF on bacterial biofilms. To identify studies that measure the effect of SDF on bacterial biofilms, the Boolean operator "AND" was used to combine the intervention and outcome keywords.

Only studies providing data at the end of the intervention were included. Exclusion criteria were as follows: (1) studies that did not investigate the effect of SDF on bacterial biofilms or microbial colonies; (2) studies that did not compare SDF to other biomarkers or control groups; (3) studies that did not report a statistical analysis of the evaluation of SDF; (4) studies that considered the effect of SDF but abstained from revealing the findings; (5) cross-over study design; (6) studies written in a language different from English; and (7) full-text unavailability (i.e., posters and conference abstracts).

2.2. Search Strategy

PubMed, Scopus, and Web of Science databases were systematically searched for articles published from the year 2013 until 2022, following the strategy described in Table 1. Furthermore, a manual search of the references of previous systematic reviews on a similar topic was conducted as well.

Table 1. Search strategy.

PubMed: ("silver diamine fluoride" OR "SDF") AND ("bacterial biofilms" OR "anti-bacterial agents"[MeSH Terms] OR "fluorides"[MeSH Terms] OR "dental caries"[MeSH Terms] OR "*Streptococcus mutans*"[MeSH Terms] OR "dental plaque"[MeSH Terms] OR "biofilms"[MeSH Terms]) AND English[lang]
Web of Sciences: ("silver diamine fluoride" OR "SDF") AND ("bacterial biofilms" OR "anti-bacterial agents" OR "fluorides" OR "dental caries" OR "*Streptococcus mutans*" OR "dental plaque" OR "biofilms") AND Language: (English)
Scopus: ("silver diamine fluoride" OR "SDF") AND ("bacterial biofilms" OR "anti-bacterial agents" OR "fluorides" OR "dental caries" OR "*Streptococcus mutans*" OR "dental plaque" OR "biofilms") AND (LIMIT-TO (DOCTYPE, "ar") OR LIMIT-TO (DOCTYPE, "re")) AND (LIMIT-TO (LANGUAGE, "English"))

This systematic review with meta-analysis was conducted according to the guidance of Preferred Reporting Items for Systematic Reviews and Meta-Analyses (PRISMA) guidelines [39], Figure 1 and the *Cochrane Handbook for Systematic Reviews of Interventions* [40]. The systematic review protocol has been registered on the International Prospective Register of Systematic Reviews (PROSPERO) with acknowledgement of the receipt number 405877.

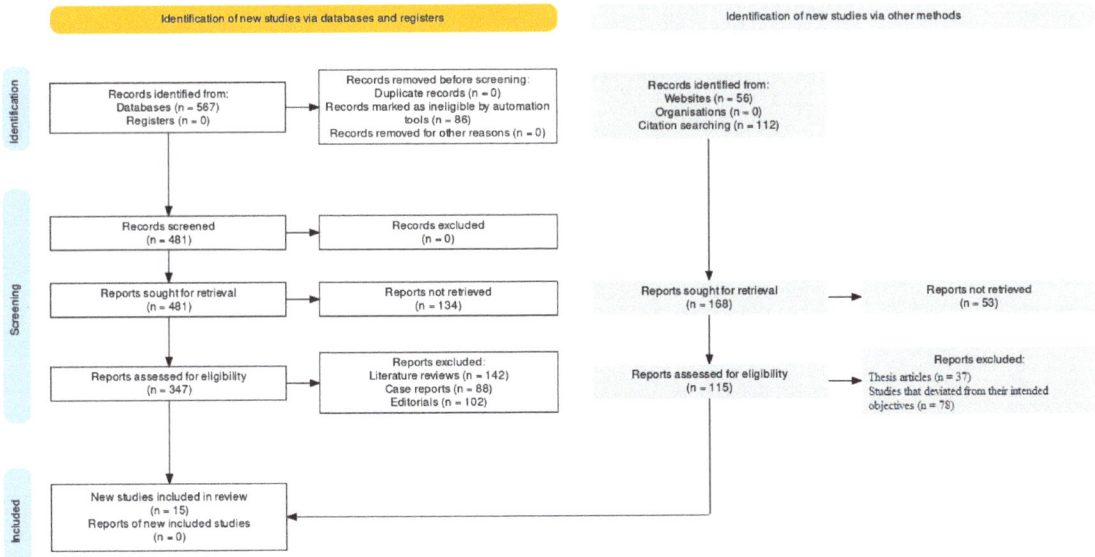

Figure 1. Representation of selection of articles through the PRISMA framework.

2.3. Data Extraction

Two reviewers (S.O. and S.C.) independently extracted data from the included studies using a customized data extraction on a Microsoft Excel sheet. In case of disagreement, the consensus was achieved through a third reviewer.

The following data were extracted: (1) first author; (2) publication year; (3) nationality; (4) type of study design; (5) type of compounds as intervention; (6) type of control (placebo or other); (7) population and the number of patients/biofilms included; (8) SDF's efficacy as an outcome; and (9) main findings.

2.4. Quality Assessment

The ROBINS-E tool was used for the assessment of bias in the selected papers for our review (Figure 2). The tool is used to evaluate the risk of bias in cohort studies, case-control studies, and before–after studies, among others [41].

2.5. Statistical Analysis

Using the data extraction form that the reviewers had compiled in a single dataset, the statistical protocol for this study was initiated by entering the data into RevMan 5, choosing the random effects statistical model for the meta-analysis, calculating the odds ratio, risk ratio, or risk difference for each study and entering the data into the RevMan 5 software (IBM, version 5.4.1, New York, NY, USA), thereby generating a forest plot to graphically display the results of the meta-analysis, assessing the heterogeneity of the studies using the I^2 statistic, interpreting the results of the meta-analysis and drawing conclusions about the effect of SDF on bacterial biofilms, conducting sensitivity analyses to examine the robustness of the meta-analysis results, interpreting and reporting the results of the sensitivity analyses (which included the forest plot, summary of the effect estimates, and interpretation of the heterogeneity and sensitivity analyses).

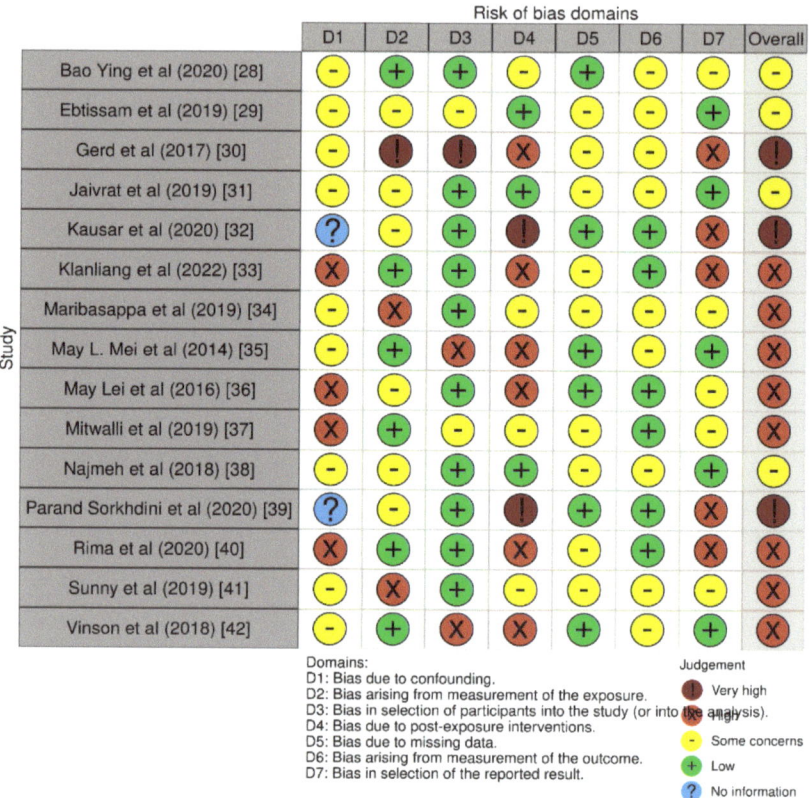

Figure 2. ROBINS-E tool for bias assessment for papers selected for the systematic review.

3. Results

After conducting an extensive search of online journals, a total of 207 documents were identified, out of which 103 papers were initially selected. After eliminating 47 similar or duplicate articles, 56 separate papers were available for further review. Subsequently, after reviewing the abstracts and titles of the submissions, a further 41 papers were excluded. Finally, 15 studies that met the inclusion and exclusion criteria were included in the systematic review and meta-analysis. These studies comprised eight in vitro studies, four case-control studies, and one in situ, ex situ, and ex vivo study each.

The results of the systematic review have been presented in Table 2, providing details of the 15 studies included in the review. The meta-analysis was performed using RevMan 5 software, and the results were presented in the form of forest plots depicting the odds ratio, risk ratio, and risk difference, as shown in Figures 3–5, respectively.

Our investigation revealed a very positive impact of SDF compared to other biomarkers mentioned in the 15 studies. The events favoring SDF demonstrated an odds ratio of 3.59 (2.13, 6.05), a risk ratio of 1.63 (1.32, 2.00), and a risk difference of 0.28 (0.16, 0.40). These findings provide strong evidence that SDF is an effective treatment for reducing bacterial biofilms in dental practice.

The implications of these findings are significant for improving oral health outcomes, particularly for individuals who may not have access to traditional dental treatments or who may have difficulty receiving such treatments. The clear correlation between the usage of SDF and the decrease in bacterial biofilms makes it a potential standard treatment option for dental caries and related conditions. Therefore, further research is recommended to explore the potential of SDF in dental practice.

The statistical analysis displayed an odds ratio of 3.59 (2.13, 6.05) for events favoring SDF compared to other biomarkers/control groups in the selected studies as represented in Figure 3. The forest plot visualized the risk difference for each study included in the meta-analysis, which represented the difference in the proportion of events favoring SDF between the SDF and control groups. The analysis found heterogeneity between studies, with a Tau^2 of 0.49 and a Chi^2 of 31.64 with 14 degrees of freedom ($p = 0.005$) and an I^2 of 56%. The significant p-value for Chi^2 indicates that this heterogeneity was unlikely to have occurred by chance. The Z-statistic for the overall effect was 4.81 ($p < 0.00001$), indicating that the odds of events favoring SDF were significantly higher in the SDF group compared to the control group. In summary, the statistical analysis suggests that SDF is associated with a higher odd of events favoring SDF compared to other biomarkers/control groups, with some degree of heterogeneity between studies. Further research may be needed to better understand this variation.

The risk ratio of 1.63 (1.32, 2.00) is displayed in Figure 4 for events favoring SDF compared to other biomarkers/control groups in the selected studies. The forest plot displayed the risk difference for each study included in the meta-analysis, representing the difference in the proportion of events favoring SDF between the SDF and control groups. The analysis found heterogeneity between studies, with a Tau^2 of 0.08 and a Chi^2 of 36.46 with 14 degrees of freedom ($p = 0.0009$) and an I^2 of 62%. The Z-statistic for the overall effect was 4.60 ($p < 0.00001$), indicating that the odds of events favoring SDF were significantly higher in the SDF group compared to the control group.

The representation of the risk difference in the form of a forest plot in Figure 5 displayed the individual studies included in the meta-analysis, the value of which was found to be 0.28 (0.16, 0.40). The results showed some heterogeneity, with a tau-squared value of 0.03 and a Chi^2 value of 48.79 with 14 degrees of freedom, resulting in a p-value of less than 0.00001. This indicated significant heterogeneity in the results. The overall effect was statistically significant, with a Z-score of 4.72 and a p-value of less than 0.00001. The analysis indicated that SDF had a significant risk difference compared to other biomarkers/control groups, and while some heterogeneity was observed, the overall effect was statistically significant.

Table 2. Variables selected and analysed for the review at the end of the data extraction protocol.

ID and Year	Study Sample (n)	Objectives	Design	Assessment Drawn
Bao Ying et al. (2020) [38]	Five children	To evaluate the antibacterial performance of SDF in dentine biofilms	In vitro	Microbial diversity fell after SDF application.
Ebtissam et al. (2019) [39]	Seventy dentin discs (made from extracted human teeth)	To evaluate the antibacterial performance of CHX and NaOCl as compared to SDF	Case control	SDF exhibited higher antibacterial efficacy as compared to the controls.
Gerd et al. (2017) [40]	100 samples of bovine dentin.	To evaluate the antibacterial performance of NaF and CHX as compared to SDF	In vitro	When compared to control, SDF dramatically reduced bacterial numbers.
Jaivrat et al. (2019) [41]	32 extracted human molars and 32 extracted human premolars	To evaluate the antibacterial performance of CHX, distilled water and PAA as compared to SDF	Case control	SDF-KI was deemed to be effective in eliminating *S. mutans*.
Kausar et al. (2020) [42]	35 *Candida* isolates	To evaluate the antifungal performance of SDF in isolation	In vitro	SDF appeared to successfully stop fungal filamentation even at extremely low doses, complementing its antibacterial activity
Klanliang et al. (2022) [43]	10 healthy individuals (aged between 26–31 years)	To evaluate the microbiological performance of SDF in dentine biofilms	In situ	Dental biofilm development was inhibited and the percentage of killed bacteria was enhanced when SDF was applied to demineralized dentin but only up to 4 days

Table 2. Cont.

ID and Year	Study Sample (n)	Objectives	Design	Assessment Drawn
Maribasappa et al. (2019) [44]	5 patients with carious lesions	To evaluate the antibacterial performance of SDF + potassium iodide (KI).	In vivo	In four of the five patients, SDF + KI totally stopped the growth of S. mutans
May L. Mei et al. (2014) [45]	12 primary upper-central carious incisors	To evaluate the physicochemical performance of SDF in carious teeth	Ex vivo	Clinical SDF application enhanced the levels of dentine remineralization
May Lei et al. (2016) [46]	6 premolars	To evaluate the antibacterial performance of SDF in two different types of restorations	In vitro	SDF application made both the types of restorations more resistant to subsequent caries.
Mitwalli et al. (2019) [47]	20 participants (who had at least one cervical carious lesion or soft cavitated root)	To evaluate the microbiological performance of SDF in carious lesions	In vitro	Several bacterium species showed a substantial decrease in relative abundance following SDF treatment.
Najmeh et al. (2018) [48]	45 extracted deciduous canines	To evaluate the antibacterial performance of fluorinated varnish as compared to SDF	In vitro	No significant differences between the antibacterial performance of both the compounds were observed
Parand Sorkhdini et al. (2020) [49]	90 human enamel samples	To evaluate the antibacterial performance of $AgNO_3$, KF and water as compared to SDF	Case control	SDF performed on a similar parlance as DW and KF that SDF was compared with.
Rima et al. (2020) [50]	Samples of bovine dentin divided into 3 groups	To evaluate the antifungal performance of SDF in isolation	In vitro	SDF appeared to successfully stop fungal filamentation even at extremely low doses, complementing its antibacterial activity
Sunny et al. (2019) [51]	159 active dentinal carious lesions from primary molars	To evaluate the antibacterial performance of AgF as compared to SDF	RCT	SDF performed on a similar parlance as NaF that SDF was compared to
Vinson et al. (2018) [52]	S. mutans biofilm in six-well tissue culture plates	To evaluate the antibacterial performance of KI as compared to SDF	In vitro	SDF + KI performed with the highest efficacy, followerd by KI and SDF alone.

Study or Subgroup	Favoring SDF Events	Total	Favoring other markers Events	Total	Weight	Odds Ratio M-H, Random, 95% CI
Bao Ying et al (2020)	9	15	6	15	6.8%	2.25 [0.52, 9.70]
Ebtissam et al (2019)	40	70	30	70	11.7%	1.78 [0.91, 3.47]
Gerd et al (2017)	23	25	48	75	6.5%	6.47 [1.41, 29.57]
Jaivrat et al (2019)	16	18	29	54	6.3%	6.90 [1.44, 32.96]
Kausar et al (2020)	31	35	27	35	7.6%	2.30 [0.62, 8.48]
Kianliang et al (2022)	8	10	3	10	4.4%	9.33 [1.19, 72.99]
Maribasappa et al (2019)	4	5	1	5	2.4%	16.00 [0.72, 354.80]
May L. Mei et al (2014)	9	12	5	12	5.5%	4.20 [0.74, 23.91]
May Lei et al (2016)	3	4	2	4	2.5%	3.00 [0.15, 59.89]
Mitwalli et al (2019)	12	20	8	20	7.8%	2.25 [0.63, 7.97]
Najmeh et al (2018)	31	45	22	45	10.4%	2.31 [0.98, 5.47]
Parand Sorkhdini et al (2020)	72	90	18	90	11.3%	16.00 [7.71, 33.22]
Rima et al (2020)	2	3	1	3	2.0%	4.00 [0.13, 119.23]
Sunny et al (2019)	22	76	16	71	11.2%	1.40 [0.66, 2.95]
Vinson et al (2018)	4	6	2	6	3.6%	4.00 [0.36, 44.11]
Total (95% CI)		434		515	100.0%	3.59 [2.13, 6.05]
Total events	286		218			

Heterogeneity: $Tau^2 = 0.49$; $Chi^2 = 31.64$, df = 14 (P = 0.005); $I^2 = 56\%$
Test for overall effect: Z = 4.81 (P < 0.00001)

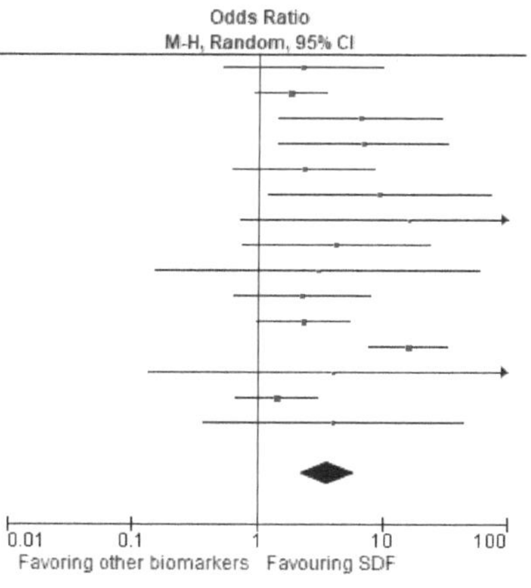

Figure 3. Odds ratio of events favoring SDF vs. other biomarkers/control groups.

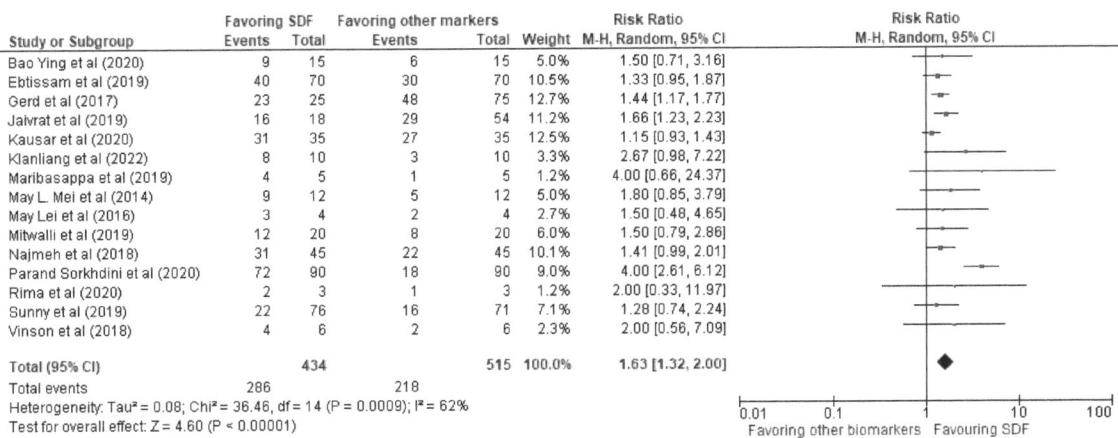

Figure 4. Risk ratio of events favoring SDF vs. other biomarkers/control groups.

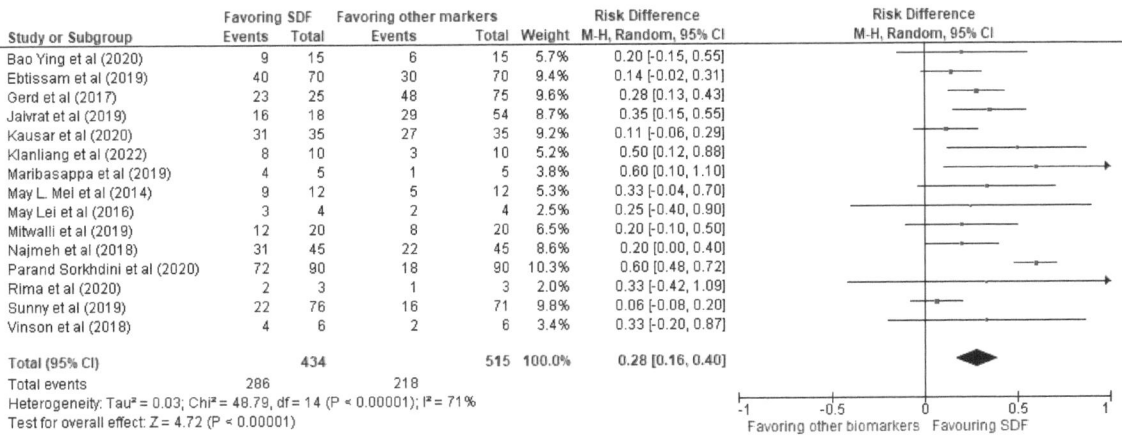

Figure 5. Risk difference of events favoring SDF vs. other biomarkers/control groups.

4. Discussion

The findings observed through the meta-analysis reveal important information about the effectiveness of SDF as a therapy for bacterial biofilms. The results of the review show that SDF, both alone and in contrast to other conventional antibacterial and antifungal substances frequently used in dentistry, has a very favorable effect on reducing bacterial biofilms. This is a significant finding because it implies that SDF may be a more effective treatment option for dental caries and related conditions, especially for people who might not have access to or struggle with conventional dental treatments. This study also emphasizes SDF's promise as a standard treatment for dental caries and associated conditions. SDF may be a useful and efficient way to improve oral health outcomes, especially in places where access to conventional dental treatments is restricted. This is supported by the clear correlation between the use of SDF and the decline in bacterial biofilms across a variety of bacterial species. This comprehensive review and meta-analysis, in addition, offer crucial direction for further study in this field. The review's conclusions suggest that additional study is required to fully investigate SDF's potential as a remedy for bacterial biofilms and associated conditions. Studies examining the long-term benefits of SDF therapy and the possibility of combining SDF with other therapies to further enhance oral health outcomes may fall under this category.

In a clinical trial [53], a single SDF application reduced the burden of care for weak, dependent patients. An annual application of SDF varnish halted the active root carious lesions in nearly 90% of cases in one of the studies [44]. Therefore, it seems that SDF applied by an expert is effective in delaying the onset and development of root caries [54]. Nevertheless, there have also been claims that SDF treatment has disadvantages, including staining/discoloration [55–57], an inflammatory impact on the dentin–pulp complex, and a decrease in bond strength [58].

When a serious caries lesion has already developed, root caries cannot be successfully treated by simply controlling plaque and using fluoride treatments [59,60]. Because dentin's decay and flaws have progressed, restorative materials must be used as a management strategy. The progression of tooth decay can be halted with SDF therapy, but it is possible that cavities will need to be filled with dental fillings. The restorative approach is regarded as a non-traumatic method that could provide patients with a sense of aesthetic gratification [61]. In order to effectively treat advanced root caries lesions, the focus has been placed on the use of restorative materials in combination with SDF administration [60].

Discoloration, one of the main problems that plagues SDF, has been the subject of numerous efforts. A study suggested following SDF usage with KI application to address the issue [62]. Another clinical study revealed that the use of KI did not, however, have a long-term impact on resolving the staining problem, and the discoloration eventually returned [44]. There have been other suggested remedies for staining, such as adding glutathione to SDF, which significantly lessened the coloring but left some pigmentation [63]. Other efforts have used different compounds with somewhat promising results [64,65], but more studies are needed in that regard.

AgNPs have garnered considerable scientific interest and significance owing to their distinct characteristics and broad-ranging applications in diverse scientific domains [66]. Their small size and large surface area-to-volume ratio contribute to heightened reactivity and unique physicochemical properties, rendering them highly versatile nanomaterials. A primary facet of the importance of silver nanoparticles lies in their remarkable antimicrobial efficacy [67]. They exhibit potent antimicrobial activity against a wide spectrum of microorganisms, encompassing bacteria, fungi, and viruses. This renders them prospective candidates for the development of antimicrobial agents, disinfectants, and coatings that impede the growth and dissemination of pathogens [66,67]. Their integration into healthcare settings, including wound dressings, medical devices, and antibacterial coatings, holds promise for mitigating the risk of infections and enhancing patient outcomes.

A couple of studies provide important insights into the synthesis and potential applications of AgNPs. In the first study [66], silver nanoparticles were synthesized using olive leaf extract as a reducing agent. The results demonstrate the feasibility of using natural extracts for the synthesis of AgNPs. This study highlights the green synthesis approach and the potential of synthesized AgNPs using olive leaf extract. In the second study [67], an aqueous extract obtained from chickpea leaves was used for the synthesis of AgNPs. The results reveal the successful synthesis of AgNPs with specific properties, including a maximum surface plasmon resonance wavelength, crystallite dimension, and size range. The inhibitory effect of AgNPs on food pathogen strains and yeast was evaluated, demonstrating high effectiveness at low concentrations against certain strains. The cytotoxic effects of AgNPs on cancerous and healthy cell lines were also investigated, showing no significant decrease in cell viability with increased AgNPs concentration. Overall, these studies [66,67] emphasize the importance of silver nanoparticles as versatile and potentially valuable nanomaterials. The green synthesis approach using natural extracts offers an eco-friendly and cost-effective method for their production. The synthesized AgNPs exhibit desirable characteristics such as specific size, shape, and inhibitory effects against pathogens. The findings support the exploration of AgNPs for various applications, including antimicrobial agents in food preservation and potential biomedical applications. However, further research is necessary to elucidate the mechanisms of action, optimize synthesis methods, and assess the long-term effects and safety of AgNPs in different contexts.

While our study provides valuable insights into the efficacy of Silver Diamine Fluoride (SDF) on bacterial biofilms, there are some limitations to consider. The studies included in the analysis were limited to those published in English, which may introduce bias into the results. It is possible that studies conducted in other languages may have different findings, which were not included in the review. Moreover, the studies included in the analysis varied in their methodology, which may have influenced the results. Some studies had smaller sample sizes or shorter follow-up periods than others, which may have affected the overall conclusions drawn from the analysis. In addition, the review only included studies published up to a certain point in time, and new research may have been published since then that could affect the conclusions drawn from the analysis. It is also important to note that the review focused specifically on the effects of SDF on bacterial biofilms and did not examine other potential benefits or drawbacks of SDF treatment. Therefore, while the findings of the review are important for understanding the potential of SDF as a treatment for dental caries and related conditions, they do not provide a comprehensive analysis of the potential benefits and drawbacks of SDF treatment.

5. Conclusions

In conclusion, our systematic review and meta-analysis has revealed a very positive impact of SDF in comparison to other biomarkers mentioned in the 15 studies that were included in this review. The events favoring SDF exhibited statistical values which indicate that, on an overall basis, our systematic review and meta-analysis provide strong evidence that SDF is an effective treatment for reducing bacterial biofilms. This finding has important implications for improving oral health outcomes, particularly for individuals who may not have access to traditional dental treatments or who may have difficulty receiving such treatments. Given the clear correlation between the usage of SDF and the decrease in bacterial biofilms, we recommend that further research be conducted to explore the potential of SDF as a standard treatment option for dental caries and related conditions.

Author Contributions: Conceptualization, H.M., N.A.I. and M.A.B.; methodology, O.M.A. and S.M.; software O.M.A. and S.M.; validation, H.M. and N.A.I.; formal analysis, O.M.A. and S.M.; investigation, N.A.I.; resources, O.M.A.; data curation, N.A.I. and M.A.B.; writing—original draft preparation, G.M. and M.C.; writing—review and editing, G.M. and M.C.; visualization, G.M. and M.C.; supervision, G.M. and M.C.; project administration, H.M.; funding acquisition, N.A.I. All authors have read and agreed to the published version of the manuscript.

Funding: This research received no external funding.

Institutional Review Board Statement: Not applicable.

Informed Consent Statement: Not applicable.

Data Availability Statement: The data presented in this study are available on request from the corresponding author. The data are not publicly available due to privacy related concerns.

Conflicts of Interest: The authors declare no conflict of interest.

Abbreviations

SDF	Silver diamine fluoride
CHX	Chlorhexidine
HA	Hydroxyapatite
SDF-KI	Silver diamine fluoride + Potassium iodide
AgNPs	Silver nanoparticles
DW	Deionized water
PAA	Polyacrylic acid (PAA)

References

1. Marsh, P.D.; Moter, A.; Devine, D.A. Dental plaque biofilms: Communities, conflict and control. *Periodontol. 2000* **2011**, *55*, 16–35. [CrossRef]
2. Maiorana, C.; Beretta, M.; Grossi, G.B.; Santoro, F.; Herford, A.S.; Nagursky, H.; Cicciù, M. Histomorphometric Evaluation of Anorganic Bovine Bone Coverage to Reduce Autogenous Grafts Resorption: Preliminary Results. *Open Dent. J.* **2011**, *5*, 71–78. [CrossRef] [PubMed]
3. Rengo, C.; Spagnuolo, G.; Ametrano, G.; Juloski, J.; Rengo, S.; Ferrari, M. Micro-Computerized Tomographic Analysis of Premolars Restored with Oval and Circular Posts. *Clin. Oral Investig.* **2014**, *18*, 571–578. [CrossRef] [PubMed]
4. Cicciù, M.; Herford, A.S.; Stoffella, E.; Cervino, G.; Cicciù, D. Protein-Signaled Guided Bone Regeneration Using Titanium Mesh and Rh-BMP2 in Oral Surgery: A Case Report Involving Left Mandibular Reconstruction after Tumor Resection. *Open Dent. J.* **2012**, *6*, 51–55. [CrossRef] [PubMed]
5. Mosaddad, S.A.; Tahmasebi, E.; Yazdanian, A.; Rezvani, M.B.; Seifalian, A.; Yazdanian, M.; Tebyanian, H. Oral microbial biofilms: An update. *Eur. J. Clin. Microbiol. Infect. Dis.* **2019**, *38*, 2005–2019. [CrossRef] [PubMed]
6. Mira, A.; Simon-Soro, A.; Curtis, M.A. Role of microbial communities in the pathogenesis of periodontal diseases and caries. *J. Clin. Periodontol.* **2017**, *44*, S23–S38. [CrossRef]
7. Marsh, P.D. Are dental diseases examples of ecological catastrophes? *Microbiology* **2003**, *149*, 279–294. [CrossRef]
8. Marsh, P.D. Dental plaque as a biofilm and a microbial community—Implications for health and disease. *BMC Oral Health* **2006**, *6*, S14. [CrossRef]
9. Marimallappa, T.R.; Pal, S.; Ashok, K.K.R.; Bhat, P.; Raghupathy, R.K. Acomparative microbiological study of polyglycolic acid and silk sutures in oral surgical procedures. *Minerva Dent. Oral Sci.* **2021**, *70*, 239–247.
10. Bowen, W.H.; Burne, R.A.; Wu, H.; Koo, H. Oral Biofilms: Pathogens, Matrix, and Polymicrobial Interactions in Microenvironments. *Trends Microbiol.* **2018**, *26*, 229–242. [CrossRef]
11. Takahashi, N.; Nyvad, B. Ecological Hypothesis of Dentin and Root Caries. *Caries Res.* **2016**, *50*, 422–431. [CrossRef] [PubMed]
12. Gati, D.; Vieira, A.R. Elderly at Greater Risk for Root Caries: A Look at the Multifactorial Risks with Emphasis on Genetics Susceptibility. *Int. J. Dent.* **2011**, *2011*, 647168. [CrossRef] [PubMed]
13. Steele, J.G.; Sheiham, A.; Marcenes, W.; Fay, N.; Walls, A.W.G. Clinical and behavioural risk indicators for root caries in older people. *Gerodontology* **2001**, *18*, 95–101. [CrossRef] [PubMed]
14. Uccioli, U.; Fonzar, A.; Lanzuolo, S.; Meloni, S.M.; Lumbau, A.I.; Cicciù, M.; Tallarico, M. Tissue Recession around a Dental Implant in Anterior Maxilla: How to Manage Soft Tissue When Things Go Wrong? *Prosthesis* **2021**, *3*, 209–220. [CrossRef]
15. Kleinberg, I. A mixed-bacteria ecological approach to understanding the role of the oral bacteria in dental caries causation: An alternative to Streptococcus mutans and the specific-plaque hypothesis. *Crit. Rev. Oral Biol. Med.* **2002**, *13*, 108–125. [CrossRef] [PubMed]
16. Tanzer, J.M.; Livingston, J.; Thompson, A.M. The Microbiology of Primary Dental Caries in Humans. *J. Dent. Educ.* **2001**, *65*, 1028–1037. [CrossRef] [PubMed]
17. Femiano, F.; Femiano, R.; Femiano, L.; Nucci, L.; Minervini, G.; Antonelli, A.; Bennardo, F.; Barone, S.; Scotti, N.; Sorice, V.; et al. A New Combined Protocol to Treat the Dentin Hypersensitivity Associated with Non-Carious Cervical Lesions: A Randomized Controlled Trial. *Appl. Sci.* **2020**, *11*, 187. [CrossRef]
18. Hamada, S.; Slade, H.D. Biology, immunology, and cariogenicity of Streptococcus mutans. *Microbiol. Rev.* **1980**, *44*, 331–384. [CrossRef]
19. Loesche, W.J. Role of Streptococcus mutans in human dental decay. *Microbiol. Rev.* **1986**, *50*, 353–380. [CrossRef]
20. Peng, J.-Y.; Tsoi, J.K.H.; Matinlinna, J.P.; Botelho, M.G. Silver deposition on demineralized dentine surface dosed by silver diammine fluoride with different saliva. *J. Investig. Clin. Dent.* **2019**, *10*, e12382. [CrossRef]
21. Chu, C.H.; Lo, E.C.M.; Lin, H.C. Effectiveness of Silver Diamine Fluoride and Sodium Fluoride Varnish in Arresting Dentin Caries in Chinese Pre-school Children. *J. Dent. Res.* **2002**, *81*, 767–770. [CrossRef] [PubMed]
22. Chu, C.-H.; Lee, A.H.C.; Zheng, L.; Mei, M.L.; Chan, G.C.-F. Arresting rampant dental caries with silver diamine fluoride in a young teenager suffering from chronic oral graft versus host disease post-bone marrow transplantation: A case report. *BMC Res. Notes* **2014**, *7*, 3. [CrossRef] [PubMed]
23. Amenta, F.; Battineni, G.; Kalyan, L.; Reddy, V.; Madithati, P.; Reddy Narapureddy, B. Personalized Medicine Perception about Health Applications (Apps) in Smartphones towards Telemedicine during COVID-19: A Cross-Sectional Study. *J. Pers. Med.* **2022**, *12*, 12.
24. Fiori, A.; Minervini, G.; Nucci, L.; d'Apuzzo, F.; Perillo, L.; Grassia, V. Predictability of crowding resolution in clear aligner treatment. *Prog. Orthod.* **2022**, *23*, 43. [CrossRef]
25. Hendre, A.D.; Taylor, G.W.; Chávez, E.M.; Hyde, S. A systematic review of silver diamine fluoride: Effectiveness and application in older adults. *Gerodontology* **2017**, *34*, 411–419. [CrossRef]
26. Tan, H.P.; Lo, E.C.M.; Dyson, J.E.; Luo, Y.; Corbet, E.F. A Randomized Trial on Root Caries Prevention in Elders. *J. Dent. Res.* **2010**, *89*, 1086–1090. [CrossRef]
27. Knight, G.M.; McIntyre, J.M.; Craig, G.G.; Mulyani Zilm, P.S.; Gully, N.J. Inability to form a biofilm of Streptococcus mutans on silver fluoride—And potassium iodide-treated demineralized dentin. *Quintessence Int.* **2009**, *40*, 155–161. [PubMed]
28. Mei, M.L.; Ito, L.; Cao, Y.; Li, Q.L.; Lo, E.C.M.; Chu, C.H. Inhibitory effect of silver diamine fluoride on dentine demineralisation and collagen degradation. *J. Dent.* **2013**, *41*, 809–817. [CrossRef]

29. Chu, C.H.; Mei, L.E.I.; Seneviratne, C.J.; Lo, E.C.M. Effects of silver diamine fluoride on dentine carious lesions induced by Streptococcus mutans and Actinomyces naeslundii biofilms. *Int. J. Paediatr. Dent.* **2012**, *22*, 2–10. [CrossRef]
30. Mei, M.L.; Nudelman, F.; Marzec, B.; Walker, J.M.; Lo, E.C.M.; Walls, A.W.; Chu, C.H. Formation of Fluorohydroxyapatite with Silver Diamine Fluoride. *J. Dent. Res.* **2017**, *96*, 1122–1128. [CrossRef]
31. Knight, G.; McIntyre, J.; Craig, G.; Mulyani Zilm, P.; Gully, N. An in vitro model to measure the effect of a silver fluoride and potassium iodide treatment on the permeability of demineralized dentine to Streptococcus mutans. *Aust. Dent. J.* **2005**, *50*, 242–245. [CrossRef] [PubMed]
32. Mei, M.L.; Li, Q.; Chu, C.-H.; Lo, E.-M.; Samaranayake, L.P. Antibacterial effects of silver diamine fluoride on multi-species cariogenic biofilm on caries. *Ann. Clin. Microbiol. Antimicrob.* **2013**, *12*, 4. [CrossRef] [PubMed]
33. Mei, M.L.; Chu, C.H.; Low, K.H.; Che, C.M.; Lo, E.C.M. Caries arresting effect of silver diamine fluoride on dentine carious lesion with S. mutans and L. acidophilus dual-species cariogenic biofilm. *Med. Oral Patol. Oral Cir. Bucal.* **2013**, *18*, e824–e831. [CrossRef] [PubMed]
34. Minervini, G.; Franco, R.; Marrapodi, M.M.; Mehta, V.; Fiorillo, L.; Badnjević, A.; Cervino, G.; Cicciù, M. The Association between COVID-19 Related Anxiety, Stress, Depression, Temporomandibular Disorders, and Headaches from Childhood to Adulthood: A Systematic Review. *Brain Sci* **2023**, *13*, 481. [CrossRef]
35. Qamar, Z.; Alghamdi, A.M.S.; Bin Haydarah, N.K.; Balateef, A.A.; Alamoudi, A.A.; Abumismar, M.A.; Shivakumar, S.; Cicciù, M.; Minervini, G. Impact of Temporomandibular Disorders on Oral Health Related Quality of Life: A Systematic Review and Meta-analysis. *J. Oral Rehabil.* **2023**. [CrossRef]
36. Watson, P.S.; Pontefract, H.A.; Devine, D.A.; Shore, R.C.; Nattress, B.R.; Kirkham, J.; Robinson, C. Penetration of Fluoride into Natural Plaque Biofilms. *J. Dent. Res.* **2005**, *84*, 451–455. [CrossRef]
37. Prada-López, I.; Quintas, V.; Vilaboa, C.; Suárez-Quintanilla, D.; Tomás, I. Devices for In situ Development of Non-disturbed Oral Biofilm. A Systematic Review. *Front Microbiol.* **2016**, *7*, 1055. [CrossRef]
38. Liu, B.-Y.; Liu, J.; Zhang, D.; Yang, Z.-L.; Feng, Y.-P.; Wang, M. Effect of silver diamine fluoride on micro-ecology of plaque from extensive caries of deciduous teeth—In vitro study. *BMC Oral Health* **2020**, *20*, 151. [CrossRef]
39. Al-Madi, E.M.; Al-Jamie, M.A.; Al-Owaid, N.M.; Almohaimede, A.A.; Al-Owid, A.M. Antibacterial efficacy of silver diamine fluoride as a root canal irrigant. *Clin. Exp. Dent. Res.* **2019**, *5*, 551–556. [CrossRef]
40. Göstemeyer, G.; Schulze, F.; Paris, S.; Schwendicke, F. Arrest of Root Carious Lesions via Sodium Fluoride, Chlorhexidine and Silver Diamine Fluoride In Vitro. *Materials* **2017**, *11*, 9. [CrossRef]
41. Gupta, J.; Thomas, M.; Radhakrishna, M.; Srikant, N.; Ginjupalli, K. Effect of silver diamine fluoride-potassium iodide and 2% chlorhexidine gluconate cavity cleansers on the bond strength and microleakage of resin-modified glass ionomer cement. *J. Conserv. Dent.* **2019**, *22*, 201. [PubMed]
42. Fakhruddin, K.S.; Egusa, H.; Ngo, H.C.; Panduwawala, C.; Pesee, S.; Venkatachalam, T.; Samaranayake, L.P. Silver diamine fluoride (SDF) used in childhood caries management has potent antifungal activity against oral Candida species. *BMC Microbiol.* **2020**, *20*, 95. [CrossRef] [PubMed]
43. Klanliang, K.; Asahi, Y.; Maezono, H.; Sotozono, M.; Kuriki, N.; Machi, H.; Ebisu, S.; Hayashi, M. An extensive description of the microbiological effects of silver diamine fluoride on dental biofilms using an oral in situ model. *Sci. Rep.* **2022**, *12*, 7435. [CrossRef] [PubMed]
44. Karched, M.; Ali, D.; Ngo, H. In vivo antimicrobial activity of silver diammine fluoride on carious lesions in dentin. *J. Oral Sci.* **2019**, *61*, 19–24. [CrossRef]
45. Mei, M.L.; Ito, L.; Cao, Y.; Lo, E.C.M.; Li, Q.L.; Chu, C.H. An ex vivo study of arrested primary teeth caries with silver diamine fluoride therapy. *J. Dent.* **2014**, *42*, 395–402. [CrossRef]
46. Mei, M.L.; Zhao, I.S.; Ito, L.; Lo, E.C.-M.; Chu, C.-H. Prevention of secondary caries by silver diamine fluoride. *Int. Dent. J.* **2016**, *66*, 71–77. [CrossRef]
47. Mitwalli, H.; Mourao, M.D.A.; Dennison, J.; Yaman, P.; Paster, B.J.; Fontana, M. Effect of Silver Diamine Fluoride Treatment on Microbial Profiles of Plaque Biofilms from Root/Cervical Caries Lesions. *Caries Res.* **2019**, *53*, 555–566. [CrossRef]
48. Mohammadi, N.; Farahmand Far, M. Effect of fluoridated varnish and silver diamine fluoride on enamel demineralization resistance in primary dentition. *J. Indian Soc. Pedod. Prev. Dent.* **2018**, *36*, 257. [CrossRef]
49. Sorkhdini, P.; Gregory, R.L.; Crystal, Y.O.; Tang, Q.; Lippert, F. Effectiveness of in vitro primary coronal caries prevention with silver diamine fluoride—Chemical vs biofilm models. *J. Dent.* **2020**, *99*, 103418. [CrossRef]
50. Alshahni, R.Z.; Alshahni, M.M.; Hiraishi, N.; Makimura, K.; Tagami, J. Effect of Silver Diamine Fluoride on Reducing Candida albicans Adhesion on Dentine. *Mycopathologia* **2020**, *185*, 691–698. [CrossRef]
51. Tirupathi, S.; Nirmala, S.V.S.G.; Rajasekhar, S.; Nuvvula, S. Comparative cariostatic efficacy of a novel Nano-silver fluoride varnish with 38% silver diamine fluoride varnish a double-blind randomized clinical trial. *J. Clin. Exp. Dent.* **2019**, *11*, e105–e112. [CrossRef] [PubMed]
52. Vinson, L.A.; Gilbert, P.R.; Sanders, B.J.; Moser, E.; Gregory, R.L. Silver Diamine Fluoride and Potassium Iodide Disruption of In Vitro Streptococcus mutans Biofilm. *J. Dent. Child.* **2018**, *85*, 120–124.
53. Li, R.; Lo, E.C.M.; Liu, B.Y.; Wong, M.C.M.; Chu, C.H. Randomized clinical trial on arresting dental root caries through silver diammine fluoride applications in community-dwelling elders. *J. Dent.* **2016**, *51*, 15–20. [CrossRef] [PubMed]

54. Wierichs, R.J.; Meyer-Lueckel, H. Systematic Review on Noninvasive Treatment of Root Caries Lesions. *J. Dent. Res.* **2015**, *94*, 261–271. [CrossRef]
55. Duangthip, D.; Chu, C.H.; Lo, E.C.M. A randomized clinical trial on arresting dentine caries in preschool children by topical fluorides—18 month results. *J. Dent.* **2016**, *44*, 57–63. [CrossRef] [PubMed]
56. Llodra, J.C.; Rodriguez, A.; Ferrer, B.; Menardia, V.; Ramos, T.; Morato, M. Efficacy of Silver Diamine Fluoride for Caries Reduction in Primary Teeth and First Permanent Molars of Schoolchildren: 36-month Clinical Trial. *J. Dent. Res.* **2005**, *84*, 721–724. [CrossRef]
57. Lau, N.; O'Daffer, A.; Yi-Frazier, J.P.; Rosenberg, A.R. Popular Evidence-Based Commercial Mental Health Apps: Analysis of Engagement, Functionality, Aesthetics, and Information Quality. *JMIR Mhealth Uhealth* **2021**, *9*, e29689. [CrossRef]
58. Greenwall-Cohen, J.; Greenwall, L.; Barry, S. Silver diamine fluoride—An overview of the literature and current clinical techniques. *Br. Dent. J.* **2020**, *228*, 831–838. [CrossRef]
59. Al Qranei, M.S.; Balhaddad, A.A.; Melo, M.A.S. The burden of root caries: Updated perspectives and advances on management strategies. *Gerodontology* **2021**, *38*, 136–153. [CrossRef]
60. Jiang, M.; Mei, M.L.; Wong, M.C.M.; Chu, C.H.; Lo, E.C.M. Effect of silver diamine fluoride solution application on the bond strength of dentine to adhesives and to glass ionomer cements: A systematic review. *BMC Oral Health* **2020**, *20*, 40. [CrossRef]
61. Jiang, M.; Wong, M.C.M.; Chu, C.H.; Dai, L.; Lo, E.C.M. Effects of restoring SDF-treated and untreated dentine caries lesions on parental satisfaction and oral health related quality of life of preschool children. *J. Dent.* **2019**, *88*, 103171. [CrossRef] [PubMed]
62. Knight, G.; McIntyre, J.; Craig, G.; Zilm, P.; Gully, N. Differences between normal and demineralized dentine pretreated with silver fluoride and potassium iodide after an in vitro challenge by Streptococcus mutans. *Aust. Dent. J.* **2007**, *52*, 16–21. [CrossRef] [PubMed]
63. Sayed, M.; Matsui, N.; Hiraishi, N.; Nikaido, T.; Burrow, M.; Tagami, J. Effect of Glutathione Biomolecule on Tooth Discoloration Associated with Silver Diammine Fluoride. *Int. J. Mol. Sci.* **2018**, *19*, 1322. [CrossRef] [PubMed]
64. Sayed, M.; Hiraishi, N.; Matin, K.; Abdou, A.; Burrow, M.; Tagami, J. Effect of silver-containing agents on the ultra-structural morphology of dentinal collagen. *Dent. Mater.* **2020**, *36*, 936–944. [CrossRef]
65. Schwass, D.R.; Lyons, K.M.; Love, R.; Tompkins, G.R.; Meledandri, C.J. Antimicrobial Activity of a Colloidal AgNP Suspension Demonstrated In Vitro against Monoculture Biofilms: Toward a Novel Tooth Disinfectant for Treating Dental Caries. *Adv. Dent. Res.* **2018**, *29*, 117–123. [CrossRef]
66. Ramazanli, V.N.; Ahmadov, I.S. Synthesis of Silver Nanoparticles by Using Extract of Olive Leaves. *Adv. Biol. Earth Sci.* **2022**, *7*, 238–244.
67. Baran, A.; Fırat Baran, M.; Keskin, C.; Hatipoğlu, A.; Yavuz, Ö.; İrtegün Kandemir, S.; Eftekhari, A. Investigation of antimicrobial and cytotoxic properties and specification of silver nanoparticles (AgNPs) derived from *Cicer arietinum* L. green leaf extract. *Front. Bioeng. Biotechnol.* **2022**, *10*, 263. [CrossRef]

Disclaimer/Publisher's Note: The statements, opinions and data contained in all publications are solely those of the individual author(s) and contributor(s) and not of MDPI and/or the editor(s). MDPI and/or the editor(s) disclaim responsibility for any injury to people or property resulting from any ideas, methods, instructions or products referred to in the content.

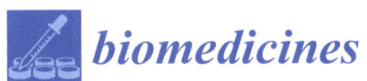

Article

The Impact of Benign Jawbone Tumors on the Temporomandibular Joint and Occlusion in Children: A Ten-Year Follow-Up Study

Emil Crasnean [1], Alina Ban [1,†], Raluca Roman [1], Cristian Dinu [1], Mihaela Băciuț [1], Vlad-Ionuț Nechita [2], Simion Bran [1,†], Florin Onișor [1,†], Teodora Badiu [1], Oana Almășan [3,*] and Mihaela Hedeșiu [1]

1 Department of Maxillofacial Surgery and Implantology, Iuliu Hațieganu University of Medicine and Pharmacy, 37 Iuliu Hossu Street, 400029 Cluj-Napoca, Romania
2 Department of Medical Informatics and Biostatistics, Iuliu Hațieganu University of Medicine and Pharmacy, 400349 Cluj-Napoca, Romania
3 Department of Prosthetic Dentistry and Dental Materials, Iuliu Hațieganu University of Medicine and Pharmacy, 32 Clinicilor Street, 400006 Cluj-Napoca, Romania
* Correspondence: oana.almasan@umfcluj.ro
† These authors contributed equally to this work.

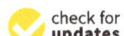

Citation: Crasnean, E.; Ban, A.; Roman, R.; Dinu, C.; Băciuț, M.; Nechita, V.-I.; Bran, S.; Onișor, F.; Badiu, T.; Almășan, O.; et al. The Impact of Benign Jawbone Tumors on the Temporomandibular Joint and Occlusion in Children: A Ten-Year Follow-Up Study. *Biomedicines* **2023**, *11*, 1210. https://doi.org/10.3390/biomedicines11041210

Academic Editors: Giuseppe Minervini and Gianmarco Abbadessa

Received: 19 March 2023
Revised: 5 April 2023
Accepted: 13 April 2023
Published: 19 April 2023

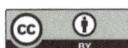

Copyright: © 2023 by the authors. Licensee MDPI, Basel, Switzerland. This article is an open access article distributed under the terms and conditions of the Creative Commons Attribution (CC BY) license (https://creativecommons.org/licenses/by/4.0/).

Abstract: This study aimed to provide a complex analysis of the modifications in craniofacial skeleton development that may arise following the diagnosis of pediatric benign jaw tumors. A prospective study was undertaken involving 53 patients younger than 18 years of age, who presented for treatment at the Department of Maxillo-Facial Surgery, University of Medicine and Pharmacy, Cluj-Napoca, with a primary benign jaw lesion between 2012 and 2022. A total of 28 odontogenic cysts (OCs), 14 odontogenic tumors (OTs), and 11 non-OTs were identified. At follow-up, dental anomalies were identified in 26 patients, and overjet changes were found in 33 children; lateral crossbite, midline shift, and edge-to-edge bite were found in 49 cases; deep or open bite were found in 23 patients. Temporomandibular disorders (TMDs) were found in 51 children, with unilateral TMJ changes identified in 7 cases and bilateral modifications found in 44 patients. Degenerative changes in the TMJ were also diagnosed in 22 pediatric patients. Although benign lesions could be associated with dental malocclusions, a direct etiological factor could be not identified. The presence of jaw tumors or their surgical treatment could, however, be linked to a change of the occlusal relationships or the onset of a TMD.

Keywords: tumor; benign; odontogenic cyst; occlusion; temporomandibular joint

1. Introduction

The jaw region is the site of numerous types of bone tumors [1]. Although pediatric patients are less affected by these lesions compared to adults, the impact of jaw tumors on children's life is significant, since they cause alterations in facial growth and development [2].

The prevalence of pediatric jawbone tumors varies in most previous studies [2,3]. The majority of jaw tumors in children are benign [4], and according to the latest WHO classification, they are recognized [5] as odontogenic (OTs) and non-odontogenic (non-OTs), depending on their origin. Several studies have highlighted that odontoma is the most frequent OT [6]. Of all odontogenic cysts (OCs), developmental cysts, such as dentigerous cysts, are more common in children [7]. Additionally, certain non-OTs such as central giant cell tumors and aneurysmal bone cysts commonly occur within the first 20 years of life [8].

Pediatric benign jawbone tumors are often asymptomatic and are typically identified incidentally during routine dental radiographs [5]. Optimal management of these patients requires interdisciplinary work-up, complex treatment planning strategies, and post-treatment follow-up into adulthood. Treatment consists of a range of surgical procedures, including curettage, surgical excision, cryosurgery, or "en bloc" resection [9]. Of all OTs, ameloblastoma remains particularly controversial in terms of treatment, primarily due to its distinct biological behavior, characterized by slow-growth, local invasiveness, and a high recurrence rate. Compared to adult counterparts, surgeries carried out in pediatric patients are generally more conservative, as both facial growth and dental development [10] need to be evaluated.

However, the influence of these tumors on the development of the craniofacial skeleton is still poorly understood. Ameloblastomas, cemento-osseous dysplasia, fibrous dysplasia, and ossifying fibroma are examples of tumors that can enlarge the jaw and have numerous or widespread sites on the maxillary bones. Because these tumors are adjacent to important anatomical structures and developing teeth, they may result in facial abnormalities or functional limitations [11]. Other extraosseous lesions, such as tori, that develop on the lingual aspect of the jaws do not affect facial growth [12].

The growth of the craniofacial skeleton influences occlusal and jaw relationships, as well as orofacial functions [13]. Cartilaginous tissues, such as the spheno-occipital synchondrosis, nasal septal cartilage, and condylar cartilage play an important role as major growth sites for the respective anatomical structures. Among these, the condylar cartilage of the mandible is the center of greatest growth in the craniofacial complex, and it is associated with the morphogenesis of the maxillofacial complex and temporomandibular joint function [14].

In contrast to the lower jaw, the upper jaw undergoes a different growth pattern. Epiphyseal proliferation and remodeling are the two ways by which the mandible develops. Epiphyseal proliferation is the primary mechanism for bone length growth throughout the first 18 years of life. Under the condyle, the mandibular epiphysis serves as a growth site that permits the intercondylar distance to increase as the skull base widens. Mandibular remodeling occurs after growth is completed to widen the mandible [15,16].

The treatment for tumors may potentially impact a child's mandibular growth centers. For both benign and malignant neoplasms, mandibular reconstruction with osteocutaneous free tissue transfer and titanium plate fixation has been shown to be beneficial [17].

Unlike the mandible, the maxilla does not have any endochondral growth sites, and its growth pattern is defined by an increase in vertical height and width. During maxillary growth, the maxilla is shifted inferiorly, causing remodeling along the suture lines, which promotes the development of vertical height [18].

The cranial base angle does not exert a significant influence on the emergence of dental malocclusions [19]. Numerous studies have investigated the connection between the cranial base, dental malocclusion, and jaw alignment. The findings indicate that jaw position is determined by the inclination and length of the cranial base. Abnormalities of the anterior cranial base are associated with a retrusive maxilla, while mandibular prognathism is related to various abnormalities of the posterior cranial base [20].

The development of the craniofacial skeleton is also influenced by intermaxillary occlusion. Without proper occlusion, midface and mandibular growth cessation could occur, resulting in facial asymmetry and functional alteration [21].

The presence of dental malocclusion can produce temporomandibular disorders (TMDs) [22]. TMDs commonly refer to a category of musculoskeletal conditions that affect the health of the temporomandibular joint (TMJ), masticatory muscles, and other tissues [23,24]. TMD prevalence in pediatric patients varies significantly, with estimates ranging between 4.2% and 68%, depending on the population under investigation and the assessment method employed [25–27]. Moreover, this prevalence appears to increase with age from childhood to adolescence [28,29]. The diagnostic criteria for TMD (DC/TMD) are based on a diagnostic protocol formulated by a group of interdisciplinary experts, including clinicians and researchers, with the goal of providing a better understanding of the diagnostics and treatment of TMD. DC/TMD protocol includes a patient's medical history and clinical examination, imaging studies (X-rays and magnetic resonance imaging), psychological testing and blood tests. During the evaluation process, particular attention is given to symptoms associated with TMD, such as myofascial pain, difficulty eating or speaking, restricted mouth opening or closing, joint noise, or headaches [30].

To the best of our knowledge, this is the first prospective study to assess the changes in craniofacial skeleton development induced by benign jaw tumors. This research aims to provide a complex analysis of the modifications in craniofacial skeleton development, including dental malposition, dysfunctional occlusal relationships, and temporomandibular changes, that may occur following the diagnosis of pediatric benign jaw tumor.

2. Materials and Methods

A follow-up longitudinal cohort study was conducted at the Department of Maxillo-Facial Surgery, University of Medicine and Pharmacy, Cluj-Napoca, Romania, on pediatric patients who underwent treatment for benign tumoral lesions, over a ten-year timeframe, between January 2012 and January 2022. The study enrolled pediatric patients under the age of 18 with a histologically confirmed diagnosis of a jawbone tumor, affecting the mandible and/or the maxilla and maxillary sinus. Accessible follow-up cone beam computed tomography (CBCT) imaging (T_1) was performed at least six months postoperatively. Patients with uncertain histopathological diagnoses, infections, soft tissue or vascular lesions, malignant jaw tumors, and salivary gland tumors and lesions were excluded from the study. Patients without CBCT images or with missing parental consent for clinical examinations or additional investigations, including follow-up, were excluded from this study. Additionally, patients with limited CBCT field of view images were excluded due to limitations in establishing a diagnosis.

The preoperative and postoperative CBCT scans were obtained using the same equipment and imaging protocol (Promax 3D Max, Planmeca, Finland). The following CBCT scan parameters were analyzed by two experienced radiologists (M.H. and R.R.): dental anomalies (tooth malposition or impaction), malocclusion (jaw relationship in the sagittal, transversal and vertical planes, inter-canine, inter-first premolar, and inter-first molar distances), temporomandibular joint condyle position, and bone morphology changes.

Inter-canine, inter-first premolar, and inter-first molar widths were measured on the preoperative and postoperative CBCT coronal images in both maxillary and mandibular jaws. Inter-canine width was measured from the cusp tips of the right and left canine. The inter-first molar width was determined as the distance between the mesiobuccal cusp tips of the right and left first permanent molars. The inter-first premolar width was measured as the distance between the tips of the buccal cusps.

The condylar position (anterior, posterior, or centric) was assessed using oblique sagittal and coronal reformatted CBCT images, according to the Pullinger et al. method [31].

Inter-rater reliability for all measurements was evaluated by two experienced independent examiners. Intra-rater reliability was assessed by conducting two separate measurements performed by the primary investigator (for the first 15 participants) at a two-week interval.

The study was approved by the Ethical Committee of the University of Medicine and Pharmacy 'Iuliu Hațieganu', Cluj-Napoca, Romania, DEP 227 (5 July 2022).

Statistical Methods

The statistical analysis was performed using the R Commander software (R Foundation for Statistical Computing, Vienna, Austria) version 4.0.5. Quantitative data distribution was assessed using the Shapiro–Wilk test, skewness, and kurtosis values. For normally distributed data, results were presented as mean and standard deviation, whereas for non-normal distribution, the median and interquartile range (IQR) were used. Comparison of quantitative data was obtained using the Wilcoxon test for pre-postoperative evaluation. For normally distributed data, the Student t-test was employed. For qualitative data, the results were presented as absolute and relative frequencies. Frequencies were compared through the Stuart–Maxwell Marginal Homogeneity Test with Monte Carlo resampling approximation.

Results were considered statistically significant if the *p*-value was lower than 0.05. The intra-and inter-rater reliability data were analyzed using the two-way random effect model and were expressed using the intra-class correlation coefficient (ICC) and its corresponding 95% confidence interval (CI).

3. Results

3.1. General Follow-Up Data

The total sample included 53 pediatric patients (29 males and 24 females) who underwent CBCT imagistic follow-up. Imaging follow-up was carried out between 6 and 118 months postoperatively (radical excision, marsupialization, biopsy, or reconstruction). Twenty-five patients underwent a preoperative CBCT examination (T_0). Other cases (28 patients) underwent different radiological investigations assessing their preoperative status.

The mean age of the follow-up pediatric patients was 15.1 ± 4.1 (with an age range from 4 years to 22 years). A total of 28 odontogenic cysts (OCs), 14 odontogenic tumors (OTs), and 11 non-OTs were identified at follow-up imaging (Table 1).

Table 1. Distribution and prevalence of follow-up pediatric jaw lesions (N = 53).

Jaw Lesion	N (%) *
Benign odontogenic tumors (OTs)	14 (26.4)
Epithelial	
Ameloblastoma	2 (3.7)
Mesenchymal	
Odontogenic fibroma	1 (1.8)
Odontogenic myxoma	5 (9.4)
Mixed	
Ameloblastic fibroma	1 (1.8)
Odontoma	5 (9.4)
Benign nonodontogenic tumors (non-OTs)	11 (20.7)
Maxillofacial bone tumors	
Osteoma	1 (1.8)
Osteoid osteoma	1 (1.8)
Desmoplastic fibroma	1 (1.8)
Fibro-osseous tumors	
Fibrous dysplasia	3 (5.6)
Giant cell lesions and bone cysts	
Giant cell granuloma	3 (5.6)
Simple bone cyst	1 (1.8)
Cherubism	1 (1.8)
Odontogenic cysts (OCs)	28 (52.8)
Inflammatory	
Radicular cyst	13 (24.5)
Developmental	
Dentigerous cyst	6 (11.3)
Odontogenic keratocysts	9 (16.9)

N—number of jaw lesions; * absolute values and percentages.

The mandible was the most common location for the tumors (64.1%). The most frequent surgical procedure performed was tumor enucleation (84.9%), followed by jaw reconstruction in 0.9% of cases. Simple biopsy was performed in 0.7 % of the patients, while marsupialization was performed only in 4 cases (0.7%).

The median time for the CBCT follow-up examination was 49.8 ± 29.2 months postoperatively. During the follow-up period, recurrence was observed only in one case of odontogenic keratocysts (1.8% of all pediatric jaw tumors) (Table 2).

Table 2. General follow-up data findings for pediatric patients with jaw tumors and lesions (N = 53).

	Total N (%)	Odontogenic Tumors (OTs) N (%)	Non-Odontogenic Tumors (Non-OTs) N (%)	Odontogenic Cysts (OCs) N (%)
Gender				
Male	29 (54.7)	7 (50)	6 (54.5)	16 (57.1)
Female	24 (45.2)	7 (50)	5 (45.4)	12 (42.8)
Size (cm)	2.9 ± 1.4	2.8 ± 0.9	3.9 ± 2	2.6 ± 1.3
Age	15.1 ± 4.1	11.7 ± 4.7	15.2 ± 2.2	16.8 ± 3.2
Tumor location				
Mandible	34 (64.1)	8 (57.1)	6 (54.5)	20 (71.4)
Maxillary	19 (35.8)	6 (42.8)	5 (45.4)	8 (28.5)
Treatment				
Simple biopsy	4 (0.7)	0 (0)	4 (36.3)	0 (0)
Excision	45 (84.9)	13 (92.8)	7 (63.6.5)	25 (89.2)
Reconstruction	5 (0.9)	3 (21.4)	1 (0.9)	1 (0.3)
Marsupialization	4 (0.7)	1 (0.7)	0 (0)	3 (10.7)
Follow-up				
Median	49.8 ± 29.2	41.7 ± 28.7	70.2 ± 29.8	45.8 ± 26.3
Range	6–118	7–100	33–118	6–118
Recurrence	1 (1.8)	0 (0)	0 (0)	1 (1.8)

Data presented as N (%) and median ± standard deviation for follow-up (months), respectively, for the follow-up age of the children.

3.2. Dental Anomalies and Jaw Relationship

At follow-up, from a total number of 53 patients, 27 patients did not exhibit any dental anomalies (50.1%). Dental relationships were found to be normal in the sagittal plane (20%), in the transversal plane (28.3%), and in the vertical plane (56.6%).

Overall, the results showed that a total of 26 pediatric patients had at least one dentoalveolar development anomaly. Dental anomalies were identified in 26 cases (49%, tooth malposition in 21 cases, impacted teeth in 5 cases); overjet changes were found in 33 patients; a total of 49 cases exhibited lateral crossbite, midline shift, and edge-to-edge bite; deep or open bite was found in 23 patients (Table 3).

3.3. Temporomandibular Joint

The centric position of the condyle was found in 65 temporomandibular joints (61.3%). Temporomandibular disorders were noted in 51 (96.2%) patients; unilateral TMJ changes were identified in 7 cases; and bilateral modification was found in 44 patients. The most frequent TMJ pathology was condyle flattening (57.5%). Degenerative changes in the temporomandibular joint were also diagnosed in 22 (20.7%) pediatric patients (Table 4).

3.4. CBCT Comparison in the Preoperative and Postoperative Status

From a total number of 53 patients, only 25 children and adolescents were assessed using preoperative and postoperative CBCT. A comparison between preoperative and postoperative dentoalveolar anomalies and TMJ is summarized in Table 5.

3.5. CBCT Dental Measurements

Comparison of CBCT dental measurements between T_0 and T_1 revealed no statistical significance (Table 6).

We also found that all intra- and inter-rater reliabilities for measurements were greater than 0.8, which is considered excellent according to Cicchetti's classification [32].

Table 3. Dental anomalies and jaw relationship in imagistic follow-up for pediatric patients with jaw tumor (N = 53).

	Total N (%) *	Odontogenic Tumors (OTs) N (%) *	Odontogenic Cysts (OCs) N (%) *	Non-Odontogenic Tumors (Non-OTs) N (%) *
Dental anomalies				
Malposition	21 (39.6)	10 (71.4)	8 (28.5)	3 (27.2)
Impacted teeth	5 (9.4)	1 (7.1)	2 (7.1)	2 (18.1)
Malocclusion				
Sagittal plane				
Normal sagittal	20 (37.7)	7 (13.2)	12 (42.8)	1 (9)
Increased Overjet	31 (58.4)	7 (50)	16 (57.1)	8 (72.7)
Negative Overjet	2 (3.7)	0 (0)	2 (7.1)	0 (0)
Transverse plane				
Normal transverse	15 (28.3)	4 (28.5)	9 (32.1)	2 (18.1)
Cross bite, scissor bite	8 (15)	2 (14.2)	4 (14.2)	2 (18.1)
Midline shift	30 (56.6)	7 (50)	15 (53.5)	8 (72.7)
Edge-to-Edge bite	11 (20.7)	3 (21.4)	7 (25)	1 (9)
Vertical plane				
Normal vertical	30 (56.6)	10 (71.4)	15 (53.5)	5 (45.4)
Deep bite	7 (13.2)	3 (21.4)	3 (10.7)	1 (9)
Open bite	16 (30.1)	3 (21.4)	5 (17.8)	8 (72.7)

N = number of patients; * absolute values and percentages; OTs—odontogenic tumors; non-OTs—nonodontogenic tumors; OCs—odontogenic cysts.

Table 4. Temporomandibular joint changes in follow-up imaging found in pediatric patients with jaw tumors (N = 106).

TMJ Changes	Total N (%) *	Odontogenic Tumors (OTs) N (%) *	Odontogenic Cysts (OCs) N (%) *	Non-Odontogenic Tumors (Non-OTS) N (%) *
Normal condyle position	65 (61.3)	18 (64.2)	35 (62.5)	12 (54.5)
Anterior condyle position	21 (19.8)	6 (21.4)	10 (17.8)	5 (22.7)
Posterior condyle position	15 (14.1)	4 (14.2)	9 (16)	2 (9)
Superior condyle position	5 (4.7)	0 (0)	2 (3.5)	3 (13.6)
Medial position	36 (33.9)	13 (46.4)	14 (25)	9 (40.1)
Lateral position	24 (22.6)	5 (17.8)	14 (25)	5 (22.7)
Condyle flattening	61 (57.5)	18 (64.2)	28 (50)	15 (68.1)
Degenerative bone changes	22 (20.7)	5 (17.8)	14 (25)	3 (13.6)

N = total number of TMJ; * absolute values and percentages; OTs—odontogenic tumors; non-OTs—nonodontogenic tumors; OCs—odontogenic cysts.

Table 5. Comparison of the preoperative and postoperative dentoalveolar anomalies and TMJ changes on CBCT examination associated with pediatric bone tumors (N = 25).

	Preoperative T_0 N(%) *	Postoperative T_1 N(%) *	p-Value (T_0, T_1)
Dental anomalies			
Malposition	16 (64)	10 (40)	0.06
Impacted teeth	7 (28)	0 (0)	0.16
Malocclusion			
Sagittal plane			
Normal Overjet	5 (20)	7 (28)	0.62
Increased Overjet	18 (72)	16 (64)	0.62
Negative Overjet	2 (8)	2 (8)	0.99

Table 5. Cont.

	Preoperative T_0 N(%) *	Postoperative T_1 N(%) *	p-Value (T_0, T_1)
Transversal plane			
Normal transversal	3 (12)	0 (0)	0.25
Cross bite, scissor bite	0 (0)	3 (12)	0.25
Edge-to-edge bite	9 (36)	7 (28)	0.67
Midline shift	13 (52)	15 (60)	0.50
Vertical plane			
Normal Vertical	6 (24)	14 (56)	0.07
Deep bite	6 (24)	5 (20)	0.99
Open bite	13 (52)	6 (24)	0.11
**TMJ changes ** **			
Sagittal plane			
Normal condyle position	29 (58)	32 (64)	0.58
Anterior condyle position	13 (26)	12 (24)	0.99
Posterior condyle position	7 (14)	6 (12)	0.99
Superior condyle position	1 (2)	0 (0)	0.99
Coronal plane			
Central position	21 (42)	18 (36)	0.59
Medial position	20 (40)	18 (36)	0.72
Lateral position	9 (18)	14 (28)	0.12
Condyle flattening	42 (84)	43 (86)	0.67
Degenerative bone changes	14 (28)	16 (32)	0.99

N—number of patients; * absolute values and percentages; **—50 TMJs from 25 patients.

Table 6. Inter-canine, inter-first premolar, and inter-first molar CBCT measurements in preoperative and postoperative assessments (N = 25).

	Preoperative (T_0) *	Postoperative (T_1) *	p-Value
Upper jaw			
Inter-canine distance	35.5 ± 3.9	36.3 ± 3	0.07
Inter-first premolar	44.1 [39.2–44.9]	43.8 [40.6–44.4]	0.38
Inter-first molar	52.3 ± 4.1	53.2 ± 3.3	0.06
Lower jaw			
Inter-canine distance	28.9 [27.6–30.3]	29.2 [20.1–30.1]	0.36
Inter-first premolar	38.5 ± 3.1	38.8 ± 2.3	0.89
Inter-first molar	50.6 ± 3.1	50.9 ± 3	0.39

* Distance measured in millimeters (mm). For data with normal distribution, results were presented as average and standard deviation; for asymmetric distribution, results were presented as median and interquartile range.

4. Discussion

The overall prevalence of the reported pediatric bone tumors varies widely depending on the type of tumoral classification applied. Our findings suggest overall male dominance and a higher incidence of mandibular cases, which is consistent with previous studies [2,33,34]. The current investigation also revealed that a majority of inflammatory pediatric jaw cysts were odontogenic tumors (OT) (52.8%), contrasting with the results identified by other studies [35].

Occurrence of lesions and tumors was most frequently observed among patients in their second decade of life. Jaw tumor development is also considered to occur predominantly within the second decade of a child's life [36–38]. The findings of this study confirm this hypothesis. This may be explained by the transitions from mixed to permanent dentition, and it is worth highlighting that the greatest proportion of the follow-up patients included in our study were adolescents (15.1 ± 4.1 years old) (Table 2).

Cancer diagnosis in children and adolescents can result in dental anomalies and disorders ranging from mild to severe [39]. Hypodontia, microdontia, enamel defect, and root malformation are the most common dental anomalies found in cancer survivors [40]. Our study highlighted the prevalence of dental malposition and impacted teeth (49%) (Table 3). These results indicate that different types of anomalies can be observed, contingent on whether the jaw tumor is malignant or benign.

In our research, it was noted that more than half of the patients (64%) presented changes in tooth position during the preoperative period, while 28% suffered from impacted teeth due to the presence of the tumor. Following surgical intervention, most of the patients received orthodontic treatment that corrected most of the dental malposition. Our research shows that dental malposition could arise in pediatric patients who did not receive orthodontic treatment following the surgical procedure (40% of patients), emphasizing the importance of an interdisciplinary approach to pediatric jawbone tumors and lesions. The predominant surgical option employed for children with impacted teeth was radical tumor excision with tooth extraction. Overall, careful consideration must be given to the surgical treatment for impacted teeth in pediatric patients to avoid potential disturbances in dental eruption and the dental alignment of permanent dentition.

Malocclusion is one of the most important dental modifications, with prevalence estimates ranging from 20% to 100%, according to various studies [41–43]. Midline deviation, deep overbite, increased overjet, and crossbite are frequently found in children and adolescents (36), and the present research reveals a comparable pattern of results. The majority of patients (72%) presented with an increased overjet during the preoperative period. Midline shift (13 patients) and edge-to-edge bite (9 patients) were the most common modifications found in the transversal plane. However, open bite was the most consistent change in the vertical plane (52%). These findings suggest that the majority of patients exhibited malocclusion in the preoperative period. Furthermore, these results demonstrate that jawbone lesions or tumors have the potential to induce or maintain dental malocclusion.

Conversely, various other factors may be associated with occlusal disorders during the preoperative period. Ectopic eruption or dental malposition could be regarded as important factors in the development of malocclusions prior to surgical treatment. Dental caries or dental pain could produce unilateral mastication, altering the distribution of occlusal forces. In addition, trauma of the primary teeth, periapical lesions of the deciduous teeth, abnormal tooth development, or different oral habits could also be key factors that contribute to dental malocclusion [44]. Our study revealed that the majority of dental occlusion modifications were corrected or improved after surgical treatment via orthodontic therapy.

On the other hand, in some cases, the emergence of new malocclusion was noted. In preoperative status, none of the patients had crossbite or scissor-bite modification. Following surgical treatment, changes in the transverse plane were identified in three patients (12%). This could be attributed to either the absence of orthodontic treatment or to a particular type of surgical treatment. Posterior crossbite is considered to be the most frequent dental malocclusion in primary and mixed dentition, occurring in 8% to 22% of the cases [45]. The main cause of postoperative crossbite could be the reduction in the width of the maxillary arch after surgical treatment. Additionally, it is worth noting that 13 patients presented with midline shifts at the preoperative evaluation, while 2 additional patients showed mandibular deviation at follow-up. This postoperative occlusal modification (mandibular deviation and crossbite) is reported to produce changes in the size of the jaws and occlusal interference according to some studies [46]. At the same time, midline shift and/or posterior crossbite have been found to cause temporomandibular dysfunction, potentially leading to disturbance of facial growth in children.

Our results cast new light on the importance of dental occlusal analysis following surgical treatment in identifying and preventing future complications. Drawing on our expertise, we contend that surgical procedures may induce dental malocclusion, especially in young patients who have not received orthodontic treatment. However, the main limitation of our research is the relatively small sample size of patients (n = 25) who underwent preoperative and postoperative imaging. To overcome this limitation and extend the generalizability of our findings, a multicenter collaboration study would be recommended.

Tumor size in our pediatric cohort ranged from 1 cm to 8 cm. This large variation may suggest that most occlusal alterations were not directly attributable to the presence of the tumor, but rather they aggravated an already existing malocclusion.

Serving as one of the growth centers of the jaw, the TMJ condylar cartilage has the capacity to adapt to the physiological changes of the occlusion. Hence, occlusal stress, trauma, the presence of tumors, and malocclusions can induce abnormal mechanical stress to the TMJ, ultimately contributing to degenerative changes and remodeling of the joint. TMJ osseous degenerative changes include sclerosis, erosion, condyle flattening, osteophyte, subchondral cysts, and narrowing of the joint space [47,48]. In our study, patients with malocclusions presented TMJ degenerative changes (Table 5). However, new cases of TMD (86%) were also identified postoperatively. Occlusal instability with posterior crossbite has been observed in 12% of our patients, although different results were obtained by Krasteva et al. [46]. Postoperatively, condyle flattening (86%) and degenerative changes (32%) were found in patients who did not have TMJ alterations before the surgical intervention. Several studies suggested that distally positioned condyles could predict the development of TMD [49]. However, in our study, only seven children exhibited posterior condyle position in preoperative status, and only one case was corrected after surgical treatment. Therefore, our results show that distal condyle positioning does not significantly impact the occurrence of TMD.

Our findings also suggest that surgical treatment of benign jaw tumors and lesions does not produce skeletal changes or transverse bimaxillary deficiency. Additionally, no statistically significant difference between maxillary and mandibular dental measurements were found at different follow-up periods (T_0–T_1) (Table 6). The treatment of small benign tumors usually involves a minimally invasive approach and does not require complex bone reconstruction [50]. However, in cases where surgical resection is required, it is mandatory to preserve the condylar and the subcondylar growth center [51], as several studies have shown that extensive or radical surgical treatment can result in developmental disorders of the jaws [21,52]. In our study, the mean size of the tumoral lesions was 2.9 ± 1.4 cm. Nevertheless, a higher number of patients with large jawbone tumors is needed to establish the possibility of transversal jaw deficiency. Therefore, a multicenter collaboration would be desirable to corroborate our results.

The use of radiotherapy and chemotherapy as adjuvant therapies in pediatric malignancies and benign tumors is rarely required. However, in certain histopathological forms such as ameloblastoma, adjuvant radiotherapy/chemotherapy may be necessary [53]. Radiotherapy can induce alterations in dental eruption, and it has been demonstrated that a dose of 10 Gy could generate irreversible changes in ameloblasts, while a dose of 30 Gy could stop dental development [54]. Animal studies have shown that chemotherapy can also produce severe dental developmental disorders [55,56]. While this type of alterations were not observed in our study, it is extremely important to identify the possible dental alterations resulting from these therapies.

When dealing with this variety of tumors and lesions in the pediatric population, it is crucial to promptly identify the signs and symptoms of a tumor, perform pre- and post-surgical imaging evaluations, and assess the dental occlusion and TMJ status both preoperatively and postoperatively. A multidisciplinary approach, including orthodontic therapy and surgical treatment, may contribute to a favorable follow-up of the occlusal changes and of the TMJ status.

5. Conclusions

Pediatric jaw tumors and lesions are rare, and the epidemiology, clinical characteristics, radiographic findings, and treatment principles of pediatric jaw tumors differ from those of adults. Our study revealed a significant prevalence of dental malposition and impacted teeth among pediatric patients with jawbone tumors and lesions. It was observed that the majority of children exhibited malocclusion at the preoperative stage. Our study has revealed that jawbone lesions or tumors could induce or aggravate dental malocclusion. We also concluded that surgical procedures might result in dental malocclusion, particularly in young patients who have not received orthodontic treatment. The occurrence of a jaw tumor or its surgical treatment may be associated to alterations of the occlusal relationships or the onset of a temporomandibular disorder. Our research demonstrated a significant correlation between malocclusions and TMJ degenerative changes in our patient cohort. Further investigations involving a larger sample size are required to establish the relationship between bimaxillary transversal deficiency and benign pediatric jawbone lesions or tumors.

Author Contributions: Conceptualization, E.C., A.B., S.B., F.O., O.A. and M.H.; methodology, E.C., A.B., R.R., C.D., M.B., S.B., F.O., O.A. and M.H.; software, C.D., M.B. and V.-I.N.; validation, E.C., A.B., R.R., C.D., M.B., S.B., F.O., V.-I.N., T.B., O.A. and M.H.; formal analysis, O.A. and M.H.; investigation, E.C., A.B., R.R., T.B., O.A. and M.H.; resources, E.C., A.B., C.D., S.B., F.O., O.A. and M.H.; data curation, E.C., C.D., T.B., F.O., O.A. and V.-I.N.; writing—original draft preparation, E.C., A.B., S.B., F.O., T.B., O.A., R.R, C.D. and M.H.; writing—review and editing, O.A., E.C., S.B., A.B. and M.H.; visualization, O.A., M.B. and M.H.; supervision, C.D., S.B., O.A. and M.H.; project administration, O.A., S.B., F.O. and M.H. All authors have read and agreed to the published version of the manuscript.

Funding: This research received no external funding.

Institutional Review Board Statement: The study was conducted in accordance with the Declaration of Helsinki and approved by the Ethics Committee of Iuliu Hațieganu University of Medicine and Pharmacy Cluj-Napoca, Romania, under the number DEP 227 (5 July 2022).

Informed Consent Statement: Informed consent was obtained from all subjects involved in the study.

Data Availability Statement: The data presented in this study are available on request from the corresponding author. The data are not publicly available due to due to restrictions: privacy and ethical.

Conflicts of Interest: The authors declare no conflict of interest.

Abbreviations

Temporomandibular joint	TMJ
Odontogenic Cysts	OCs
Odontogenic Tumors	OTs
Non-odontogenic Tumors	non-OTs
Temporomandibular disorders	TMDs
Diagnostic Criteria for temporomandibular disorders	DC/TMD
Cone Beam Computed Tomography	CBCT

References

1. Akhiwu, B.I.; Osunde, D.O.; Akhiwu, H.O.; Aliyu, I.; Omeje, K.U.; Ojukwu, B.; Ameh, P.O.; Adebola, R.A.; Ladeinde, A.L. Paediatric Jaw Tumours: Experiences and Findings from a Resource Limited Tertiary Health Care Center. *Pan Afr. Med. J.* **2020**, *36*, 111. [CrossRef] [PubMed]
2. Perry, K.S.; Tkaczuk, A.T.; Caccamese, J.F.; Ord, R.A.; Pereira, K.D. Tumors of the Pediatric Maxillofacial Skeleton: A 20-Year Clinical Study. *JAMA Otolaryngol. Head Neck Surg.* **2015**, *141*, 40–44. [CrossRef] [PubMed]
3. Mamabolo, M.; Noffke, C.; Raubenheimer, E. Odontogenic Tumours Manifesting in the First Two Decades of Life in a Rural African Population Sample: A 26 Year Retrospective Analysis. *Dentomaxillofac. Radiol.* **2011**, *40*, 331–337. [CrossRef] [PubMed]
4. Tkaczuk, A.T.; Bhatti, M.; Caccamese, J.F.; Ord, R.A.; Pereira, K.D. Cystic Lesions of the Jaw in Children: A 15-Year Experience. *JAMA Otolaryngol. Head Neck Surg.* **2015**, *141*, 834–839. [CrossRef]
5. Vered, M.; Wright, J.M. Update from the 5th Edition of the World Health Organization Classification of Head and Neck Tumors: Odontogenic and Maxillofacial Bone Tumours. *Head Neck Pathol.* **2022**, *16*, 63–75. [CrossRef] [PubMed]
6. Brierley, D.J.; Chee, C.K.M.; Speight, P.M. A Review of Paediatric Oral and Maxillofacial Pathology. *Int. J. Paediatr. Dent.* **2013**, *23*, 319–329. [CrossRef] [PubMed]
7. Arce, K.; Streff, C.S.; Ettinger, K.S. Pediatric Odontogenic Cysts of the Jaws. *Oral Maxillofac. Surg. Clin. N. Am.* **2016**, *28*, 21–30. [CrossRef] [PubMed]
8. Jones, R.S.; Dillon, J. Nonodontogenic Cysts of the Jaws and Treatment in the Pediatric Population. *Oral Maxillofac. Surg. Clin. N. Am.* **2016**, *28*, 31–44. [CrossRef]
9. Koraitim, M.; Medra, A.M.; Salloum, A.M.; Shehata, E.A. Pediatric Aggressive Benign Mandibular Tumors: Clinical Features and Management. *J. Craniofac. Surg.* **2022**, *33*, e265–e267. [CrossRef]

10. Kutcipal, E. Pediatric Oral and Maxillofacial Surgery. *Dent. Clin. N. Am.* **2013**, *57*, 83–98. [CrossRef]
11. Burke, A.; Collins, M.; Boyce, A. Fibrous Dysplasia of Bone: Craniofacial and Dental Implications. *Oral Dis.* **2017**, *23*, 697–708. [CrossRef] [PubMed]
12. Stefanelli, S.; Mundada, P.; Rougemont, A.-L.; Lenoir, V.; Scolozzi, P.; Merlini, L.; Becker, M. Masses of Developmental and Genetic Origin Affecting the Paediatric Craniofacial Skeleton. *Insights Imaging* **2018**, *9*, 571–589. [CrossRef] [PubMed]
13. Yamashiro, T. Mechanisms of growth, development and disease of the craniofacial skeleton. *Clin. Calcium* **2016**, *26*, 140–145.
14. Stocum, D.L.; Roberts, W.E. Part I: Development and Physiology of the Temporomandibular Joint. *Curr. Osteoporos. Rep.* **2018**, *16*, 360–368. [CrossRef] [PubMed]
15. Manlove, A.E.; Romeo, G.; Venugopalan, S.R. Craniofacial Growth: Current Theories and Influence on Management. *Oral Maxillofac. Surg. Clin. N. Am.* **2020**, *32*, 167–175. [CrossRef] [PubMed]
16. Costello, B.J.; Rivera, R.D.; Shand, J.; Mooney, M. Growth and Development Considerations for Craniomaxillofacial Surgery. *Oral Maxillofac. Surg. Clin. N. Am.* **2012**, *24*, 377–396. [CrossRef]
17. Bak, M.; Jacobson, A.S.; Buchbinder, D.; Urken, M.L. Contemporary Reconstruction of the Mandible. *Oral Oncol.* **2010**, *46*, 71–76. [CrossRef]
18. Al-Jewair, T.S.; Preston, C.B.; Flores-Mir, C.; Ziarnowski, P. Correlation between Craniofacial Growth and Upper and Lower Body Heights in Subjects with Class I Occlusion. *Dent. Press J. Orthod.* **2018**, *23*, 37–45. [CrossRef]
19. Nie, X. Cranial Base in Craniofacial Development: Developmental Features, Influence on Facial Growth, Anomaly, and Molecular Basis. *Acta Odontol. Scand.* **2005**, *63*, 127–135. [CrossRef]
20. Andria, L.M.; Leite, L.P.; Prevatte, T.M.; King, L.B. Correlation of the Cranial Base Angle and Its Components with Other Dental/Skeletal Variables and Treatment Time. *Angle Orthod.* **2004**, *74*, 361–366. [CrossRef]
21. Fowler, N.M.; Futran, N.D. Utilization of Free Tissue Transfer for Pediatric Oromandibular Reconstruction. *Facial Plast. Surg. Clin. N. Am.* **2014**, *22*, 549–557. [CrossRef]
22. Kalladka, M.; Young, A.; Thomas, D.; Heir, G.M.; Quek, S.Y.P.; Khan, J. The Relation of Temporomandibular Disorders and Dental Occlusion: A Narrative Review. *Quintessence Int.* **2022**, *53*, 450–459. [CrossRef] [PubMed]
23. Schiffman, E.; Ohrbach, R.; Truelove, E.; Look, J.; Anderson, G.; Goulet, J.-P.; List, T.; Svensson, P.; Gonzalez, Y.; Lobbezoo, F.; et al. Diagnostic Criteria for Temporomandibular Disorders (DC/TMD) for Clinical and Research Applications: Recommendations of the International RDC/TMD Consortium Network and Orofacial Pain Special Interest Group. *J. Oral Facial Pain Headache* **2014**, *28*, 6–27. [CrossRef] [PubMed]
24. Almășan, O.; Kui, A.; Duncea, I.; Manea, A.; Buduru, S. Temporomandibular Joint Disk Displacements in Class II Malocclusion and Cervical Spine Alterations: Systematic Review and Report of a Hypodivergent Case with MRI Bone and Soft Tissue Changes. *Life* **2022**, *12*, 908. [CrossRef] [PubMed]
25. Perrotta, S.; Bucci, R.; Simeon, V.; Martina, S.; Michelotti, A.; Valletta, R. Prevalence of Malocclusion, Oral Parafunctions and Temporomandibular Disorder-pain in Italian Schoolchildren: An Epidemiological Study. *J. Oral Rehabil.* **2019**, *46*, 611–616. [CrossRef] [PubMed]
26. Paduano, S.; Bucci, R.; Rongo, R.; Silva, R.; Michelotti, A. Prevalence of Temporomandibular Disorders and Oral Parafunctions in Adolescents from Public Schools in Southern Italy. *CRANIO®* **2020**, *38*, 370–375. [CrossRef]
27. Rauch, A.; Schierz, O.; Körner, A.; Kiess, W.; Hirsch, C. Prevalence of Anamnestic Symptoms and Clinical Signs of Temporomandibular Disorders in Adolescents—Results of the Epidemiologic LIFE Child Study. *J. Oral Rehabil.* **2020**, *47*, 425–431. [CrossRef]
28. Al-Khotani, A.; Naimi-Akbar, A.; Albadawi, E.; Ernberg, M.; Hedenberg-Magnusson, B.; Christidis, N. Prevalence of Diagnosed Temporomandibular Disorders among Saudi Arabian Children and Adolescents. *J. Headache Pain* **2016**, *17*, 41. [CrossRef]
29. Marpaung, C.; Lobbezoo, F.; van Selms, M.K.A. Temporomandibular Disorders among Dutch Adolescents: Prevalence and Biological, Psychological, and Social Risk Indicators. *Pain Res. Manag.* **2018**, *2018*, 5053709. [CrossRef]
30. Minervini, G.; Franco, R.; Marrapodi, M.M.; Fiorillo, L.; Cervino, G.; Cicciù, M. Prevalence of Temporomandibular Disorders in Children and Adolescents Evaluated with Diagnostic Criteria for Temporomandibular Disorders: A Systematic Review with Meta-analysis. *J. Oral Rehabil.* **2023**, joor.13446. [CrossRef]
31. Pullinger, A.; Hollender, L. Variation in Condyle-Fossa Relationships According to Different Methods of Evaluation in Tomograms. *Oral Surg. Oral Med. Oral Pathol.* **1986**, *62*, 719–727. [CrossRef] [PubMed]
32. Cicchetti, D.V.; Sharma, Y.; Cotlier, E. Assessment of Observer Variability in the Classification of Human Cataracts. *Yale J. Biol. Med.* **1982**, *55*, 81–88. [PubMed]
33. Urs, A.B.; Arora, S.; Singh, H. Intra-Osseous Jaw Lesions in Paediatric Patients: A Retrospective Study. *J. Clin. Diagn. Res.* **2014**, *8*, 216–220. [CrossRef] [PubMed]
34. Chen, Y.; Zhang, J.; Han, Y.; Troulis, M.J.; August, M. Benign Pediatric Jaw Lesions at Massachusetts General Hospital Over 13 Years. *J. Oral Maxillofac. Surg.* **2020**, *78*, 1124–1135. [CrossRef] [PubMed]
35. Kaplan, I.; Gal, G.; Anavi, Y.; Manor, R.; Calderon, S. Glandular Odontogenic Cyst: Treatment and Recurrence. *J. Oral Maxillofac. Surg.* **2005**, *63*, 435–441. [CrossRef] [PubMed]
36. Lawal, A.O.; Adisa, A.O.; Popoola, B.O. Odontogenic Tumours in Children and Adolescents: A Review of Forty-Eight Cases. *Ann. Ib. Postgrad. Med.* **2013**, *11*, 7–11.

37. Taiwo, A.O.; Braimah, R.O.; Ibikunle, A.A.; Obileye, M.F.; Jiya, N.M.; Sahabi, S.M.; Jaja, I.K. Oral and Maxillofacial Tumours in Children and Adolescents: Clinicopathologic Audit of 75 Cases in an Academic Medical Centre, Sokoto, Northwest Nigeria. *Afr. J. Paediatr. Surg.* **2017**, *14*, 37–42. [CrossRef]
38. Tanaka, N.; Murata, A.; Yamaguchi, A.; Kohama, G. Clinical Features and Management of Oral and Maxillofacial Tumors in Children. *Oral Surg. Oral Med. Oral Pathol. Oral Radiol. Endod.* **1999**, *88*, 11–15. [CrossRef]
39. Carrillo, C.M.; Corrêa, F.N.P.; Lopes, N.N.F.; Fava, M.; Odone Filho, V. Dental Anomalies in Children Submitted to Antineoplastic Therapy. *Clinics* **2014**, *69*, 433–437. [CrossRef]
40. Kılınç, G.; Bulut, G.; Ertuğrul, F.; Ören, H.; Demirağ, B.; Demiral, A.; Aksoylar, S.; Kamer, E.S.; Ellidokuz, H.; Olgun, N. Long-Term Dental Anomalies after Pediatric Cancer Treatment in Children. *Turk. J. Haematol.* **2019**, *36*, 155–161. [CrossRef]
41. Akbari, M.; Lankarani, K.B.; Honarvar, B.; Tabrizi, R.; Mirhadi, H.; Moosazadeh, M. Prevalence of Malocclusion among Iranian Children: A Systematic Review and Meta-Analysis. *Dent. Res. J.* **2016**, *13*, 387–395. [CrossRef]
42. Alvarado, K.; López, L.; Hanke, R.; Picón, F.; Rivas-Tumanyan, S. Prevalence of Malocclusion and Distribution of Occlusal Characteristics in 13- to 18-Year-Old Adolescents Attending Selected High Schools in the Municipality of San Juan, PR (2012–2013). *Puerto Rico Health Sci. J.* **2017**, *36*, 61–66.
43. Mtaya, M.; Brudvik, P.; Astrøm, A.N. Prevalence of Malocclusion and Its Relationship with Socio-Demographic Factors, Dental Caries, and Oral Hygiene in 12- to 14-Year-Old Tanzanian Schoolchildren. *Eur. J. Orthod.* **2009**, *31*, 467–476. [CrossRef] [PubMed]
44. Zou, J.; Meng, M.; Law, C.S.; Rao, Y.; Zhou, X. Common Dental Diseases in Children and Malocclusion. *Int. J. Oral Sci.* **2018**, *10*, 7. [CrossRef]
45. da Silva Andrade, A.; Gameiro, G.H.; Derossi, M.; Gavião, M.B.D. Posterior Crossbite and Functional Changes. A Systematic Review. *Angle Orthod.* **2009**, *79*, 380–386. [CrossRef]
46. Krasteva, S.A. Epidemiological Study of Laterognathia, Mandibular Deviation and Posterior Crossbite in Children Aged 7-17 Years from Plovdiv. *Folia Med.* **2013**, *55*, 66–72. [CrossRef]
47. Alexiou, K.; Stamatakis, H.; Tsiklakis, K. Evaluation of the Severity of Temporomandibular Joint Osteoarthritic Changes Related to Age Using Cone Beam Computed Tomography. *Dentomaxillofac. Radiol.* **2009**, *38*, 141–147. [CrossRef]
48. Ahmad, M.; Hollender, L.; Anderson, Q.; Kartha, K.; Ohrbach, R.; Truelove, E.L.; John, M.T.; Schiffman, E.L. Research Diagnostic Criteria for Temporomandibular Disorders (RDC/TMD): Development of Image Analysis Criteria and Examiner Reliability for Image Analysis. *Oral Surg. Oral Med. Oral Pathol. Oral Radiol. Endod.* **2009**, *107*, 844–860. [CrossRef]
49. Pereira, L.J.; Gavião, M.B.D. Tomographic Evaluation of TMJ in Adolescents with Temporomandibular Disorders. *Braz. Oral Res.* **2004**, *18*, 208–214. [CrossRef]
50. Dimachkieh, A.L.; Chelius, D.C. Complex Head and Neck Resection, Reconstruction, and Rehabilitation in Children. *Otolaryngol. Clin. N. Am.* **2022**, *55*, 1205–1214. [CrossRef]
51. Markiewicz, M.R.; Ruiz, R.L.; Pirgousis, P.; Bryan Bell, R.; Dierks, E.J.; Edwards, S.P.; Fernandes, R. Microvascular Free Tissue Transfer for Head and Neck Reconstruction in Children: Part I. *J. Craniofac. Surg.* **2016**, *27*, 846–856. [CrossRef] [PubMed]
52. Benoit, M.M.; Vargas, S.O.; Bhattacharyya, N.; McGill, T.A.; Robson, C.D.; Ferraro, N.; Didas, A.E.; Labow, B.I.; Upton, J.; Taghinia, A.; et al. The Presentation and Management of Mandibular Tumors in the Pediatric Population. *Laryngoscope* **2013**, *123*, 2035–2042. [CrossRef] [PubMed]
53. McClary, A.C.; West, R.B.; McClary, A.C.; Pollack, J.R.; Fischbein, N.J.; Holsinger, C.F.; Sunwoo, J.; Colevas, A.D.; Sirjani, D. Ameloblastoma: A Clinical Review and Trends in Management. *Eur. Arch. Otorhinolaryngol.* **2016**, *273*, 1649–1661. [CrossRef] [PubMed]
54. Chang, P.-C.; Lin, S.-Y. A Long-Term Follow-Up of Dental and Craniofacial Disturbances after Cancer Therapy in a Pediatric Rhabdomyosarcoma Patient: Case Report. *Int. J. Environ. Res. Public Health* **2021**, *18*, 12158. [CrossRef]
55. Näsman, M.; Hammarström, L. Influence of the Antineoplastic Agent Cyclophosphamide on Dental Development in Rat Molars. *Acta Odontol. Scand.* **1996**, *54*, 287–294. [CrossRef]
56. Näsman, M.; Hultenby, K.; Forsberg, C.M. A Scanning Electron Microscopy Study of Disturbances in the Developing Rat Molar Induced by Cyclophosphamide. *Acta Odontol. Scand.* **1997**, *55*, 186–191. [CrossRef]

Disclaimer/Publisher's Note: The statements, opinions and data contained in all publications are solely those of the individual author(s) and contributor(s) and not of MDPI and/or the editor(s). MDPI and/or the editor(s) disclaim responsibility for any injury to people or property resulting from any ideas, methods, instructions or products referred to in the content.

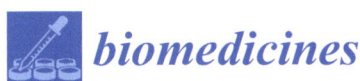

Article

Effect of Various Protocols of Pre-Emptive Pulpal Laser Analgesia on Enamel Surface Morphology Using Scanning Electron Microscopy: An Ex Vivo Study

Ani Belcheva [1,2,*], Elitsa Veneva [1] and Reem Hanna [2,3,4,*]

1. Department of Pediatric Dentistry, Faculty of Dental Medicine, Medical University-Plovdiv, 3 Hristo Botev Blvd, 4000 Plovdiv, Bulgaria
2. Department of Surgical Sciences and Integrated Diagnostics, Laser Therapy Centre, University of Genoa, Viale Benedetto XV, 6, 16132 Genoa, Italy
3. Department of Oral Surgery, King's College Hospital NHS Foundation Trust, Denmark Hill, London SE5 9RS, UK
4. Department of Restorative Dental Sciences, UCL-Eastman Dental Institute, Faculty of Medical Sciences, Rockefeller Building, London WC1E 6DE, UK
* Correspondence: ani.belcheva@mu-plovdiv.bg (A.B.); reemhanna@hotmail.com (R.H.)

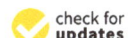

Citation: Belcheva, A.; Veneva, E.; Hanna, R. Effect of Various Protocols of Pre-Emptive Pulpal Laser Analgesia on Enamel Surface Morphology Using Scanning Electron Microscopy: An Ex Vivo Study. *Biomedicines* 2023, 11, 1077. https://doi.org/10.3390/biomedicines11041077

Academic Editors: Giuseppe Minervini and Gianmarco Abbadessa

Received: 5 March 2023
Revised: 23 March 2023
Accepted: 28 March 2023
Published: 3 April 2023

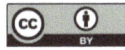

Copyright: © 2023 by the authors. Licensee MDPI, Basel, Switzerland. This article is an open access article distributed under the terms and conditions of the Creative Commons Attribution (CC BY) license (https://creativecommons.org/licenses/by/4.0/).

Abstract: Achieving local anaesthesia for various clinical dental applications is a challenge that we encounter in our daily practice. Pre-emptive pulpal laser analgesia (PPLA) treatment strategy could be a promising non-pharmacological modality. Hence, our ex vivo laboratory study is aimed at evaluating the changes in enamel surface morphology when irradiated with various published PPLA protocols using scanning electron microscopy (SEM). To do so, 24 extracted healthy human permanent premolar teeth were collected, and each tooth was divided into equal halves randomised into six groups. The following laser parameter protocols based on published protocols of clinical Er:YAG laser-induced PPLA were randomly assigned for each group: 0.2 W/10 Hz/3 J/cm^2 (Group A—100% water spray; Group B—no water); 0.6 W/15 Hz/10 J/cm^2 (Group C—100% water spray; Group D—no water); 0.75 W/15 Hz/12 J/cm^2 (Group E—100% water spray; Group F—no water); 1 W/20 Hz/17 J/cm^2 (Group G—100% water spray; Group H—no water). Each sample was irradiated at an angle of 90° to the dental pulp, with a sweeping speed of 2 mm/s for a 30 s exposure time. Our results have shown, for the first time, no alteration to the mineralised tooth structure when irradiated with the following protocols: 0.2 W/10 Hz/3 J/cm^2 with 100% water spray or without water spray with an irradiated area fixed at a 10 mm tip-to-tissue distance, sweeping motion with 2 mm/s speed of movement; average power output of 0.6 W/15 Hz/10 J/cm^2, maximum water cooling of 100%, tip-to-tooth distance fixed at 10 mm, 30 s exposure time, sweeping motion with 2 mm/s speed of movement. The authors concluded that the current available proposed PPLA protocols in the literature might cause an alteration to the enamel surface. Hence, future clinical studies are warranted to validate our study's PPLA protocols.

Keywords: light-induced therapy; scanning electron microscopy; light-responsive molecule; anaesthesia; photodiagnostics; enamel ablation; photobiology; Er:YAG; enamel–light interaction; pulp anaesthesia; restorative dentistry

1. Introduction

Achieving local anaesthesia for various clinical applications is a challenge that we encounter in our daily practice. In this context, pre-emptive pulpal laser analgesia (PPLA) treatment strategy could be a promising non-pharmacological modality, considering its non-thermogenic biomodulation of the dental pulp responsiveness by reducing the pulpal nociceptive nerve impulse formation; it is obtainable in a low-energy-level irradiation form [1,2]. Hence, PPLA can be utilised in various clinical applications, especially in restorative dentistry, where Er:YAG (2940-nm) is one of the most commonly utilised wavelengths.

Fluence plays a crucial role in achieving an optimal outcome of Er:YAG laser-induced PPLA [3,4], as well the photo-acoustic effect of pulsed lasers [3].

Nevertheless, currently, there is no established consensus for a standardised PPLA protocol due to either a lack of reliable laser parameters or unreported essential laser parameters. Many concepts have been hypothesised, with one related to the utilisation of low fluences of laser pulses altering the cell membrane behaviour of the pulpal nerve fibres by coinciding with their natural resonance frequency (15–20 Hz) [5]. This leads to hyperpolarisation and loss of the nociceptive impulse conduction.

Walsh [1] suggested that in order to achieve an effective analgesia, the use of sub-ablative pulse energies at an appropriate frequency is essential, and the following protocols for the erbium lasers and Nd:YAG, respectively, were proposed: 60–120 mJ/pulse (defocused, with water spray), at a frequency between 10 and 30 Hz (preferably 20 Hz), applied for at least 30 s; 50–100 mJ/pulse (defocused, without water spray), at a frequency of 20 Hz, once again applied for 30 s at each of the line angles of the tooth.

Many studies have agreed that in order to achieve a good PPLA, it is necessary to take advantage of low energy and fluences with a circular irradiation motion of the tooth's neck area at a distance of 3–10 mm [6–10]. Nevertheless, the current literature shows conflicting findings. A study by Bjordal et al. [11] utilised 7.5 J/cm^2, whereas another study, conducted by Angelieri et al. [12], proposed greater levels of fluence within the range 5–20 J/cm^2 for severe pain. A fluence of 35 J/cm^2 was suggested by another group of investigators to reduce orthodontic pain, since a level of only 5 J/cm^2 was not found to be effective; however, in the currently available literature, conflicting results are reported for similar protocols [13].

Moreover, the morphology and nature of the tooth structure in terms of enamel and dentine need to be taken into consideration during the formulation of PPLA protocol. An evaluation of laser irradiation's effect on surface enamel must be based on the knowledge of its natural morphology. In humans, the outermost layer of the enamel surface is composed of columns of hydroxyapatite crystals arranged parallel to each other and perpendicular to the enamel periphery, designated prismless enamel [13].

The prismless enamel was initially identified as an area that has no prism boundaries due to the parallel arrangement of the crystals and has a thickness of about 5–25 μm [13]. However, this definition is not functional due to the frequent sporadic presence of unclear and/or incorrect prism structures in areas otherwise considered aprismatic [14–17]. Given the variety in frequency, structure and thickness of the prismless enamel in human teeth [18], the development of an index evaluating laser-induced effect on the enamel surface appears to be obsolete. On the basis of this theoretical rationale, we have identified object-based analysis as the most appropriate for the means of our investigation.

PPLA settings are fundamental to induce laser analgesic effects. However, there is a lack of research determining the optimal mid-infrared (IR) energy and parametry to produce more predictable protocol and reliable laser analgesic-based treatment protocol. Hence, we conducted our ex vivo study aiming to examine and evaluate the effects of the currently available protocols for Er:YAG laser-induced PPLA on enamel surface morphology via scanning electron microscopy (SEM). The null hypothesis of our study was to validate that the currently available protocols for Er:YAG laser-induced PPLA initiate morphological changes on the enamel surface. In this context, the study's objectives are as follows: (1). To establish the most suitable Er:YAG-induced PPLA protocol with effective fluence without enamel morphology changes for future clinical studies; (2). To determine whether low or high fluence has an influence on enamel surface morphology.

2. Materials and Methods

2.1. Study Design

This was a randomised ex vivo laboratory study, where 24 sound human premolar teeth free of racks, erosion, caries or any structural defect were collected. Then, each tooth was divided into equal halves and the 48 enamel surfaces were randomly assigned into eight groups (Groups A–I) according to the laser protocols illustrated in Table 1. The randomisation process was achieved via a computer-generated permuted block sequence in matched pairs design. All the collected teeth were extracted for orthodontic purposes. Informed written consent was obtained from all the patients and patients' legal guardians for the purposes of utilising their teeth in research and publications.

Table 1. The distribution of the pre-emptive pulp laser analgesia (PPLA) parameters according to the experimental group of the study treatment protocol.

Laser Parameters	Group A	Group B	Group C	Group D	Group E	Group F	Group G	Group I
Average power (W)	0.2	0.2	0.6	0.6	0.75	0.75	1	1
Pulse frequency (Hz)	10	10	15	15	15	15	20	20
Energy per pulse (mJ)	20	20	40	40	50	50	50	50
Fluence (J/cm^2)	3	3	10	10	12	12	17	17
Water spray (%)	100	0	100	0	100	0	100	0
Tip-to-tissue distance	10 mm							
Speed of movement	2 mm/s							
Tip type and diameter	1.3 × 6.3 mm sapphire tip							
Irradiation time	30 s/sample							

2.2. Preparation of the Enamel Samples

All the 24 extracted teeth were stored in 0.1% thymol solution prior to commencing the experiments. Then, the teeth were sectioned mesio-distally into two equal halves (48 surfaces), using a diamond-tipped sectorial blade of an "Minosekar-2, Imer" sawing machine. The device is located at the Bulgarian Academy of Sciences, Institute of Physical Chemistry "Rostislaw Kaischew", Sofia, Bulgaria.

2.3. Experimental Design

The enamel surfaces of each tooth that was divided into two halves were irradiated with the same power output, and one half was subjected to 100% water spray cooling, whereas the other half was not. This approach provided a sample from each tooth in two groups of the same power settings while differing in their water-cooling status. This was an equivalent and within-subject control design.

Table 1 summarises the settings of the laser parameters for each group, which were adjusted and modified to adapt properly to each device given its limitations. Pulsed Er:YAG (2940-nm) (LiteTouch™, Light Instruments LTD CAM building, 2nd floor, 4 HaTnufa St. Industrial Zone Yokneam, 2066717, P.O. Box 223, Yokneam 2069203, Israel) was utilised in this study.

The rationale behind choosing different parameter settings recommended for clinical Er:YAG laser-induced PPLA was equivalent to and supported by the literature clinical parameters for Er:YAG laser induction pulpal analgesia of Walsh et al. [3], which were as follows: "subablative pulse energies between 60–120 mJ/pulse (defocused, with water spray), at a frequency ranged between 1–30 Hz (preferably 20 Hz), applied for at least 30 s".

A study by Walsh et al. [3] highlighted that the optimal effect can be achieved at a pulse frequency of 20 Hz, which appears to align with the resonance frequency needed to temporarily disrupt the action of the Na/K pump, whereas the sweeping motion was at approximately 2–3 mm/second (s), during which 20–30 s exposure time at each line angle can distribute the effect evenly across the dental pulp [3].

2.4. Laser Irradiation Process

A non-contact hand-piece with a sapphire tip 1.3 × 6.3 mm in diameter was held fixed at a 10 mm distance from the tooth neck by using a spacer designed specifically for the purpose of the present study (Figure 1). The photonic energy of 2940 nm was utilised to irradiate the cervical enamel surface above the cemento-enamel junction (CEJ) perpendicularly towards the dental pulp of each half at a sweeping speed of 2 mm/s for 30 s, in order to evaluate the optimal sub-ablative effect of various literature-recommended PPLA parameters and irradiation areas such as the neck and occlusal surfaces of the teeth [10,19]. Our study PPLA protocol was formulated based on this.

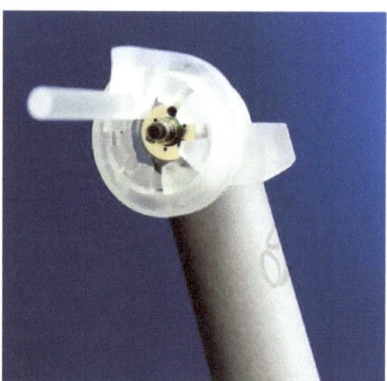

Figure 1. Adjustable rotating spacer, providing tip-to-tissue distance of 10 mm from 1.3 × 6.3 mm sapphire tip, used in this study.

2.5. Scanning Electron Microscopy (SEM)

2.5.1. SEM Description

SEM device that was utilised in our study was a JEOL JSM 6390 with an attachment (INCA Oxford) for elemental analysis, allowing the determination of the surface structure, morphology and elemental composition of any materials. The JSM-6390 is a high-performance SEM with a high resolution of 3.0 nm [20]. The customizable GUI interface allows the instrument to be intuitively operated, and the software ensures optimum operation settings. The JSM-6390 specimen chamber can accommodate a specimen of up to 6 inches in diameter. Standard automated features include auto focus/auto stigmator, auto gun (saturation, bias and alignment) and automatic contrast and brightness. The JSM-6390 is used in many varied applications with several options that increase its versatility. SEM has SE (secondary electron), BSE (backscattered electron) and CL (cathodoluminescence) imaging capabilities, and can provide standard-based analyses of major and some minor elements through EDS (energy dispersive spectrometry) [21]. The manufacturer of the SEM-JEOL JSM 6390 is JEOL Ltd. The company's main office is located in 3-1-2 Musashino, Akishima, Tokyo 196-8558, Japan.

2.5.2. SEM Preparation

After completion of the samples' irradiation, the prepared samples of each group, as described in Section 2.1, were examined using SEM. Subsequently, the samples were fixed in 2.5% glutaraldehyde solution for 12 h (4 °C), dehydrated (25–100% ethanol in increasing concentrations), dried and then spatter-coated with gold [18]. Finally, all the enamel surfaces were analysed with SEM at ×50, ×100, ×500 and ×1000 magnifications. The SEM preparation, examination and analysis were performed by two independent experienced chemists (SA and IS) at the Department of Physics and Chemistry, Bulgarian Academy of Science, Sofia, Bulgaria. The examined samples were rated on the basis of the absence or presence of surface impact cratering, scaly surfaces or exposed enamel prisms.

3. Results

All the SEM analyses were performed after the Er:YAG laser-induced analgesic treatments were completed. Under ×50 magnification, the micrographs of all the samples showed striae of Retzius, where few of them were either masked focally with debris or showed fine cracks and lamella on their surfaces. The debris was found only in the samples that was irradiated without water cooling.

The laser-irradiated samples in the following groups were examined using SEM, and showed no alteration to the mineralised tooth structure: Group A, Group B (Figure 2a,b), Group C (Figure 3a,b), Group E (Figure 5a,b) and Group G (Figure 7a,b). Nevertheless, samples that were irradiated without water at the lowest used energy of 0.2 W at a frequency of 10 Hz with a fluence of 3 J/cm^2 were observed to be sub-ablative in Group B, when a 10 mm laser tip-to-tissue distance was employed. Equally, the samples of Groups A and B were irradiated with the protocol 0.2 W/10 Hz/3 J/cm^2, but those in Group A exposed to 100% water spray showed an absence of surface cratering or melting, whereas the samples in Group B exposed to no water cooling had striae of Retzius clearly visible, which is well illustrated in Figure 2a,b.

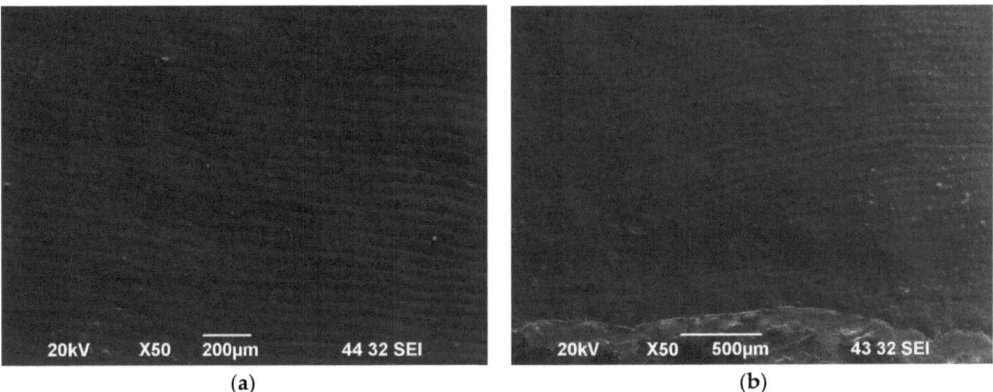

Figure 2. SEM images of enamel surfaces irradiated with 0.2 W/10 Hz/20 mJ/3 J/cm^2 under ×50 magnification. Group A (**a**) was irradiated without water spray cooling and Group B (**b**) had maximum water spray applied, with both showing an intact enamel surface morphology with striae of Retzius.

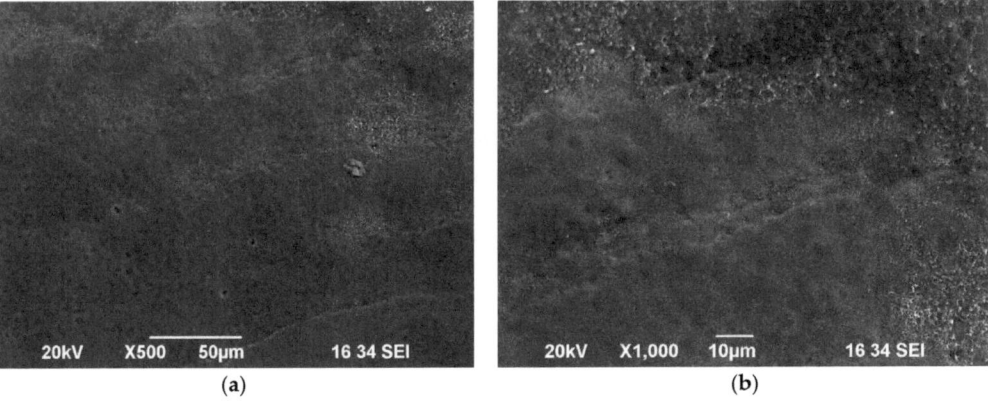

Figure 3. SEM images of tooth surface irradiated with 0.6 W/15 Hz/40 mJ/10 J/cm^2 with 100% water spray—Group C—under ×500 magnification (**a**) and ×1000 magnification (**b**). Observation of intact enamel surface morphology, showing striae of Retzius.

Interestingly, when samples of Group C were irradiated with the protocol 0.6 W/15 Hz/10 J/cm^2 with a maximum water spray level of 100%, this resulted in a lack of alteration in the enamel surface morphology—no impact craters or melting surfaces were observed (Figure 3a,b). However, when the same energy settings were applied without water cooling in Group D (Figure 4a,b), the SEM investigation showed the presence of impact craters and scaly surfaces. In this context, it is noteworthy that in order to achieve a sub-ablative laser action at a distance of 10 mm from the target tissue, a maximum water of 100% should be applied with the following protocol: 0.6 W/15 Hz/10 J/cm^2.

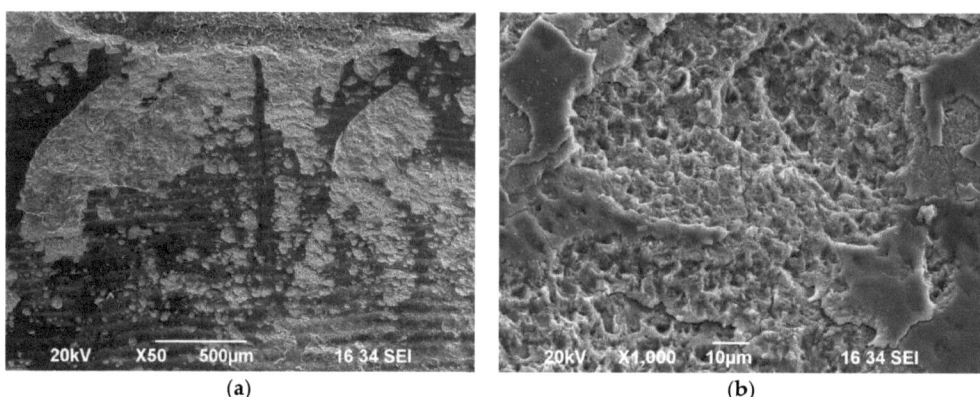

Figure 4. SEM images of enamel surface morphology following irradiation with 0.6 W/15 Hz/40 mJ/10 J/cm^2 without water spray cooling—Group D—under ×50 magnification (**a**) and ×1000 magnification (**b**), showing presence of impact craters and scaly surface.

Laser-induced impact craters and scaly ablated morphology on the enamel surface were observed as well in Group E (Figure 5a,b) and Group F (Figure 6a,b) samples irradiated with the following laser settings: 0.75 W/15 Hz/12 J/cm^2 with or without maximum water cooling, at a distance of 10 mm from target area. Hence, it can be considered as an ablative protocol.

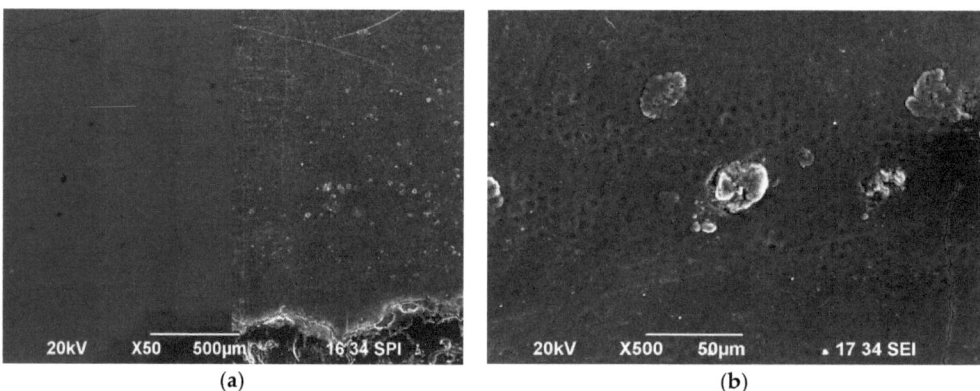

Figure 5. SEM images of enamel surface morphology following irradiation with 0.75 W/15 Hz/50 mJ/12 J/cm^2 with maximum water spray cooling—Group E—under ×50 magnification (**a**) and ×500 magnification (**b**), showing presence of scattered impact craters.

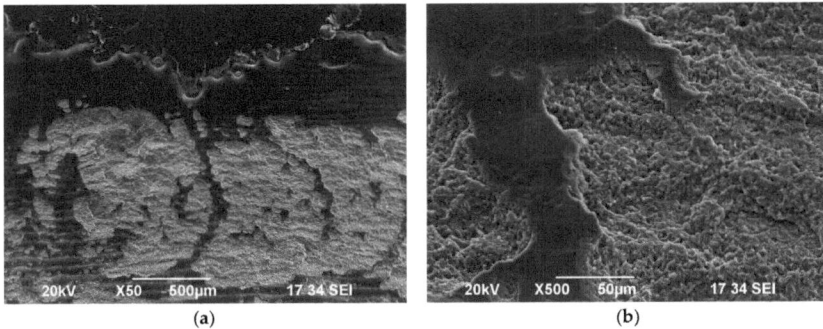

Figure 6. SEM images of enamel surface morphology following irradiation with 0.75 W/15 Hz/50 mJ/12 J/cm^2 without water spray—Group F—under ×50 magnification (a) and ×500 magnification (b), showing scaly surface and wide-diameter impact craters.

The presence of wide scaly surfaces with impact craters and exposed prisms was observed in the samples of Group G (Figure 7a,b) and Group H (Figure 8a,b). Additionally, the impact craters appeared to be of a wider diameter and at a greater depth compared to the Group G samples irradiated with water when the samples in Group H were irradiated with the following laser protocol without water spray: 1 W/20 Hz/17 J/cm^2.

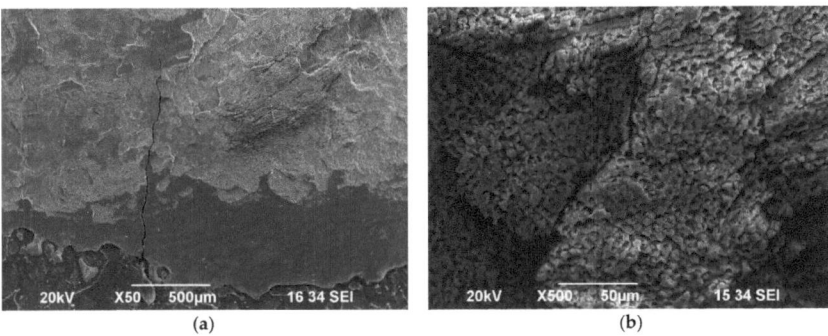

Figure 7. SEM images of enamel surface morphology following irradiation with 1 W/20 Hz/50 mJ/17 J/cm^2 with maximum water spray cooling—Group G—under ×50 magnification (a) and ×500 magnification, (b) showing scaly surface and impact craters with exposed prisms.

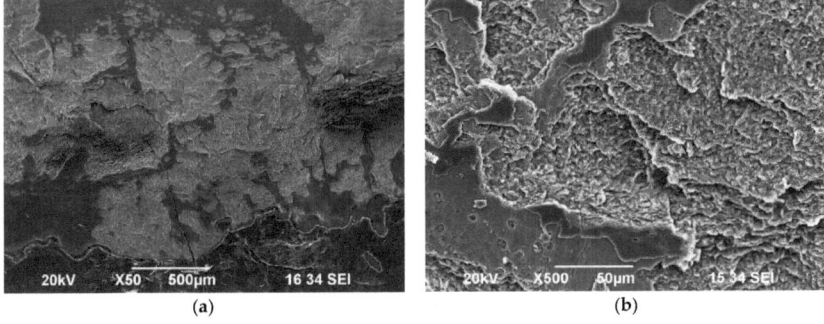

Figure 8. SEM images of enamel surface morphology following irradiation with 1 W/20 Hz/50 mJ/17 J/cm^2 with no water spray cooling—Group H—under ×100 magnification (a) and under ×500 magnification (b), showing scaly surface and wide-diameter impact craters with exposed prisms.

4. Discussion

The data of our ex vivo study demonstrated for the first time that the current published clinical PPLA protocols can cause enamel morphological changes.

The concept of laser-induced analgesia, "photobiomodulation (PBM) of pulpal reactivity", is developed, contributing to a minimal-to-none use of local anaesthesia, resulting in a reduction in the discomfort experienced by patients during dental restorative intervention, especially cavity preparation.

Many studies have documented that PBM is effective within the optical window of (600–1100 nm) [9,22]. Hence, the mechanism of PBM pulpal reactivity of pulsed mid-IR lasers (Nd:YAG, Er:YAG and Er, Cr:YSGG) is different and employed for a low-level effect in PPLA [10,19,23].

The present study utilised an Er:YAG laser (2940 nm), which coincides with the peak absorption of water. The hydroxyl groups in the hydroxyapatite crystals can absorb some of the generated irradiation, but to a lesser extent.

Walsh [1] developed the first hypothesis about laser analgesia protocol by irradiating the cervical part of the tooth. They proposed the following Er:YAG PPLA protocol: pulse frequency 15–20 Hz; pulse energy 80–120 mJ; water spray setup "on"; focused or slightly defocused beam; contact or non-contact handpiece. This work was followed by a publication in 2008 [3] highlighting that energy should be directed at the CEJ towards the dental pulp through the enamel or dentine by moving the laser hand-piece in a sweeping motion approximately 2–3 mm/s for 20–30 s (exposure time). However, the tip-to-tissue distance was not reported. The authors claimed that the optimal effect was gained at a pulse frequency of 20 Hz, which appeared to align with the resonance frequency needed to temporarily disrupt Na/K pump action. The scientific literature led us to conclude that to the best of our knowledge, there is a lack of scientific evidence of the real bio-resonance frequency of the nerve fibres in the pulp.

Interestingly, a clinical trial conducted by Genovese et al. [10] utilised Er:YAG to evaluate the pain self-reported by paediatric patients on a visual analogue scale (VAS) during cavity preparation, in which the following laser protocol was utilised: power output: 0.5 W and then increased to 2 W, pulse frequency: 20 Hz, pulse energy: 75 mJ, laser tip-to-tissue distance: 3 mm, defocused mode on the gingival margin (1–3 mm) and then slowly moved for 2 min. The usage of water cooling during the procedure was not reported. Additionally, there was a lack of substantial information on the duration and the steps in which the energy was applied, how it was increased and whether any water was used as a cooling agent during the manipulation. Due to the lack of reported laser parameters and protocol, it is difficult to reproduce this protocol for future studies.

Many studies investigated the clinical efficacy of various modifications of the laser analgesia technique with the help of an electrical pulp tester (EPT), using a 904 nm GaAs diode laser [9] or 1064 nm Nd: YAG [6] without previous verification of the proposed protocols' safety.

To the best of our knowledge, a study conducted by Chan et al. [7] showed the first SEM investigation on teeth irradiated with the following modified laser analgesia protocol of Nd:YAG: average power: 1.1 ± 0.2 W, power density: 3.9 ± 0.7 W/cm^2, spot area: 0.28 cm^2, pulse frequency: 15 Hz, fluence: 0.260 ± 0.047 J/cm^2. They concluded that no alteration to the mineralised tooth structure was induced [8]. However, in a previous clinical study conducted by Chan et al., using the same laser settings reported, the tip was placed approximately 1 mm from the tooth surface. Nevertheless, the tip-to-tissue distance was not reported in this investigation.

A clinical study conducted by Poli et al. [19] developed the following modified laser analgesic protocol using Er,Cr:YSGG (2780 nm): power output increased from 0.1 W to 1 W (15% water, 20% air), fluence: between 6 and 59 J/cm^2, tip-to-tissue distance: 10 mm, buccal and lingual cervical areas irradiated for 3 min and 30 s. They evaluated self-reported pain during cavity preparation and EPT threshold. However, their study did not provide any information about the morphological alterations on the enamel surface, despite the fact that the laser energy was applied on the neck of the tooth and on the occlusal surface using a Rabbit technique, which is based on utilising high-energy laser-induced analgesia [4]. However, our results have demonstrated that the structural changes were consistent with the applied fluence and water level. Our laser protocol of 0.6 W at a fluence of 10 J/cm^2 with maximum water cooling demonstrated a sub-ablative laser action achieved at a distance of 10 mm. However, higher power settings and lower water-cooling levels corresponded to an increase in the enamel roughness and impact surface cratering. Hence, laser parameters equal to or greater than the average power of 0.75 W, fluence 12 J/cm^2 (without or with maximum water cooling) provide an ablation, leading to morphological changes in the enamel surface, which is in disagreement with Poli et al.'s protocol [19].

Our results have shown through SEM that the structural changes in the enamel surfaces were consistent with the applied energy densities and with 100% of water or without water spray. Higher power settings with no water cooling corresponded to an increase in the enamel roughness and impact surface cratering. Laser parameters equal to or greater than an average power of 0.75 W and fluence of 12 J/cm^2 (without or with maximum water cooling) provided an ablation, which led to morphological changes in the enamel surface. On the other hand, there was no alteration to the mineralised tooth structure with the experimental parameters with 100% water spray or without water spray when the following protocol was applied on the irradiated area fixed at a 10 mm tip-to-tissue distance: 0.2 W/10 Hz/3 J/cm^2. Our data have shown that a fluence between 10 and 12 J/cm^2 was considered optimal without any enamel morphological changes.

Our study aimed to find the highest possible sub-ablative energy and water settings, given the limitations of our laser device, without damaging the enamel surface. Our results have shown that the following PPLA protocol was non-ablative to the cervical enamel surface with or without water: 0.2 W/10 Hz/3 J/cm^2, laser tip-to-tissue distance of 10 mm. Additionally, a sub-ablative laser action at a distance of 10 mm can be achieved when the following protocol is utilised: 0.6 W/15 Hz/10 J/cm^2 with maximum water cooling. However, the higher energy levels of the protocols 0.75 W/15 Hz/12 J/cm^2 and 1 W/20 Hz/17 J/cm^2 have proven to be ablative even when the maximum water spray was used, showing a scaly surface and impact craters with exposed enamel prisms in the SEM investigation.

In light of the above-mentioned statements and our present study, our null hypothesis was not rejected.

5. Conclusions

The data of our ex vivo study confirm for the first time that the following Er:YAG sub-ablative PPLA protocol causes no morphological changes in the enamel surface: average power output: 0.6 W, fluence: 10 J/cm^2, maximum water cooling of 100%, tip-to-tooth tissue: 10 mm, 30 s exposure time, 1.3 × 6.3 mm sapphire tip, sweeping motion with 2 mm/s speed of movement. Additional clinical studies utilising our protocols are warranted to validate Er:YAG laser analgesic effects for painless laser-assisted restorative treatments.

Author Contributions: Conceptualization, A.B.; methodology, A.B. and E.V.; software, A.B.; validation, A.B. and R.H.; formal analysis, A.B. and E.V.; investigation, A.B.; resources, A.B.; data curation, E.V., R.H. and A.B.; writing—original draft preparation, A.B. and E.V.; writing—review and editing, R.H. and A.B.; visualization, R.H. and A.B.; supervision, A.B. and R.H.; project administration, A.B.; funding acquisition, A.B. All authors have read and agreed to the published version of the manuscript.

Funding: This research received no external funding.

Institutional Review Board Statement: This study was conducted in accordance with the Declaration of Helsinki, principles of good clinical practice and Bulgarian laws and ordinances for the management of clinical and scientific investigations with the participation of people. This study was approved by the Commission of Scientific Ethics of the Medical University of Plovdiv No. P-3322/20.12.2017 for studies involving humans.

Informed Consent Statement: Informed written consent was obtained from orthodontic patients and patients' parents/guardians to allow their healthy permanent premolar teeth extracted for orthodontic purposes to be utilised in our ex vivo laboratory study. Additionally, informed written consent was obtained for publication. A copy of the consent forms was given to the patients and patients' parents., while another copy was collected by the study investigators/Department of Paediatric Dentistry, Medical University-Plovdiv.

Data Availability Statement: All the data are available in the text.

Conflicts of Interest: The authors declare no conflict of interest.

References

1. Walsh, L.J. *Technical Brief: Laser Analgesia with the ER: YAG Laser*; University of Queensland: Brisbane, Australia, 1990; pp. 1–11.
2. Neychev, D.; Chenchev, I.; Simitchiev, K. Analysis of postoperative pain after extraction of impacted mandibular third molars and administration of preemptive analgesia. *J. IMAB* **2017**, *23*, 1697–1701. [CrossRef]
3. Walsh, L.J. Laser Analgesia with Pulsed Infrared Lasers: Theory and Practice. *J. Oral Laser Appl.* **2008**, *8*, 7–16.
4. Chen, W. The Clinical applications for the Er, Cr: YSGG laser system. *Chen Laser Inst.* **2011**, *12*, 42–86.
5. Fulop, A.M.; Dhimmer, S.; Deluca, J.R.; Johanson, D.D.; Lenz, R.V.; Patel, K.B.; Douris, P.C.; Enwemeka, C.S. A meta-analysis of the efficacy of laser phototherapy on pain relief. *Clin. J. Pain* **2010**, *26*, 729–736. [CrossRef] [PubMed]
6. Whitters, C.J.; Hall, A.; Creanor, S.L.; Moseley, H.; Gilmour, W.H.; Strang, R.; Saunders, W.P.; Orchardson, R. A clinical study of pulsed Nd: YAG laser-induced pulpal analgesia. *J. Dent.* **1995**, *23*, 145–150. [CrossRef]
7. Chan, A.; Armati, P.; Moorthy, A.P.P. Pulsed Nd:YAG Laser Induces Pulpal Analgesia: A Randomized Clinical Trial. *J. Dent. Res.* **2012**, *91*, S79–S84. [CrossRef]
8. Chan, A.; Punnia-Moorthy, A.; Armati, P. Low-power pulsed Nd: YAG laser irradiation for pre-emptive anaesthesia: A morphological and histological study. *Laser Ther.* **2014**, *23*, 255–262. [CrossRef]
9. Liang, R.; George, R.; Walsh, L.J. Pulpal response following photo-biomodulation with a 904-nm diode laser: A double-blind clinical study. *Lasers Med. Sci.* **2016**, *31*, 1811–1817. [CrossRef]
10. Genovese, M.D.; Olivi, G. Laser in paediatric dentistry: Patient acceptance of hard and soft tissue therapy. *Eur. J. Paediatr. Dent.* **2008**, *9*, 13–17.
11. Veneva, E.; Belcheva, A. Placebo-controlled subjective and objective evalautio of laser analgesia efficacy—A case report. *J. IMAB* **2019**, *25*, 2343–2348. [CrossRef]
12. Angelieri, F.; Sousa, M.V.D.S.; Kanashiro, L.K.; Siquera, D.F.; Maltagliati, L.A. Effects of low intensity laser on pain sensitivity during orthodontic movement. *Dent. Press J. Orthod.* **2011**, *16*, 95–102. [CrossRef]
13. Deana, N.F.; Zaror, C.; Sandoval, P.; Alves, N. Effectiveness of Low-Level Laser Therapy in Reducing Orthodontic Pain: A Systematic Review and Meta-Analysis. *Pain Res. Manag.* **2017**, *2017*, 8560652. [CrossRef]
14. Kodaka, T. Originak article scenning. Electron microscopic observations of surface prismless enamel formed by. Minute crystals in some humna permanent teeth. *Anat. Sci. Int.* **2003**, *78*, 79–84. [CrossRef]
15. Li, C.; Risnes, S. SEM observations of retzius lines and prism cross-striations in human dental enamel after different acid etching regimes. *Arch. Oral Biol.* **2004**, *49*, 45–52. [CrossRef]
16. Kodaka, T.; Kuroiwa, M.; Higashi, S. Structural and Distribution Patterns of Surface 'Prismless' Enamel in Human Permanent Teeth. *Caries Res.* **1991**, *25*, 7–20. [CrossRef] [PubMed]
17. Risnes, S.; Saeed, M.; Sehic, A. Scannng Electron Microscopy (SEM) Methods fordental Enamel. *Methods Mol. Biol.* **2019**, *1922*, 293–308. [CrossRef]
18. Fava, M.; Watanabe, I.S.; Fava-de-moraes, F.; da Costa, L.R. Prismless enamel in human non-erupted deciduous molar teeth: A scanning electron microscopic study. *Rev. Odontol. Univ. São Paulo* **1997**, *11*, 239–243. [CrossRef]
19. Poli, R.; Parker, S. Achieving Dental Analgesia with the Erbium Chromium Yttrium Scandium Gallium Garnet Laser (2780 nm): A Protocol for Painless Conservative Treatment. *Photomed. Laser Surg.* **2015**, *33*, 364–371. [CrossRef] [PubMed]
20. Feng, X.; Garboczi, E.J.; Bentz, D.P.; Stutzman, P.E.; Mason, T.O. Estimation of the degree of hydration of blended cement pastes by a scanning electron microscope point-counting procedure. *Cem. Concr. Res.* **2004**, *34*, 1787–1793. [CrossRef]
21. Durdziński, P.T.; Dunant, C.F.; Ben-Haha, M.; Scrivener, K.L. A new quantification method based on SEM-EDS to assess fly ash composition and study the reaction of its individual components in hydrating cement paste. *Cem. Concr. Res.* **2015**, *73*, 111–122. [CrossRef]
22. Chung, H.; Dai, T.; Sharma, S.K.; Huang, Y.Y.; Carroll, J.D.; Hamblin, M.R. The nuts and bolts of low-level laser (light) therapy. *Ann. Biomed. Eng.* **2012**, *40*, 516–533. [CrossRef]
23. Elicherla, S.; Sahithi, V.; Saikiran, K.; Nunna, M.; Challa, R.; Nuvvula, S. Local anesthesia in pediatric dentistry: A literature review on current alternative techniques and approaches. *JSAAPD* **2021**, *4*, 148–154. [CrossRef]

Disclaimer/Publisher's Note: The statements, opinions and data contained in all publications are solely those of the individual author(s) and contributor(s) and not of MDPI and/or the editor(s). MDPI and/or the editor(s) disclaim responsibility for any injury to people or property resulting from any ideas, methods, instructions or products referred to in the content.

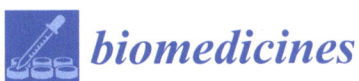

Article

Application of Biodegradable Magnesium Membrane Shield Technique for Immediate Dentoalveolar Bone Regeneration

Akiva Elad [1], Patrick Rider [2], Svenja Rogge [2], Frank Witte [3], Dražen Tadić [2], Željka Perić Kačarević [4,*] and Larissa Steigmann [5]

1. Private Practice, Tel Aviv 6473313, Israel
2. Botiss Biomaterials GmbH, 15806 Zossen, Germany
3. Department of Prosthodontics, Geriatric Dentistry and Craniomandibular Disorders, Aßmannshauser Straße 4–6, 14197 Berlin, Germany
4. Department of Anatomy Histology and Embryology, Faculty of Dental Medicine and Health, Josip Juraj Strossmayer University of Osijek, 31000 Osijek, Croatia
5. Department of Oral Medicine, Infection, and Immunity, Division of Periodontology, Harvard School of Dental Medicine, Boston, MA 02115, USA
* Correspondence: zpkacarevic@fdmz.hr; Tel.: +49-40-7410-532-51; Fax: +49-40-7410-554-67

Abstract: For the first time, the clinical application of the first CE registered magnesium membrane is reported. Due to the material characteristics of magnesium metal, new treatment methodologies become possible. This has led to the development of a new technique: the magnesium membrane shield technique, used to rebuild the buccal or palatal walls of compromised extraction sockets. Four clinical cases are reported, demonstrating the handling options of this new technique for providing a successful regenerative outcome. Using the technique, immediate implant placement is possible with a provisional implant in the aesthetic zone. It can also be used for rebuilding both the buccal and palatal walls simultaneously. For instances where additional mechanical support is required, the membrane can be bent into a double layer, which additionally provides a rounder edge for interfacing with the soft tissue. In all reported clinical cases, there was a good bone tissue regeneration and soft tissue healing. In some instances, the new bone had formed a thick cortical bone visible in cone beam computed tomography (CBCT) radiographs of the regenerated sites, which is known to be remodeled in the post treatment period. Overall, the magnesium membrane shield technique is presented as an alternative treatment option for compromised extraction sockets.

Keywords: socket preservation; ridge preservation; NOVAMag membrane; resorbable metal

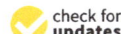

Citation: Elad, A.; Rider, P.; Rogge, S.; Witte, F.; Tadić, D.; Kačarević, Ž.P.; Steigmann, L. Application of Biodegradable Magnesium Membrane Shield Technique for Immediate Dentoalveolar Bone Regeneration. *Biomedicines* **2023**, *11*, 744. https://doi.org/10.3390/biomedicines11030744

Academic Editors: Giuseppe Minervini and Gianmarco Abbadessa

Received: 13 February 2023
Revised: 20 February 2023
Accepted: 22 February 2023
Published: 1 March 2023

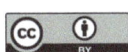

Copyright: © 2023 by the authors. Licensee MDPI, Basel, Switzerland. This article is an open access article distributed under the terms and conditions of the Creative Commons Attribution (CC BY) license (https://creativecommons.org/licenses/by/4.0/).

1. Introduction

Alveolar ridge atrophy is the unavoidable consequence of tooth loss after extraction [1]. This progressive and irreversible phenomenon can give rise to esthetic, functional, and prosthodontic challenges as well as interfere with an ideal implant placement for tooth replacement. Hence, proactive surgical intervention at the time of extraction may help providing desired surgical and prosthetic outcomes. Several techniques that allow dental extraction, implantation, and even if desired provisionalization, have been described in the literature.

Immediate dentoalveolar restoration (IDR) [2] suggests using cortico-cancellous bone graft harvested from the maxillary tuberosity, which is shaped to the defect size and is inserted between the implant and the soft tissue in a flapless approach. However, this requires a secondary surgical site to harvest donor hard tissue for rebuilding the buccal cortical wall, which increases patient pain and morbidity. Additionally, manipulation of the graft must be performed quickly to maintain its vitality.

The socket shield technique (SST) suggests partial root retention on the buccal aspect during tooth extraction with subsequent immediate implant placement [3]. This technique is technically demanding and time intensive, and the feasibility of SST had yet to established as the potential clinical benefits of SST lack strong scientific evidence [4].

An alternative treatment procedure could be designed around the characteristics and biological effects of a new material. Instead of using an autologous bone or tooth that can be challenging and time consuming to be shaped to fit the defect, a bioresorbable synthetic material could enable shorter surgery time due to easier handling.

Magnesium metal has only recently been introduced as a regenerative dental material, with the first two magnesium medical devices receiving CE approval in 2021 [5,6]. As a material choice, magnesium is already well established for orthopedic and cardiovascular applications [7], but has yet to be reported on for its clinical application in regenerative dentistry. Magnesium has a combination of properties that make it unique as a regenerative dental material: synthetic, mechanically strong but malleable, and completely resorbable [8]. Additionally, magnesium metal degrades into magnesium ions that are naturally occurring in the body and are used in many important functions, such as the maintenance, growth, and regeneration of bone [9]. Mg ions are known to promote cortical bone growth via periosteal stem cells through the release of calcitonin gene-related peptide (CGRP) from sensory nerve endings in the periosteum [10].

The magnesium membrane has previously been demonstrated to have increased soft tissue adhesion. In vitro studies have shown that gingival human fibroblast cells (Primary HGF-1 cells) will adhere and form confluent layers on the magnesium membrane surface, as well as migrate over the surface following a scratch test [11]. These results were further proven in an in vivo beagle dog model, using membranes implanted into palatal defects, which demonstrated 90% wound closure after 72 h. This can be expected, as previous studies have reported on the role of Mg ions in promoting the adhesion of oral soft tissue cells to titanium substratum, and has even been demonstrated to be more beneficial than Ca ions, a known mediator of cell to substratum adhesion [12–14].

Once implanted, the magnesium metal begins to degrade until it is completely resorbed by the body. Therefore, there is no need to extract it during a second surgical procedure. During the degradation of the magnesium metal, the metallic structure is transformed into magnesium salts and a small volume of hydrogen gas is released [15]. The composition of the magnesium salts contain elements that are naturally present within the bone matrix, have a good biocompatibility, and can become enveloped in new bone [16]. The magnesium salts keep the original shape and position of the membrane until they are resorbed by the body, whereas the small volume of hydrogen gas initially provides a slight tenting of the soft tissue. Both of these degradation by-products continue to maintain a separation of the soft and hard tissues [5,17]. As reported for other magnesium implants, once the magnesium metal has degraded, no more hydrogen gas is released and the space created by the gas spontaneously resolves [18,19]. Magnesium implants have already been proven to provide an excellent biocompatibility in applications such as cardiovascular stents [20,21] and orthopedic screws [22,23].

Magnesium ions that are resorbed by the body during the degradation process, are already prevalent within the body and are found within almost every single cell [24]. As magnesium ions are already well established within the body, there are pathological pathways for the excretion of excessive levels of magnesium ions [24].

An in vivo performance study in Beagle dogs, demonstrated that the magnesium membrane was able to provide a similar result to that of a collagen membrane when used to augment four-wall defects in combination with bovine bone graft [17]. A similar ratio of new bone volume to soft tissue volume was found at all timepoints when comparing the magnesium membrane and collagen membrane treatment groups, demonstrating that the magnesium membrane was just as effective as the collagen membrane at maintaining a barrier and enabling the bone within the defect to regenerate. In the veterinarian report, neither the magnesium membrane nor the collagen membrane group presented signs of a chronic inflammation reaction such as prolonged redness, swelling, pain, and loss of function.

In the performance study, one week post implantation, the magnesium membrane had a slightly higher inflammatory reaction; however, this quickly subsided, and by week 8, the subsequent timepoint in the study, the inflammatory reaction was similar to that of the collagen membrane. Both membranes followed a comparable inflammatory process, involving the same type and number of immune cells [5]. A similar inflammatory response of the magnesium membrane and collagen membrane has also been reported in another in vivo study, comparing a physical vapor deposition (PVD) coated magnesium membrane, a non-coated magnesium membrane and a collagen membrane implanted subcutaneously in BALB/C mice [25]. The coated magnesium membrane induced the highest level of inflammation; however, the uncoated magnesium membrane and the collagen membrane were associated with similar levels of inflammation. Both the collagen and un-coated magnesium membrane had balanced levels of M1 and M2 macrophages, in a ratio promoting the integration of the material.

Due to the magnesium membrane's mechanical strength [5], it also has the possibility to be used as a cortical plate. Despite being mechanically strong, the magnesium membrane can be cut and bent to shape to perfectly match the contours of the defect, potentially making it more clinically manageable than using an autogenic or allogenic bone cortical plate. Once in position, the membrane provides a barrier between soft and hard tissues and fully resorbs after the critical healing period [17]. As the degradation process is gradual, defect stability is maintained during the critical healing phase whilst new bony tissue infiltrates the defect site [5,17].

The aim of this paper is to report on the first clinical application of the magnesium metal membrane and demonstrate the application of a completely new technique. The magnesium membrane shield technique is used to rebuild the buccal wall and offers a novel clinical option due to the material properties of magnesium. The magnesium membrane is presented as an alternative material choice to the current gold-standard use of a cortico-cancellous bone plate or tooth root, with an aim to reduce invasiveness and the surgical limitations of the alternative techniques.

2. Materials and Methods

For each case, a minimally invasive buccal and palatal flap elevation was performed, followed by a thorough debridement of the extraction site. A periosteal releasing incision was performed on the buccal flap, 1 mm apical to the lower border of the defect. An immediate implant was placed with a high insertion torque. A sterile magnesium membrane (NOVAMag® membrane, botiss biomaterials GmbH, Berlin, Germany) with an initial thickness of 140 µm and dimensions 30 × 40 mm was prepared. The membrane was trimmed to size using the NOVAMag® scissors (Carl Martin GmbH, Solingen, Germany) (Figure 1A), ensuring smooth rounded edges to avoid sharp points that could perforate the soft tissue. The rim of the membrane is flattened using the NOVAMag® sculptor (Carl Martin GmbH, Solingen, Germany) (Figure 1B). The membrane was then either placed as a singular layer, or bent in half into a double layer of the membrane to improve its mechanical stability. The shape of the membrane was then bent according to contours of the defect using the NOVAMag® sculptor (Figure 1C). The membrane was then inserted into the socket as an extension of the buccal plate. The defect was filled with allogenic granular bone substitute (maxgraft®, botiss biomaterials GmbH, Berlin, Germany) and a collagen membrane (Jason® membrane, botiss biomaterials GmbH, Berlin, Germany) placed over the top of the augmentation and the flaps were sutured (Figure 1D,E). Closed wound healing is recommended with the magnesium membrane, as exposure can cause an accelerated resorption time. Suturing was performed with Nylon 5-0 sutures, using single interrupted and vertical mattress suturing techniques. Then, implants were immediately loaded (Figure 1F).

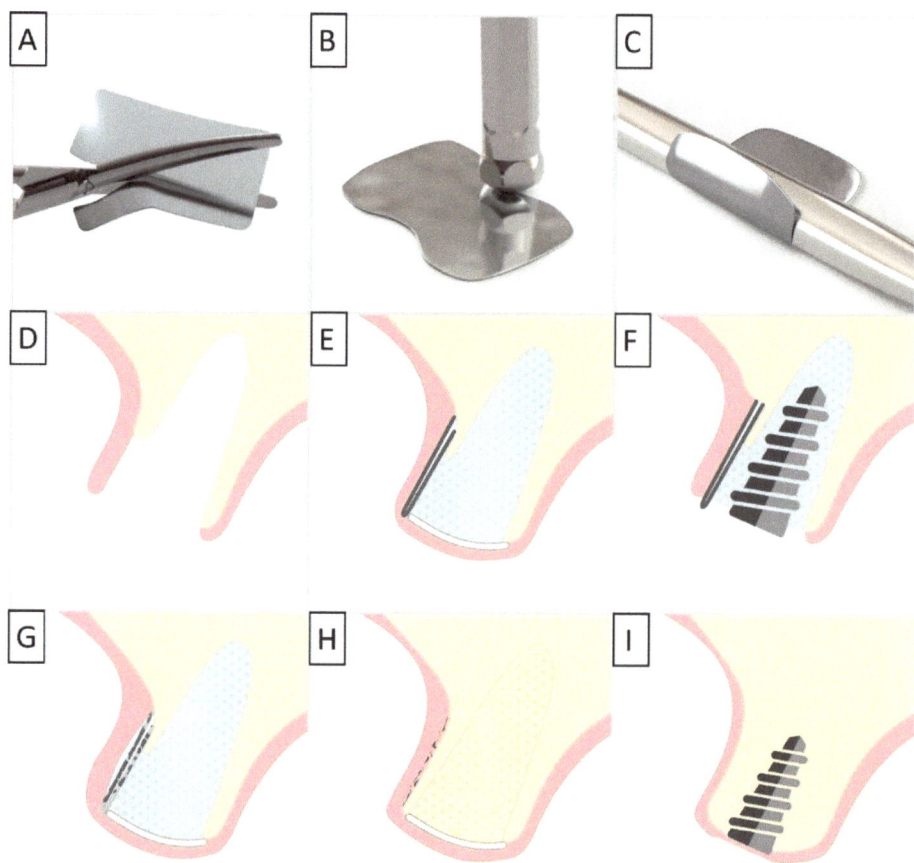

Figure 1. For the magnesium shield technique, the magnesium membrane is first cut to shape using the NOVAMag® scissors (**A**). The rim of the membrane is then flattened using the NOVAMag® sculpture (**B**) and bent into shape (**C**). In a compromised extraction socket (**D**), the membrane is either place as a single layer or bent into a double layer, before being positioned to rebuild either the buccal or palatal wall. The membrane is held in position by the periosteum and the defect space is filled with the graft material. A collagen membrane is placed on the top of the ridge (**E**). Using the technique, it is also possible to immediately place implants with a provisional restoration (**F**). Once implanted, the magnesium membrane will begin to degrade, transforming into magnesium salts that maintain the soft tissue barrier, and hydrogen gas will be released that provides a tenting of the soft tissue, which also extends the barrier effect, since cells cannot cross the gas cavity (**G**). After the magnesium metal has transformed into magnesium salts, no more gas is released, and the soft tissue returns into position over the newly formed bone and magnesium salts (**H**). After the critical healing period, the magnesium membrane is completely resorbed (**I**).

Post-operatively, the patients were instructed to rinse with chlorhexidine solution twice a day for 2 weeks.

3. Results

3.1. Case 1

The patient was a 65-year-old female in good general health condition. The patient presented with tooth 24, root canal treatment, post, core build up, and an old porcelain-fused-to-metal (PFM) crown. A vertical root fracture was present with an associated severe bone loss, including loss of both buccal and palatal plates.

The non-traumatic extraction of tooth 24. was performed, (Figure 2). The magnesium membrane shield technique was performed as described in Section 2, aiming to rebuild both buccal and palatal plates. In this instance, the magnesium membrane was used as a single layer on both the buccal and palatal sides.

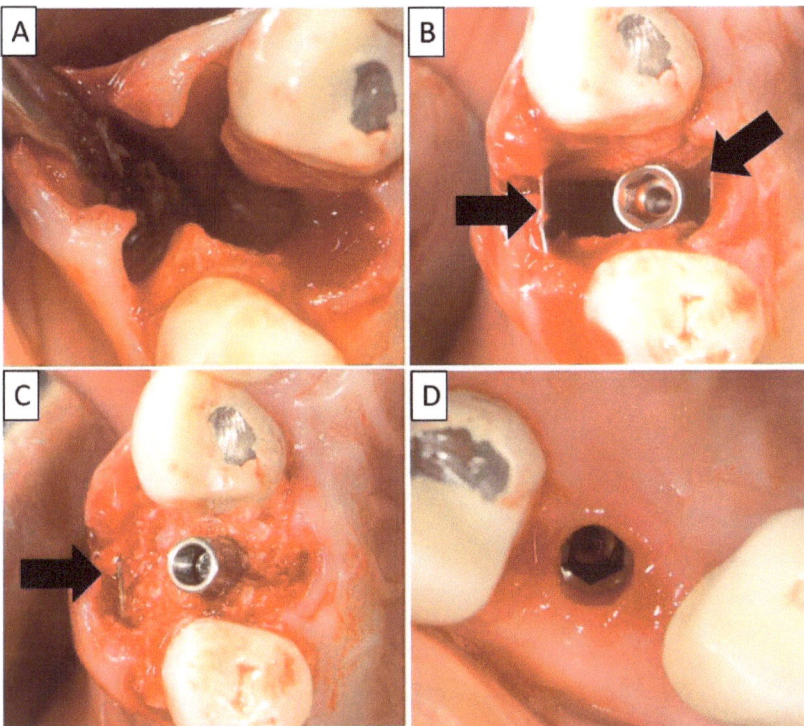

Figure 2. (**A**) Alveolar socket following atraumatic extraction and curettage. Severe bone loss of both buccal and palatal plates. (**B**) Buccal and palatial plates were created using the magnesium membrane shield technique. (**C**) Application of allograft. (**D**) Four months post operatively there was an excellent regeneration of bone defect, including fully regenerated cortical and palatal plates. The implant was stable and there was a good healing of the soft tissues. Black arrows are used to indicate the position of the magnesium membrane.

Four months post operatively, regenerated bone was present, including fully regenerated cortical and palatal plates (Figure 3). The implant was stable and there was a good healing of the soft tissues.

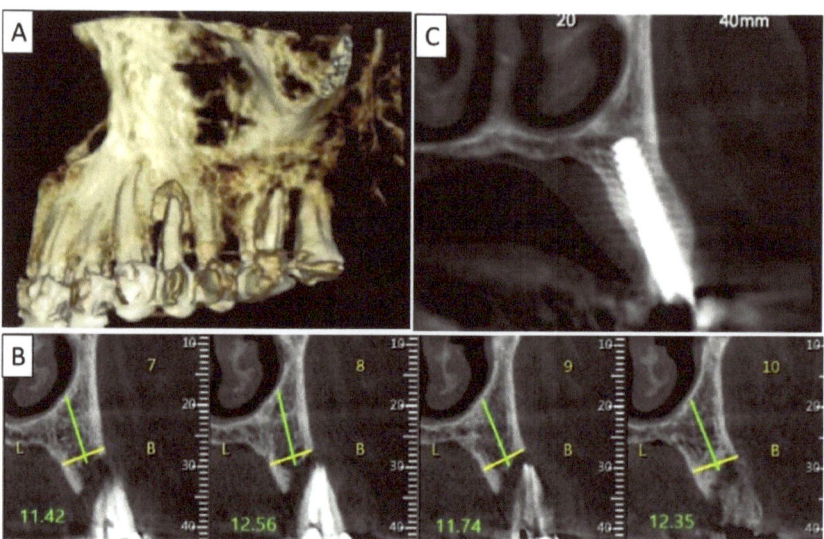

Figure 3. (**A**) Lateral volumetric cone beam computed tomography (CBCT) shows significant loss of buccal and palatal bone mass around tooth 24. (**B**) Coronal CBCT slice of the same area of tooth 24 revealing missed buccal and palatal bone and associated apical radiolucency. (**C**) The coronal CBCT section shows the implant in the area of tooth 24 and the obtained completely regenerated cortical and palatal plates.

3.2. Case 2

The patient was a 68-year-old male in good general health condition. The patient presented with tooth 25, root canal treatment, crown destroyed at the tissue level and a vertical root fracture with associated severe bone loss including loss of buccal plate. The palatal plate remained intact.

A non-traumatic extraction of tooth 25 was performed (Figure 4), followed by bone augmentation using the magnesium membrane shield technique to rebuild the buccal wall as described in Section 2. In this instance, the magnesium membrane was bent into a double layer.

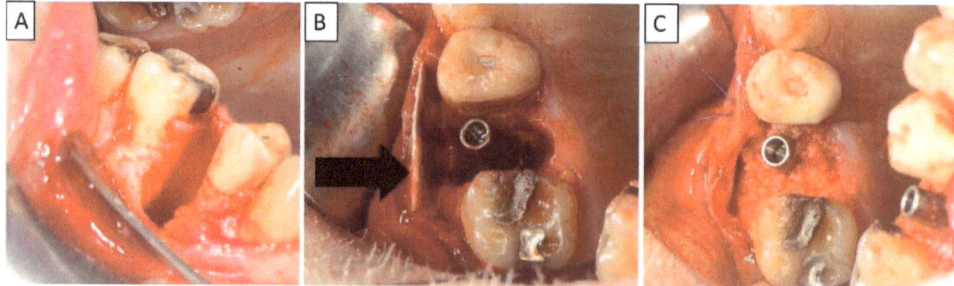

Figure 4. (**A**) Alveolar socket following atraumatic extraction and curettage. Severe bone loss of buccal plate. (**B**) Buccal plate was created using the magnesium membrane shield technique. (**C**) Application of allograft together with magnesium membrane. The black arrow indicates the position of the magnesium membrane.

Four months post operatively, there was a good regeneration of bone within the defect including a fully regenerated cortical buccal plate (Figure 5). The implant was stable and the was a good healing of the soft tissues.

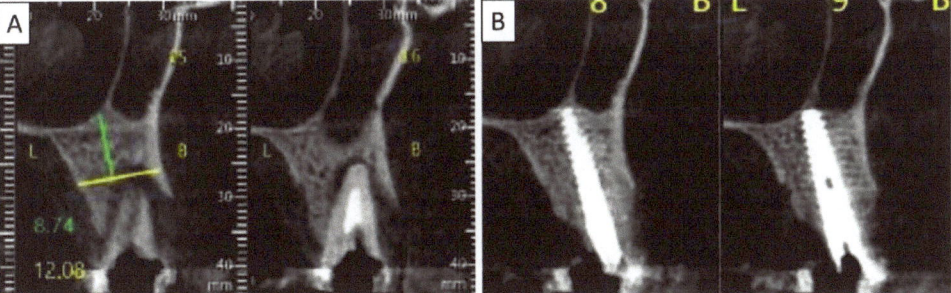

Figure 5. (**A**) Coronal CBCT section shows tooth 25 with vertical root fracture and destroyed buccal bony wall and intact palatine. (**B**) The coronal CBCT section shows the placed implant in the region of tooth 25 and the complete regeneration of the cortical wall.

3.3. Case 3

A 62-year-old male patient in good general health condition. Patient presented with tooth 21, vital tooth, horizontal oblique root fracture with associated severe bone loss including loss of buccal cortical plate. Palatal cortical plate remained intact.

Nontraumatic extraction of tooth 21 (Figure 6), followed by bone augmentation using the magnesium membrane shield technique to rebuild the buccal wall as described in Section 2. The implant was immediately covered with a provisional crown due to its location in the aesthetic zone.

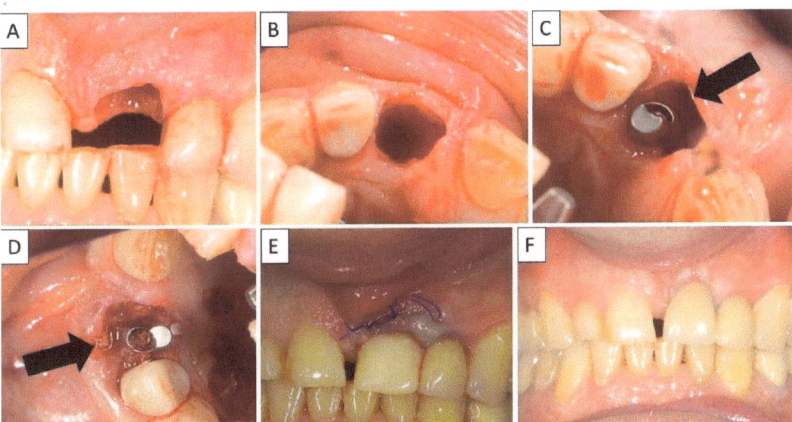

Figure 6. (**A**,**B**) Alveolar socket following atraumatic extraction. Severe bone loss of buccal plate. (**C**) Buccal plate was created using the magnesium membrane double layer technique. (**D**) Application of allograft. (**E**) closing sutures and immediate provision. (**F**) four months postoperatively there was an excellent regeneration of bone defect, including fully regenerated cortical and palatal plates. The implant was stable and there was a good healing of the soft tissues. Black arrows are used to indicate the position of the magnesium membrane.

Four months post operatively, there was an excellent regeneration of bone defect including a fully regenerated cortical buccal plate (Figure 7). The implant was stable, and a good healing of the soft tissues was observed in the postoperative phase.

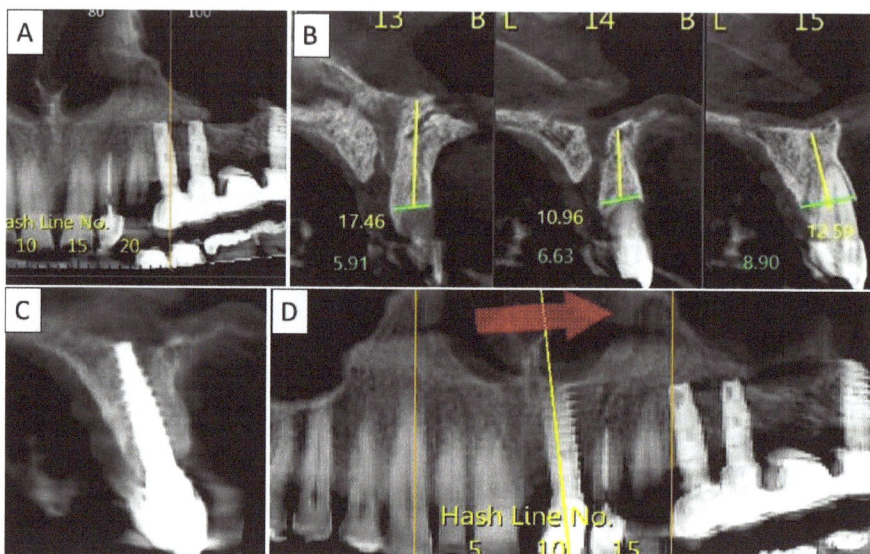

Figure 7. (**A**) Panoramic CBCT section shows bone loss around tooth 21. (**B**) Sagittal CBCT section of the area around tooth 21 shows extensive buccal bone loss. (**C**) A sagittal CBCT section shows the implant placed at site 21 with a restored cortical buccal plate. (**D**) Panoramic CBCT section shows bone formation around the implant in area 21.

3.4. Case 4

A 60-year-old female patient in good general health condition. Patient presented with tooth 15, root canal treatment, post core and PFM crown and vertical root fracture with associated severe bone loss including loss of buccal cortical plate. Palatal cortical plate was intact.

Nontraumatic extraction of tooth 15 (Figure 8), followed by bone augmentation using the magnesium membrane shield technique to rebuild the buccal wall as described in Section 2.

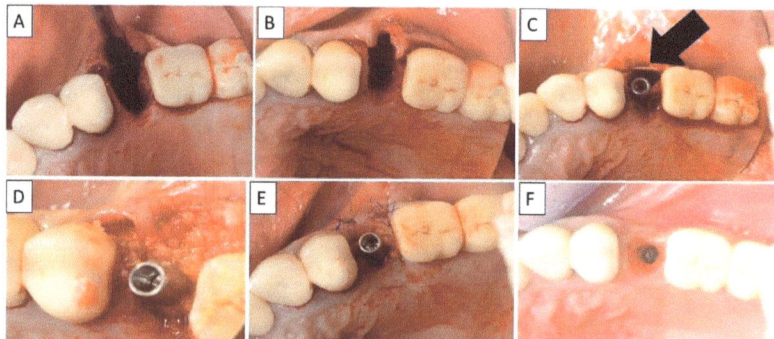

Figure 8. (**A**,**B**) Alveolar socket following atraumatic extraction and curettage. Severe bone loss on buccal wall. (**C**) Buccal wall was created using the magnesium membrane shield technique. (**D**) Application of allograft. (**E**) Closing sutures and immediate provision. (**F**) Four months post operatively there was a regeneration of bone defect, including fully regenerated cortical bone. The implant was stable and there was a good healing of the soft tissues. The black arrow indicates the position of the magnesium membrane.

Four months post operatively, there was an excellent regeneration of bone defect including a fully regenerated cortical buccal plate (Figure 9). The implant was stable and there was a good healing of the soft tissues.

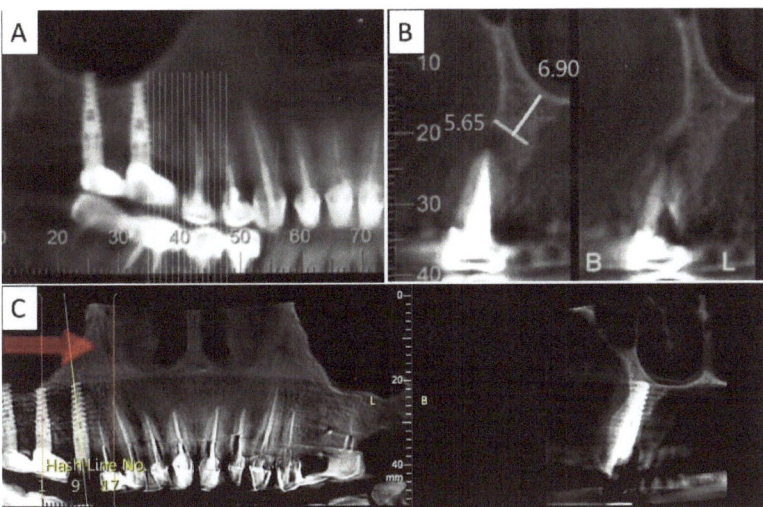

Figure 9. (**A**) Panoramic CBCT section shows associated apical radiolucency of tooth 15. (**B**) Coronal CBCT section shows tooth 15 with vertical root fracture and destroyed buccal bony wall and intact palatine. (**C**) Panoramic CBCT section shows bone formation around the implant in area 15. The coronal CBCT section shows the implant placed in the region of tooth 15.

4. Discussion

In regenerative dentistry, there is a wide choice of available materials that can be applied for hard tissue augmentation [26]. In order to overcome the negative consequences of tooth extraction, different techniques of alveolar ridge preservation have been proposed to retain the original ridge dimension, including immediate or delayed implant placement, and buccal overbuilding with bone grafting materials. The loss of buccal and palatal bone in periodontally compromised teeth or during extraction are a common clinical scenario that surgeons are faced with [27]. Each patient needs to be diagnosed separately and an appropriate choice of material must be chosen. Especially in the case of buccal and/or palatal bone loss, the clinician needs to make a choice of the most suitable material, sometimes having to prioritize mechanically strong materials over resorbable or more clinically manageable materials [28].

Large size bone defects that have lost both vertical and horizontal dimensions usually require a choice of membrane or plate that will provide mechanical stability during bone regeneration of the extraction socket space. This is to counteract the external forces on the defect space created by the overlying soft tissue. The choice of materials include titanium or titanium reinforced membranes [29], collagen membranes [30], or autologous grafts [2,3].

Titanium based materials provide high mechanical stability to enable bone regeneration, which is beneficial for vertical bone gain [28]. However, as titanium is non-resorbable, it is required to be removed in a second surgery, or potentially needs a more invasive surgery upon re-entry by requiring a larger flap to be opened to access the membrane.

Collagen membranes are the most frequently used membranes in regenerative dentistry and have an excellent biocompatibility [31], but are often unstable and can deform or even collapse under loading with the soft tissue entering the bone defect [32,33].

Autologous cortical plates are mechanical strong and have an excellent biocompatibility, but require a second surgical site, increasing patient pain and morbidity. Whilst the use of a tooth root, as in SST, is technically demanding and labor intensive [34].

The development of a magnesium membrane provides a material option that is resorbable yet offers mechanical stability during the critical healing phase [5,17]. Magnesium metal releases magnesium ions during degradation that are naturally present in the body and play an essential role in many important processes within the body [35]. This includes aspects of bone regeneration such as bone cell proliferation, migration, and alkaline phosphatase activity [9]. As the magnesium metal is malleable, it potentially provides an easier adaption to the contours of the defect than is possible with a cortical bone graft. Even though the membrane is malleable, the handling of the membrane must be taken into consideration. The membrane needs to be shaped and cut during surgery in a procedure that is more technically demanding than the application of a collagen membrane and is more comparable to that of a titanium mesh. To aid with the procedure, specialized tools (e.g., NOVAMag® scissor, NOVAMag® sculptor) have been developed for cutting and bending the membrane to shape, reducing the risk of sharp edges that could rupture the mucosa.

Titanium meshes provide mechanical stiffness to support the defect, but do not provide a barrier function for bone regeneration [28]. From a biophysiological perspective, it is suggested that for larger sized defects, maintaining regenerative space and having good osteogenic properties is more beneficial than maintaining a cell occlusivity between the soft and hard tissues [28]. In contrast, the magnesium membrane maintains its mechanical strength during the initial critical healing period [5], but has also been demonstrated in in vivo studies to provide a stable barrier between the soft and the hard tissue [17]. Additionally, as the magnesium metal degrades and is transformed into magnesium salts that are resorbed, nutrient flow into the defect space is possible. Therefore, there is no need to perforate the membrane with holes, which could otherwise negatively affect the degradation rate of the membrane and compromise the soft tissue barrier.

In addition, it has been shown in a previous study by Rider et al. that during the degradation of the magnesium metal, hydrogen gas is released, which has been shown to provide a tenting of the soft tissue [17]. This provides an additional barrier to separate the soft from the hard tissues during the critical healing period.

Alternatively, autogenic or allogenic cortical plate grafts can be used to provide a stable mechanical support [2]; however, these too have their disadvantages. Autogenic grafts require a second surgical site and are associated with donor site morbidity. Additionally, surgical times are prolonged, which can increase the risk of infection. Both autogenic and allogenic cortical plate grafts must be shaped during surgery, which can be technically demanding. In SST [3], partial root retention is used to support the buccal plate and avoid negative tissue alteration post extraction, in a procedure that is technically demanding and time consuming. Magnesium membranes offer a synthetic alternative, as shown by the cases provided in this study, to restore the buccal and the palatal plate during extraction healing with immediate implant placement and even placing provisional restauration if indicated.

The four clinical cases demonstrate the use of a magnesium membrane to provide the necessary stability for bone regeneration and integration of the dental implant.

In each instance, the magnesium membrane was handled slightly differently, but the principle of the magnesium shield technique remained the same. In the first case, the specific requirements of the defect meant that both the buccal and palatal walls had to be built using the magnesium membrane shield technique. Used as a single layer and placed inside the periosteum with the addition of a collagen membrane over the top of the ridge, enough mechanical support was provided on the two opposing sides of the defect to enable regeneration of the bone and support the implant. Potentially this method could be used to treat a much larger sized defect and improve the vertical bone gain.

In the second and fourth case, the membrane was bent into a double layer to provide additional mechanical strength to support the defect space. By bending the membrane into a double layer, a rounded edge is produced that is better for interacting with the soft tissue. If needed, the membrane could also be secured in place using fixation screws in a similar application to the Khoury technique, replacing the need to harvest an autologous cortical bone plate.

In the third case, the membrane was placed in a single layer on the buccal side and the implant was immediately treated with provisional restoration due to its location in the aesthetic zone. A major benefit of using the magnesium membrane shield technique in the aesthetic zone is that there is no need for a large flap created during the augmentation surgery. At 4 months, there was a good implant stability and soft tissue healing.

Due to the handling properties of the membrane, it was easily adapted to the contours of the defect during surgery. All patients had a good recovery, and the healing of the sites was uneventful. In the CBCT images taken 4 months post implantation, cortical bone is visible on the newly formed trabecular bone, indicating a high quality of bone.

In each of the described cases, the magnesium membrane was held in position by being placed under the periosteum. However, depending on the indication, it might be necessary to secure the membrane in place using a fixation system. The membrane has reportedly been secured using titanium fixation screws [5,17], and can also be secured with magnesium alloy fixation screws [6,36], thereby creating a regenerative approach using only fully resorbable materials.

The use of the magnesium membrane shield technique to treat compromised extraction sockets has demonstrated the potential implantation possibilities that have been created by the development of the magnesium membrane. It provides a new material choice that is synthetic, mechanically strong, promoting cortical bone formation, malleable and completely resorbable, a unique combination of properties for regenerative dentistry. These properties are especially beneficial for supporting the defect space and the final regenerative result.

5. Conclusions

For the first time, a magnesium membrane has been reported on for its clinical application in regenerative dentistry. Due to its unique material properties, a new technique is possible: the magnesium membrane shield technique, whereby a magnesium membrane is used to rebuild the buccal or oral walls in compromised sockets. There are already several techniques available for rebuilding or preserving the alveolar ridge post-tooth extraction, but in comparison to the current material choices, magnesium has many beneficial properties: it is completely resorbable and does not need to be extracted; it is synthetic and therefore does not need to be sourced from an additional surgical site, as is the case for autologous cortical bone; it promotes cortical bone growth; it is mechanically strong and able to stabilize the defect space; it is malleable and can be shaped to the contours of the defect in a less technically demanding process than IDS or SST. Four clinical cases demonstrating the use of the magnesium membrane shield technique have shown excellent bone tissue regeneration and, in some instances, the new bone has formed a thick cortical bone layer.

Author Contributions: A.E. conceived, designed, and performed the patient treatment; P.R., Ž.P.K., S.R., D.T., F.W., L.S. and A.E. analyzed the data and wrote the article; A.E., P.R., S.R., D.T., F.W., Ž.P.K. and L.S. proofread the manuscript and helped with the final editing. All authors have read and agreed to the published version of the manuscript.

Funding: The author(s) received no financial support for the research, authorship and/or publication of this article.

Informed Consent Statement: Informed consent was obtained from all subjects involved in the study.

Data Availability Statement: Data sharing is not applicable to this article.

Acknowledgments: In the Acknowledgement section, authors must include individuals and organizations that have made substantive contributions to the research or the manuscript. An exception is where funding was provided, which should be included in Funding Sources.

Conflicts of Interest: The authors P.R., Ž.P.K., S.R. and D.T. are employees of botiss biomaterials GmbH.

References

1. Araujo, M.G.; Lindhe, J. Dimensional ridge alterations following tooth extraction. An experimental study in the dog. *J. Clin. Periodontol.* **2005**, *32*, 212–218. [CrossRef] [PubMed]
2. Da Rosa, J.C.; Rosa, A.C.; da Rosa, D.M.; Zardo, C.M. Immediate Dentoalveolar Restoration of compromised sockets: A novel technique. *Eur. J. Esthet. Dent.* **2013**, *8*, 432–443.
3. Hürzeler, M.B.; Zuhr, O.; Schupbach, P.; Rebele, S.F.; Emmanouilidis, N.; Fickl, S. The socket-shield technique: A proof-of-principle report. *J. Clin. Periodontol.* **2010**, *37*, 855–862. [CrossRef] [PubMed]
4. Lin, X.; Gao, Y.; Ding, X.; Zheng, X. Socket shield technique: A systemic review and meta-analysis. *J. Prosthodont. Res. Jpn. Prosthodont. Soc.* **2022**, *66*, 226–235. [CrossRef] [PubMed]
5. Rider, P.; Kačarević, Ž.P.; Elad, A.; Tadic, D.; Rothamel, D.; Sauer, G. Biodegradable magnesium barrier membrane used for guided bone regeneration in dental surgery. *Bioact. Mater.* **2022**, *14*, 152–168. [CrossRef]
6. Kačarević, Ž.P.; Rider, P.; Elad, A.; Tadic, D.; Rothamel, D.; Sauer, G. Biodegradable magnesium fixation screw for barrier membranes used in guided bone regeneration. *Bioact. Mater.* **2022**, *14*, 15–30. [CrossRef]
7. Zheng, Y.F.; Gu, X.N.; Witte, F. Biodegradable metals. *Mater. Sci. Eng. R Rep.* **2014**, *77*, 1–34. [CrossRef]
8. Azadani, M.N.; Zahedi, A.; Bowoto, O.K.; Oladapo, B.I. A review of current challenges and prospects of magnesium and its alloy for bone implant applications. *Prog. Biomater.* **2022**, *11*, 1–26. [CrossRef]
9. Glenske, K.; Donkiewicz, P.; Köwitsch, A.; Milosevic-Oljaca, N.; Rider, P.; Rofall, S. Applications of metals for bone regeneration. *Int. J. Mol. Sci.* **2018**, *19*, 826. [CrossRef]
10. Zhang, Y.; Xu, J.; Ruan, Y.C.; Yu, M.K.; O'Laughlin, M.; Wise, H.; Qin, L. Implant-derived magnesium induces local neuronal production of CGRP to improve bone-fracture healing in rats. *Nat. Med.* **2016**, *22*, 1160–1169. [CrossRef]
11. Amberg, R.; Elad, A.; Rothamel, D.; Fienitz, T.; Szakacs, G.; Heilmann, S.; Witte, F. Design of a migration assay for human gingival fibroblasts on biodegradable magnesium surfaces. *Acta Biomater.* **2018**, *79*, 158–167. [CrossRef]
12. Okawachi, H.; Ayukawa, Y.; Atsuta, I.; Furuhashi, A.; Sakaguchi, M.; Yamane, K.; Koyano, K. Effect of titanium surface calcium and magnesium on adhesive activity of epithelial-like cells and fibroblasts. *Biointerphases* **2012**, *7*, 27. [CrossRef] [PubMed]
13. Sugimoto, Y.; Hagiwara, A. Cell locomotion on differently charged substrates: Effects of substrate charge on locomotive speed of fibroblastic cells. *Exp. Cell Res.* **1979**, *120*, 245–252. [CrossRef] [PubMed]
14. Wang, L.; Luo, Q.; Zhang, X.; Qiu, J.; Qian, S.; Liu, X. Co-implantation of magnesium and zinc ions into titanium regulates the behaviors of human gingival fibroblasts. *Bioact. Mater.* **2021**, *6*, 64–74. [CrossRef] [PubMed]
15. Atrens, A.; Song, G.L.; Liu, M.; Shi, Z.; Cao, F.; Dargusch, M.S. Review of recent developments in the field of magnesium corrosion. *Adv. Eng. Mater.* **2015**, *17*, 400–453. [CrossRef]
16. Jung, O.; Hesse, B.; Stojanovic, S.; Seim, C.; Weitkamp, T.; Batinic, M. Biocompatibility analyses of hf-passivated magnesium screws for guided bone regeneration (Gbr). *Int. J. Mol. Sci.* **2021**, *22*, 12567. [CrossRef]
17. Rider, P.; Kačarević, Ž.P.; Elad, A.; Rothamel, D.; Sauer, G.; Bornert, F.; Witte, F. Analysis of a Pure Magnesium Membrane Degradation Process and Its Functionality When Used in a Guided Bone Regeneration Model in Beagle Dogs. *Materials* **2022**, *15*, 3106. [CrossRef]
18. Biber, R.; Pauser, J.; Brem, M.; Bail, H.J. Bioabsorbable metal screws in traumatology: A promising innovation. *Trauma Case Rep.* **2017**, *8*, 11–15. [CrossRef]
19. Atkinson, H.D.; Khan, S.; Lashgari, Y.; Ziegler, A. Hallux valgus correction utilising a modified short scarf osteotomy with a magnesium biodegradable or titanium compression screws—A comparative study of clinical outcomes. *BMC Musculoskelet. Disord.* **2019**, *20*, 334. [CrossRef]
20. Haude, M.; Ince, H.; Kische, S.; Abizaid, A.; Tölg, R.; Alves Lemos, P. Safety and clinical performance of a drug eluting absorbable metal scaffold in the treatment of subjects with de novo lesions in native coronary arteries: Pooled 12-month outcomes of BIOSOLVE-II and BIOSOLVE-III. *Catheter. Cardiovasc. Interv.* **2018**, *92*, E502–E511. [CrossRef] [PubMed]
21. Sotomi, Y.; Onuma, Y.; Collet, C.; Tenekecioglu, E.; Virmani, R.; Kleiman, N.S.; Serruys, P.W. Bioresorbable scaffold: The emerging reality and future directions. *Circ. Res.* **2017**, *120*, 1341–1352. [CrossRef]
22. Willbold, E.; Weizbauer, A.; Loos, A.; Seitz, J.M.; Angrisani, N.; Windhagen, H.; Reifenrath, J. Magnesium alloys: A stony pathway from intensive research to clinical reality. Different test methods and approval-related considerations. *J. Biomed. Mater. Res.—Part A* **2017**, *105*, 329–347. [CrossRef] [PubMed]
23. Seitz, J.M.; Lucas, A.; Kirschner, M. Magnesium-Based Compression Screws: A Novelty in the Clinical Use of Implants. *JOM* **2016**, *68*, 1177–1182. [CrossRef]
24. Gröber, U.; Schmidt, J.; Kisters, K. Magnesium in prevention and therapy. *Nutrients* **2015**, *7*, 8199–8226. [CrossRef] [PubMed]

25. Steigmann, L.; Jung, O.; Kieferle, W.; Stojanovic, S.; Proehl, A.; Görke, O. Biocompatibility and Immune Response of a Newly Developed Volume-Stable Magnesium-Based Barrier Membrane in Combination with a PVD Coating for Guided Bone Regeneration (GBR). *Biomedicines* **2020**, *8*, 636. [CrossRef]
26. Elgali, I.; Omar, O.; Dahlin, C.; Thomsen, P. Guided bone regeneration: Materials and biological mechanisms revisited. *Eur. J. Oral Sci.* **2017**, *125*, 315–337. [CrossRef] [PubMed]
27. Kim, J.J.; Amara, H.B.; Chung, I.; Koo, K.T. Compromised extraction sockets: A new classification and prevalence involving both soft and hard tissue loss. *J. Periodontal Implant Sci.* **2021**, *51*, 100–113. [CrossRef]
28. Xie, Y.; Li, S.; Zhang, T.; Wang, C.; Cai, X. Titanium mesh for bone augmentation in oral implantology: Current application and progress. *Int. J. Oral Sci.* **2020**, *12*, 37. [CrossRef] [PubMed]
29. Pinho, M.N.; Novaes, A.B., Jr.; Taba, M., Jr.; Grisi, M.F.; de Souza, S.L.; Palioto, D.B. Titanium Membranes in Prevention of Alveolar Collapse After Tooth Extraction. *Implant Dent.* **2006**, *15*, 53–61. [CrossRef]
30. Guarnieri, R.; Stefanelli, L.; De Angelis, F.; Mencio, F.; Pompa, G.; Di Carlo, S. Extraction Socket Preservation Using Porcine-Derived Collagen Membrane Alone or Associated with Porcine-Derived Bone. Clinical Results of Randomized Controlled Study. *J. Oral Maxillofac. Res.* **2017**, *8*, e5. [CrossRef] [PubMed]
31. Wessing, B.; Lettner, S.; Zechner, W. Guided Bone Regeneration with Collagen Membranes and Particulate Graft Materials: A Systematic Review and Meta-Analysis. *Int. J. Oral Maxillofac. Implants* **2018**, *33*, 87–100. [CrossRef]
32. Naenni, N.; Sapata, V.; Bienz, S.P.; Leventis, M.; Jung, R.E.; Hämmerle, C.H.; Thoma, D.S. Effect of flapless ridge preservation with two different alloplastic materials in sockets with buccal dehiscence defects—Volumetric and linear changes. *Clin. Oral Investig.* **2018**, *22*, 2187–2197. [CrossRef]
33. Mir-Mari, J.; Wui, H.; Jung, R.E.; Hämmerle, C.H.; Benic, G.I. Influence of blinded wound closure on the volume stability of different GBR materials: An in vitro cone-beam computed tomographic examination. *Clin. Oral Implants Res.* **2016**, *27*, 258–265. [CrossRef] [PubMed]
34. Chen, J.T. A Novel Application of Dynamic Navigation System in Socket Shield Technique. *J. Oral Implantol.* **2019**, *45*, 409–415. [CrossRef] [PubMed]
35. Jahnen-Dechent, W.; Ketteler, M. Magnesium basics. *CKJ Clin. Kidney J.* **2012**, *5* (Suppl. S1), i3–i14. [CrossRef] [PubMed]
36. Rider, P.; Kačarević, Ž.P.; Elad, A.; Rothamel, D.; Sauer, G.; Bornert, F. Biodegradation of a Magnesium Alloy Fixation Screw Used in a Guided Bone Regeneration Model in Beagle Dogs. *Materials* **2022**, *15*, 4111. [CrossRef]

Disclaimer/Publisher's Note: The statements, opinions and data contained in all publications are solely those of the individual author(s) and contributor(s) and not of MDPI and/or the editor(s). MDPI and/or the editor(s) disclaim responsibility for any injury to people or property resulting from any ideas, methods, instructions or products referred to in the content.

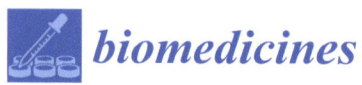 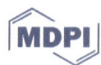

Article

A New Implantation Method for Orthodontic Anchor Screws: Basic Research for Clinical Applications

Reiko Tokuyama-Toda [1], Hirochika Umeki [1], Shinji Ide [1], Fumitaka Kobayashi [2], Shunnosuke Tooyama [2], Mai Umehara [1], Susumu Tadokoro [1], Hiroshi Tomonari [2] and Kazuhito Satomura [1,*]

[1] Department of Oral Medicine and Stomatology, School of Dental Medicine, Tsurumi University, 2-1-3, Tsurumi, Tsurumi-Ku, Yokohama 230-8501, Kanagawa, Japan
[2] Department of Orthodontics, School of Dental Medicine, Tsurumi University, 2-1-3, Tsurumi, Tsurumi-Ku, Yokohama 230-8501, Kanagawa, Japan
* Correspondence: satomura-k@tsurumi-u.ac.jp; Tel.: +81-45-580-8326

Abstract: This study aimed to determine whether the positional relationship between the underside of the screw head and the surface of the alveolar bone could alter the stress on the two surfaces and affect the stability of implanted anchor screws. First, in order to confirm the extent of the gap between the mini-screw and the bone surface, a mini-screw was placed in the palate of rabbits and examined histologically. As a result, in the conventional screw implantation procedure, oral mucosa between the base of the screw head and the bone creates a spatial gap. Removal of the oral mucosa eliminates this gap. Then, we compared the positional difference of the screw in a contact and gap group by analyzing stress distribution on the bone and screw. Analysis using the finite element method showed that more stress was loaded on both the bone and screw in the gap group than in the contact group. Cortical bone thickness did not affect stress in either group. The effects of different load strengths were similar between groups. A surgical procedure in which mucosal coverings are removed so that implanted anchor mini-screws are in contact with the bone surface was found to reduce the stress load on both the bone and screw. This procedure can be used to prevent undesirable dislodgement of implanted mini-screws.

Keywords: FEM analysis; implantation method; mini-screw; orthodontic anchor screws; von Mises stress

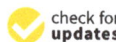

Citation: Tokuyama-Toda, R.; Umeki, H.; Ide, S.; Kobayashi, F.; Tooyama, S.; Umehara, M.; Tadokoro, S.; Tomonari, H.; Satomura, K. A New Implantation Method for Orthodontic Anchor Screws: Basic Research for Clinical Applications. *Biomedicines* **2023**, *11*, 665. https://doi.org/10.3390/biomedicines11030665

Academic Editors: Gianmarco Abbadessa and Giuseppe Minervini

Received: 16 January 2023
Revised: 13 February 2023
Accepted: 20 February 2023
Published: 22 February 2023

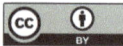

Copyright: © 2023 by the authors. Licensee MDPI, Basel, Switzerland. This article is an open access article distributed under the terms and conditions of the Creative Commons Attribution (CC BY) license (https://creativecommons.org/licenses/by/4.0/).

1. Introduction

Orthodontic anchor screws are an efficient and robust means of fixation in orthodontic treatment [1–4]. Since the mini-screw anchor system became widely used in clinical practice, it has been noted that there is occasional incidence of these screws falling out. To address this and develop means of prevention, several studies have investigated the biomechanics of mini-screw fixation. This has led to various improvements in the form of modifications to the shape [5–7] and length [8] of screws, consideration of bone condition at the fixation site [9–13], and optimization of screw angle and torque [14–18] during implantation. Nonetheless, mini-screws still fail in some cases, usually as a result of inflammation, infection, and shedding [19–25]. In this study, we investigated whether the position in which the screw is embedded affected its likelihood of falling out. Advantages of the mini-screw include its ability to penetrate the oral mucosa and its easy implantation into the bone, with no drilling required, making it a safe and convenient option [26–28]. However, when a mini-screw is implanted in the alveolar bone using this procedure, the oral mucosa lies between the underside of the screw head and the alveolar bone, causing a small separation between the screw and bone. When a load is applied in this situation, the alveolar bone is likely to be placed under more stress than it would if there were no gap between the screw and bone. Therefore, in this study, we used a rabbit mini-screw implantation model to compare the distance between the underside of the screw head and the alveolar bone surface, with and without intervening oral mucosa. The determined distances between the mini-screw and the bone surface were reproduced, and the distribution of stress on the alveolar bone and the mini-screw when clinically realistic orthodontic force was applied to the mini-screw was analyzed using the finite element method (FEM).

2. Materials and Methods

2.1. Animal Selection and Handling

Our animal care procedures and experimental protocols were approved by the Committee on the Ethics of Animal Experiments of Tsurumi University (permit number: 19A005). Surgical procedures were performed under sodium pentobarbital anesthesia, and all efforts were made to minimize the suffering of our laboratory animals. Ten male Japanese white rabbits (2.5–3.0 kg) were obtained from Tokyo Laboratory Animals Science Co., Ltd. (Tokyo, Japan). They were fed a normal diet and maintained under a 12 h light–dark cycle at 22 °C.

2.2. Implantation of Orthodontic Anchor Screws: Histological Examination to Confirm the Distance between the Bone Surface and the Mini-Screw

Mini-screws were implanted in the palatal bones of two groups of Japanese white rabbits to compare implantation preceded by removal of the oral mucosa with the conventional procedure without removal of the mucosa. In the removal group, the rabbits were given local anesthetic of 2% lidocaine. A 3 mm-diameter biopsy punch (Kai Industries, Gifu, Japan) was then used to remove a circular piece of the left palatal mucosa corresponding to the size of the screw head from each rabbit. A mini-screw was implanted in the same place without drilling, and it was confirmed that the initial fixation was good (n = 10). In members of the group that underwent the conventional procedure (the penetration group), 2% lidocaine local anesthetic was administered, and the mini-screw was then implanted in the right palate by penetrating the oral mucosa without drilling. It was confirmed that the initial fixation was good (n = 10). The mini-screw used with both groups had a diameter of 1.6 mm and a length of 5 mm (Jeil, Republic of Korea, Code 16-JK-005). The next day, maxillary tissue from around the mini-screw was obtained from each rabbit for histological analysis. The excised tissue was fixed with 10% neutral buffered formalin and embedded in methyl methacrylate (MMA) resin (Exakt, Germany). Polished 40–50 µm-thick sections were made and stained with hematoxylin and eosin (H&E).

2.3. Histometric Analysis

A histometric analysis was performed using the 10 tissue sections obtained from each group. The distances between the underside of the screw head and the bone surface were measured, and the average value for each group was calculated. The results were then analyzed using the FEM.

2.4. FEM Analysis Modeling

A three-dimensional bone block model with an integrated mini-screw was constructed using Optistruct v2020 (Altair Engineering, Troy, MI, USA), a computer-aided design support program. The cortical bone was simplified and simulated to a thickness of 1.0 mm or 2.0 mm, factoring in the buccal alveolar bone and palatal slope in which the mini-screw had been clinically placed. The shape of the mini-screw was set based on Jeil's 16-JK-006 (Figure 1).

The interface between the cortex and the cancellous bone was assumed to be fully bonded, that is, to have continuous elements sharing the same nodes along the interface. A node-to-node contact condition was modeled on the interface between the mini-screw and the bone block to imitate a stage without osseointegration. All materials in the model were homogeneous, isotropic, and linearly elastic. The mini-screw was assumed to be pure titanium, with Young's modulus of 110 gigapascals (GPa) and Poisson's ratio of 0.33 [29]. For healthy bone quality, Young's moduli of the cortical and cancellous bones were 18 GPa [29] and 1.37 GPa [8], respectively, and Poisson's ratios were 0.3 for both (Table 1).

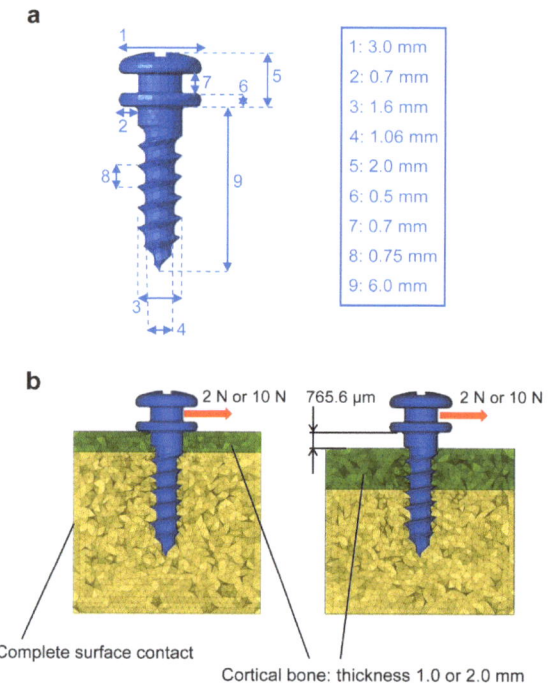

Figure 1. Setting the shape of an anchor screw shape and the conditions for finite element method analysis for a comparison of anchor screws with and without mucosa between the screw and bone. (**a**) Setting of the anchor screw shape. The shape of the mini-screw was set based on Jeil's 16-JK-006. (**b**) Setting of the conditions for analysis using finite element method. Assuming the presence of the cortical and cancellous bone, the cortical bone was set to thicknesses of either 1.0 mm or 2.0 mm. The load was set to either 2.0 or 10.0 Newtons. The gap between the underside of the screw head and the bone surface was 0 μm in the removal group and 765.6 μm in the penetration group.

Table 1. Material property values.

Component	Material	Young's Modulus [MPa]	Poisson's Ratio	Density [ton/mm^3]
Mini-screw	Titanium alloy	110,000	0.33	4.5×10^{-9}
Cortical bone	—	18,000	0.3	0.9×10^{-9}
Cancellous bone	—	13,700	0.3	0.9×10^{-9}

A static load was applied to the head of the mini-screw along the *x*-axis perpendicular to its long axis to simulate orthodontic force. The nodal solution of the von Mises stress in the bone and the mini-screw were calculated for each model with the FEM program. To determine the loading effects, two force magnitudes were applied to mimic various clinical conditions. A loading force of 2.0 Newtons (N) was used to mimic the load in space closure using a NiTi coil spring or elastomeric chains. A load of 10.0 N was used to mimic orthopedic force, such as mini-screw-assisted rapid palatal expansion. The load direction was set perpendicular to the long axis of the mini-screw. The distance between the underside of the screw head and the bone surface was set to 0 μm for the removal group and 765.6 μm for the penetration group based on the results obtained earlier

(Table 2). FEM analysis was performed under the above conditions to examine the effects on the surrounding bone and on the mini-screw itself when the same force was applied to each group.

Table 2. Analysis case list.

Case	Load [N]	Cortical Bone Thickness [mm]	Screw-Bone Distance [μm]	Element Count Screw	Cortical Bone	Cancellous Bone
1–1	2.0	1.0	0.0	6601	17,957	124,262
1–2	2.0	1.0	765.6	6601	19,365	111,551
1–3	2.0	2.0	0.0	6601	38,807	88,182
1–4	2.0	2.0	765.6	6601	32,821	98,220
2–1	10.0	1.0	0.0	6601	17,957	124,262
2–2	10.0	1.0	765.6	6601	19,365	111,551
2–3	10.0	2.0	0.0	6601	38,807	88,182
2–4	10.0	2.0	765.6	6601	32,821	98,220

Note. Element type: Tetra-quadratic element.

2.5. Statistical Analysis

All data were expressed as the mean ± standard deviation (SD). Statistical analyses were performed using the Kruskal–Wallis H test and Scheffe's test. p values of <0.05 were considered statistically significant by using StatMate V.

3. Results

3.1. Distance between the Underside of the Screw Head and the Bone Surface Obtained from Histological Examination in Animal Experiments

The distances between the underside of the screw head and the bone surface in the removal and penetration group were compared. In the penetration group, there was an average gap of 765.6 μm. In the removal group, the underside of the screw head was in contact with the bone surface (0 μm) (Figure 2).

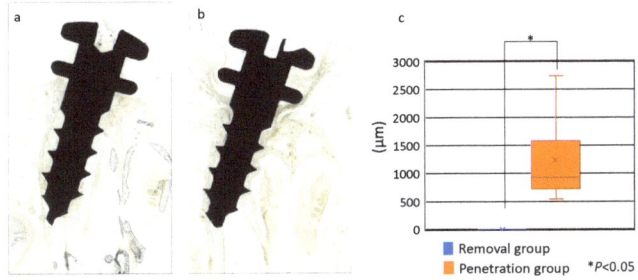

Figure 2. The distances between the underside of the screw head and the surface of the bone resulting from different methods of mini-screw implantation. (**a**) Removal group. (**b**) Penetration group. (**c**) The gap was an average of 0 μm in the removal group (n = 10) and 765.6 μm in the penetration group (n = 10).

3.2. FEM Analysis

Figure 3 shows the peak von Mises stress on the bone at a load of 2.0 N. FEM analysis showed that the peak von Mises stress on the surrounding bone at 1.0 mm of the cortical bone was 3.3 MPa and 11.3 MPa in the removal and penetration group, respectively. Even with a cortical bone thickness of 2.0 mm, there was no significant difference in the peak von Mises stress value.

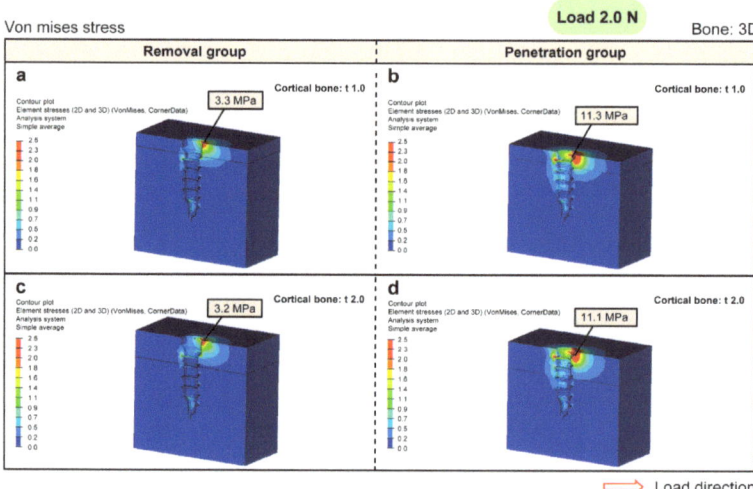

Figure 3. The peak von Mises stress on mini-screw-implanted bone with a load of 2.0 Newtons (3D view). (**a,c**) Removal group. (**b,d**) Penetration group. (**a,b**) Cortical bone thickness of 1.0 mm. (**c,d**) Cortical bone thickness of 2.0 mm. The peak von Mises stress on the surrounding bone with 1.0 mm of the cortical bone was 3.3 megapascals (MPa) in the removal group and 11.3 MPa in the penetration group. The peak von Mises stress on the surrounding bone with 2.0 mm of the cortical bone was 3.2 MPa in the removal group and 11.1 MPa in the penetration group.

Figure 4 shows an aerial view of the screw head for this condition. It was found that the von Mises stress on the surrounding bone was lower in the removal group than in the penetration group.

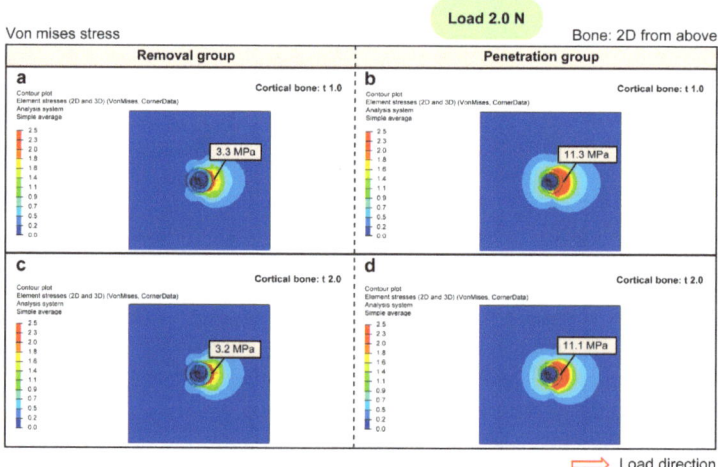

Figure 4. The peak von Mises stress on mini-screw-implanted bone with a load of 2.0 Newtons (2D view from above). (**a,c**) Removal group. (**b,d**) Penetration group. (**a,b**) Cortical bone thickness of 1.0 mm. (**c,d**) Cortical bone thickness of 2.0 mm. The peak von Mises stress on the surrounding bone with 1.0 mm of the cortical bone was 3.3 megapascals (MPa) in the removal group and 11.3 MPa in the penetration group. With 2.0 mm of the cortical bone, it was 3.2 MPa in the removal group and 11.1 MPa in the penetration group.

Figure 5 shows the result of separating the von Mises stress into tension and compression. The compression was 3.9 MPa and 9.3 MPa in the removal and penetration group, respectively, indicating that, even with the same load of 2.0 N, the effect on the surrounding bone was much greater in the penetration group.

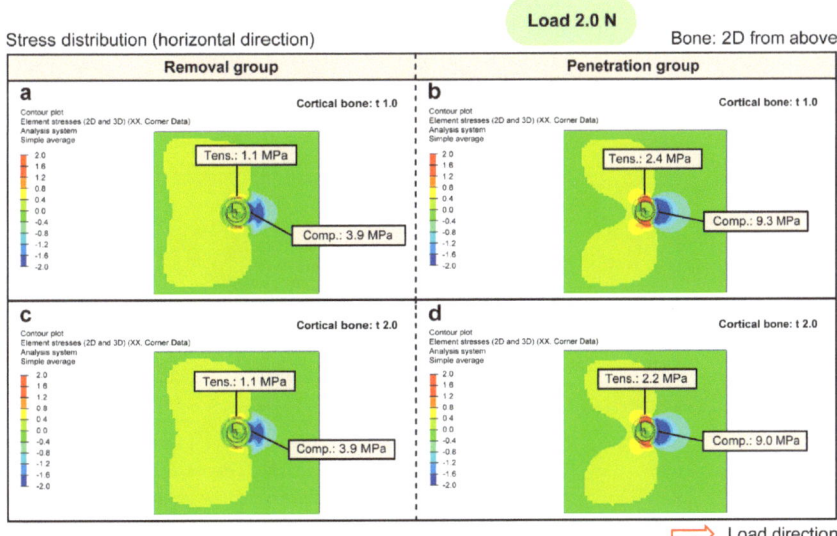

Figure 5. Deconstructing von Mises stress into the tension and compression on mini-screw implanted bone with a load of 2.0 Newtons (2D view from above). (**a**,**c**) Removal group. (**b**,**d**) Penetration group. (**a**,**b**) Cortical bone thickness of 1.0 mm. (**c**,**d**) Cortical bone thickness of 2.0 mm. With 1.0 mm of the cortical bone, the peak compression was 3.9 megapascals (MPa) and tension was 1.1 MPa in the removal group; compression was 9.3 MPa and tension was 2.4 MPa in the penetration group. With 2.0 mm of the cortical bone, the peak compression was 3.9 MPa and tension was 1.1 MPa in the removal group; compression was 9.0 MPa and tension was 2.2 MPa in the penetration group.

Figure 6 shows the peak von Mises stress on the mini-screw at a load of 2.0 N. The von Mises stress on the mini-screw itself was also lower in the removal group than in the penetration group.

The peak von Mises stress on the bone with a load of 10.0 N is shown in Figure 7. The peak von Mises stress on the surrounding bone at 1.0 mm of the cortical bone was 14.6 MPa and 54.8 MPa in the removal and penetration group, respectively. Even with a cortical bone thickness of 2.0 mm, there was no significant difference in the peak value of von Mises stress.

Figure 8 shows an aerial view of the screw head for this condition. As with the load of 2.0 N, it was found that the von Mises stress on the surrounding bone was lower in the removal group than in the penetration group.

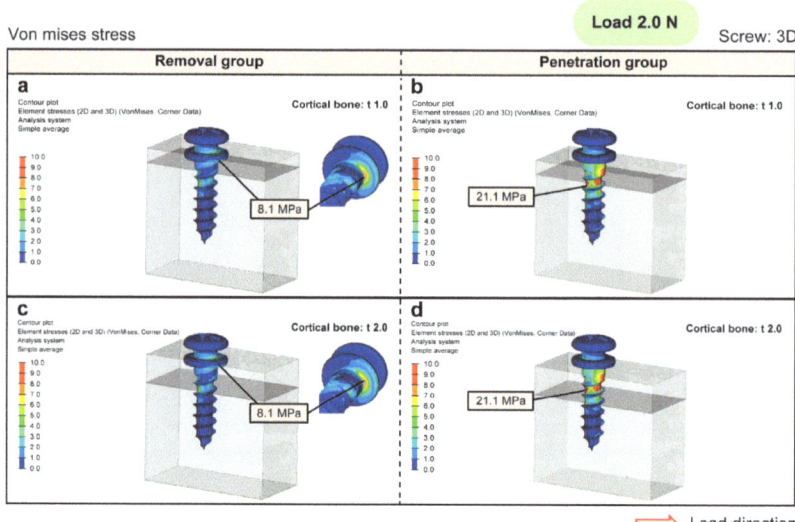

Figure 6. The peak von Mises stress for a mini-screw implanted in the bone with a load of 2.0 Newtons (3D view). (**a,c**) Removal group. (**b,d**) Penetration group. (**a,b**) Cortical bone thickness of 1.0 mm. (**c,d**) Cortical bone thickness of 2.0 mm. The peak von Mises stress on the mini-screw with 1.0 mm of the cortical bone was 8.1 megapascals (MPa) in the removal group and 21.1 MPa in the penetration group. The peak von Mises stress on the mini-screw with 2.0 mm of the cortical bone was 8.1 MPa in the removal group and 21.1 MPa in the penetration group.

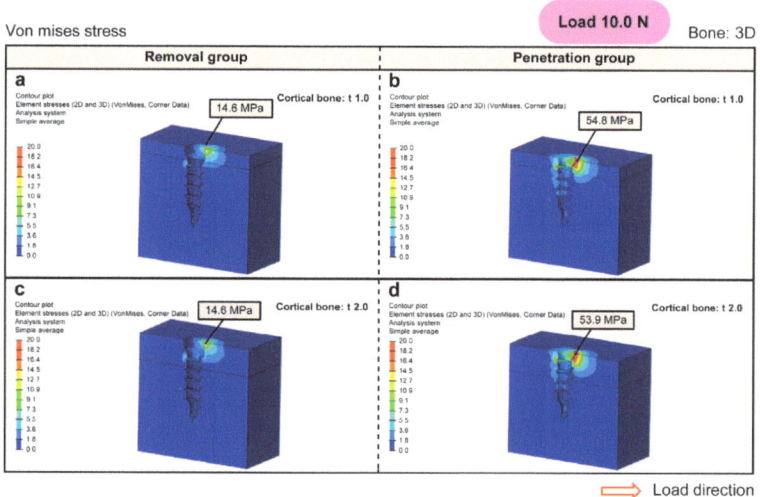

Figure 7. The peak von Mises stress on a mini-screw-implanted bone with a load of 10.0 Newtons (3D view). (**a,c**) Removal group. (**b,d**) Penetration group. (**a,b**) Cortical bone thickness of 1.0 mm. (**c,d**) Cortical bone thickness of 2.0 mm. The peak von Mises stress on the surrounding bone with 1.0 mm of the cortical bone was 14.6 megapascals (MPa) in the removal group and 54.8 MPa in the penetration group. The peak von Mises stress on the surrounding bone with 2.0 mm of the cortical bone was 14.6 MPa in the removal group and 53.9 MPa in the penetration group.

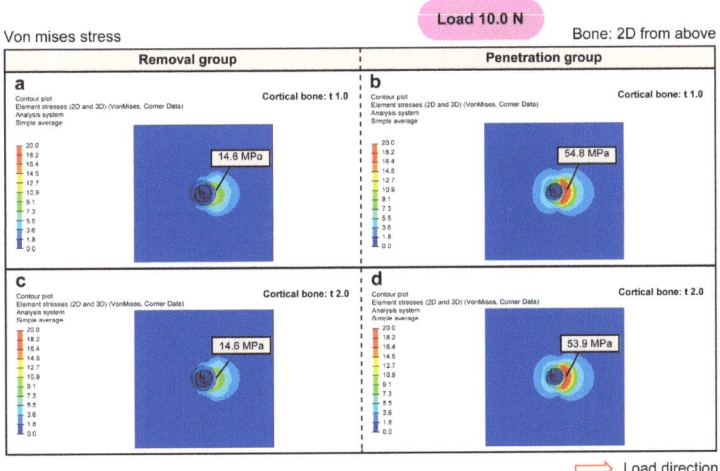

Figure 8. The peak von Mises stress on a mini-screw-implanted bone with a load of 10.0 Newtons (2D view from above). (**a**,**c**) Removal group. (**b**,**d**) Penetration group. (**a**,**b**) Cortical bone thickness of 1.0 mm. (**c**,**d**) Cortical bone thickness of 2.0 mm. The peak von Mises stress on the surrounding bone with 1.0 mm of the cortical bone was 14.6 megapascals (MPa) in the removal group and 54.8 MPa in the penetration group. The peak von Mises stress on the surrounding bone with 2.0 mm of the cortical bone was 14.6 MPa in the removal group and 53.9 MPa in the penetration group.

Figure 9 shows the result of separating the von Mises stress into tension and compression. The compression was 17.7 MPa and 47.0 MPa in the removal and penetration group, respectively, indicating that, even with the same load of 10.0 N, the effect on the surrounding bone was greater in the penetration group.

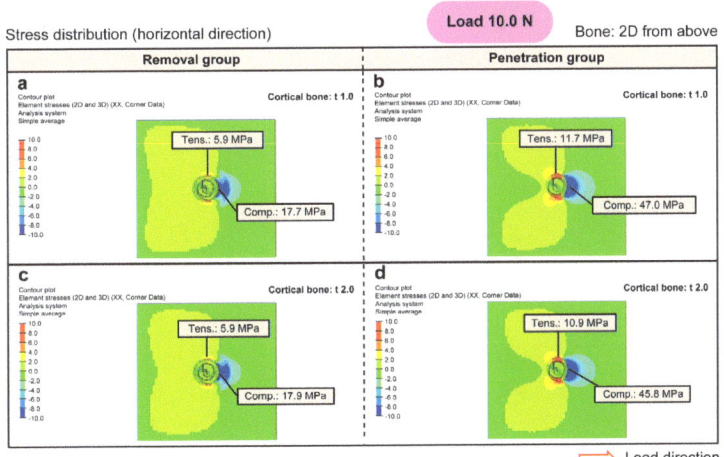

Figure 9. Deconstructing von Mises stress into the tension and compression on mini-screw implanted bone with a load of 10.0 Newtons (2D view from above). (**a**,**c**) Removal group. (**b**,**d**) Penetration group. (**a**,**b**) Cortical bone thickness is 1.0 mm. (**c**,**d**) Cortical bone thickness is 2.0 mm. With 1.0 mm of the cortical bone, the peak compression was 17.7 megapascals (MPa) and tension was 5.9 MPa in the removal group; compression was 47.0 MPa and tension was 11.7 MPa in the penetration group. With 2.0 mm of the cortical bone, the peak compression was 17.9 MPa and tension was 5.9 MPa in the removal group; compression was 45.8 MPa and tension was 10.9 MPa in the penetration group.

Figure 10 shows the peak von Mises stress on the mini-screw at a load of 10.0 N. Again, the von Mises stress on the mini-screw was lower in the removal group than in the penetration group. These results are summarized in Figure 11.

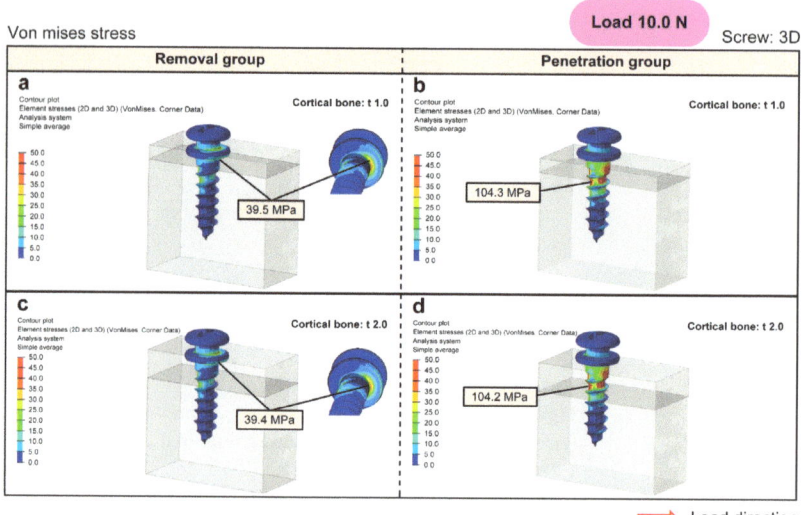

Figure 10. The peak von Mises stress on the mini-screw at a load of 10.0 N (3D view). (**a,c**) Removal group. (**b,d**) Penetration group. (**a,b**) Cortical bone thickness of 1.0 mm. (**c,d**) Cortical bone thickness of 2.0 mm. The peak von Mises stress on the mini-screw with 1.0 mm of the cortical bone was 39.5 megapascals (MPa) in the removal group and 104.3 MPa in the penetration group. The peak von Mises stress on the mini-screw with 2.0 mm of the cortical bone was 39.4 MPa in the removal group and 104.2 MPa in the penetration group.

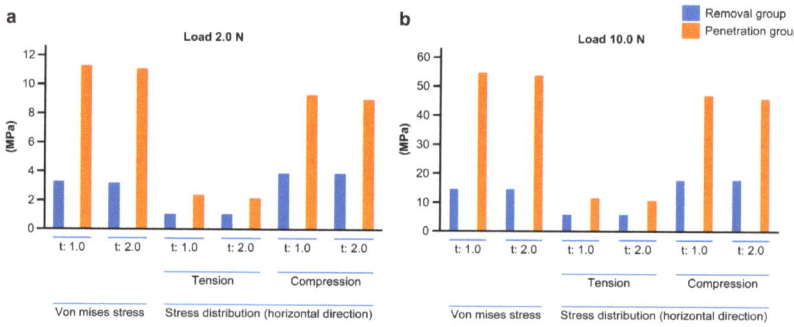

Figure 11. Summary of results of a comparison of mini-screw implantation into the bone with and without removal of the oral mucosa. (**a**) A load of 2.0 Newtons. (**b**) A load of 10.0 Newtons.

4. Discussion

Since the mini-screw first came to be used as a fixation anchor in orthodontic treatment, various studies on the optimization of its implantation have been reported [5–17]. However, clinically undesirable cases in which screws drop out or break still occur, and the cause of this is unclear. In this study, we have focused on the gap between the underside of the screw head and the bone surface in the conventional implantation procedure and hypothesized that this gap may be a critical factor in the dropping out of screws. Using the FEM, we investigated the possibility that excessive stress results from the gap between the underside of the screw head and the bone surface, causing screws to fall out.

First, to confirm the existence of such a gap, mini-screws were implanted in the palatal bones of rabbits, with and without the removal of the oral mucosa at the site of screw placement before implantation. We found that, with the mucosa left in place, there was an average gap of 765 μm between the underside of the screw head and the bone surface. In the rabbits with the excised mucosa, no gap was present. By removing the local mucous membrane, the screw can be implanted so that the underside of the screw head comes into full contact with the bone surface.

The results of the FEM analysis are summarized in Figure 11. FEM analysis confirmed that there was greater von Mises stress in the penetration group than in the removal group with both a 2.0 N and 10.0 N load. The results were similar regardless of whether the cortical bone thickness was 1.0 mm or 2.0 mm. Concentration of stress was observed in the bone around the screw on the side to which the load was applied, and a stress peak was observed on the bone surface. When this stress was divided into tension and compression, greater compression was observed in the load direction and greater tension at 90° to the site. The tendency of these stresses was the same regardless of whether the load was 2.0 N or 10.0 N. However, the peak von Mises stress exceeded 50 MPa in the penetration group, especially at 10.0 N, suggesting that the extent of the stress is sufficient for bone resorption to occur. In comparison, the peak von Mises stress was suppressed to about 15 MPa in the removal group, in which the new implantation method proposed in this study was used. Even when the load was 2.0 N, the stress peak in the removal group was suppressed to about 1/4 of that seen in the penetration group. These results suggest that for screws with mucosal intervention, the greater the load, the greater the stress on the surrounding bone and the possibility of bone resorption. Thus, if the mucous membrane is removed and the screw is placed in contact with the bone surface, the stress on the surrounding bone is reduced and bone resorption is suppressed, preventing the screw from falling out.

The stress on the screw itself in the removal group was suppressed to about 1/2–1/3 of that seen in the penetration group at both 2.0 N and 10.0 N. In the penetration group, the stress to the screw itself was as large as 100 MPa at 10.0 N. Considering these results, in treatments where a large load is expected, such as mini-screw-assisted rapid expansion, it may be possible to help prevent screws from falling out by using screws with thicker diameters or embedding deeper.

The FEM analysis of the gap between the underside of the screw head and the bone surface was based on the results of an animal study, and the soft tissue thickness of human oral mucosa varies depending on the anatomical insertion site of the mini-screw [19,23,25,30–32], as well as the patient's age and general condition [31,33]. Moreover, some changes in the surrounding mucosa and bone may occur due to the mechanical load. In light of these facts, the results in this study may not precisely reflect clinical conditions. Nonetheless, it is clear that soft tissue does intervene between the base of the anchor mini-screw head and the bone surface when it is implanted using the conventional procedure. It is also apparent that this can cause excessive stress to the surrounding bone tissue, leading to bone resorption and, eventually, to the screw falling out. Therefore, we strongly recommend the new procedure for implanting orthodontic anchor screws. The underside of the anchor screw should contact the bone surface directly, without oral mucosal intervention.

Indeed, the cause of the orthodontic anchor screw falling out is not limited to bone resorption. Screws sometimes fall out immediately after they are placed. The cause of these instances remains unclear. As previously reported, the cause may sometimes be infection or inflammation [19–25]. In this study, we proposed a new implantation method that can prevent mini-screws used as anchors in orthodontic treatment from falling out. Although further investigation is needed, this implantation method without mucosal intervention may be able to suppress excessive inflammation around the screw immediately after implantation. It is also possible that compression of the mucous membrane between the bottom of the screw head and the bone may cause the inflammation and infection of surrounding tissue. These issues should be investigated in future studies.

We compared the conventional mini-screw implantation method with the new implantation method, in which the mucosa was removed. We have shown that the new method can reduce various forces on bones. However, these studies were conducted using animal experiments and are only stress analyses by FEM. We believe that more research is needed before this new technique can be applied to clinical practice as a better alternative to traditional methods. Specifically, we believe that prospective studies should be conducted in two groups of patients: traditional and new. We are preparing to conduct a trial in the near future.

5. Conclusions

This study proposes a new procedure for implanting orthodontic anchor screws, in which the underside of the screw head is in direct contact with the bone surface, without mucosa between the two. This procedure helps to prevent excess stress on the surrounding bone and the loosening or falling out of screws.

Author Contributions: R.T.-T. conceived, designed, and performed experiments, analyzed the data, and wrote the manuscript. H.U. performed experiments. S.I. performed experiments. F.K. performed experiments. S.T. (Shunnosuke Tooyama) performed experiments. M.U. performed experiments. S.T. (Susumu Tadokoro) performed experiments. H.T. conceived and designed the experiments and provided specimens. K.S. conceived and designed the experiments and provided specimens. All authors have read and agreed to the published version of the manuscript.

Funding: This research was funded by JSPS KAKENHI, grant numbers 20K10150, 20K10104, 19K19251, 18K17210, 20K10238, 21K19617, and 17H04411.

Institutional Review Board Statement: This study was conducted in accordance with the principles of the Council of International Organizations for Medical Sciences (CIOMS) and Japanese government regulations on animal experimentation. Our animal care procedures and experimental protocols were approved by the Committee on the Ethics of Animal Experiments of Tsurumi University (permit number: 19A005), 12 April 2019.

Informed Consent Statement: Not applicable.

Data Availability Statement: The data that support the findings of this study are available from the corresponding author upon reasonable request.

Acknowledgments: 20K10150 is Reiko Tokuyama, 20K10104 is Nagataka Toyoda, 19K19251 is Hirochika Umeki, 18K17210 is Susumu Tadokoro, 20K10238 is Hiroshi Tomonari, and 21K19617 and 17H04411 are Kazuhito Satomura.

Conflicts of Interest: The authors declare no conflict of interest.

References

1. Kanomi, R. Mini-Implant for Orthodontic Anchorage. *J. Clin. Orthod.* **1997**, *31*, 763–767. [PubMed]
2. Costa, A.; Raffainl, M.; Melsen, B. Miniscrews as Orthodontic Anchorage: A Preliminary Report. *Int. J. Adult Orthod. Orthognath. Surg.* **1998**, *13*, 201–209.
3. Giancotti, A.; Arcuri, C.; Barlattani, A. Treatment of Ectopic Mandibular Second Molar with Titanium Miniscrews. *Am. J. Orthod. Dentofac. Orthop.* **2004**, *126*, 113–117. [CrossRef] [PubMed]
4. Park, H.S.; Kwon, O.W.; Sung, J.H. Micro-implant Anchorage for Forced Eruption of Impacted Canines. *J. Clin. Orthod.* **2004**, *38*, 297–302. [PubMed]
5. Wilmes, B.; Ottenstreuer, S.; Su, Y.Y.; Drescher, D. Impact of Implant Design on Primary Stability of Orthodontic Mini-Implants. *J. Orofac. Orthop.* **2008**, *69*, 42–50. [CrossRef]
6. Ye, Y.; Yi, W.; Fan, S.; Zhao, L.; Yu, Y.; Lu, Y.; Yao, Q.; Wang, W.; Chang, S. Effect of Thread Depth and Thread Pitch on the Primary Stability of Miniscrews Receiving a Torque Load: A Finite Element Analysis. *J. Orofac. Orthop.* **2021**, *online ahead of print*. [CrossRef]
7. Ye, Y.S.; Yi, W.M.; Zhuang, P.L.; Liu, M.; Yu, Y.S.; Lu, Y.J.; Yao, Q.H.; Wang, W.; Chang, S.H. Thread Shape Affects the Stress Distribution of Torque Force on Miniscrews: A Finite Element Analysis. *Comput. Methods Biomech. Biomed. Eng.* **2020**, *23*, 1034–1040. [CrossRef]

8. Gracco, A.; Cirignaco, A.; Cozzani, M.; Boccaccio, A.; Pappalettere, C.; Vitale, G. Numerical/Experimental Analysis of the Stress Field around Miniscrews for Orthodontic Anchorage. *Eur. J. Orthod.* **2009**, *31*, 12–20. [CrossRef]
9. Lombardo, L.; Gracco, A.; Zampini, F.; Stefanoni, F.; Mollica, F. Optimal Palatal Configuration for Miniscrew Applications. *Angle Orthod.* **2010**, *80*, 145–152. [CrossRef]
10. Melsen, B.; Verna, C. Miniscrew Implants: The Aarhus Anchorage System. *Semin. Orthod.* **2005**, *11*, 24–31. [CrossRef]
11. Motoyoshi, M.; Inaba, M.; Ono, A.; Ueno, S.; Shimizu, N. The Effect of Cortical Bone Thickness on the Stability of Orthodontic Mini-Implants and on the Stress Distribution in Surrounding Bone. *Int. J. Oral Maxillofac. Surg.* **2009**, *38*, 13–18. [CrossRef]
12. Motoyoshi, M.; Yoshida, T.; Ono, A.; Shimizu, N. Effect of Cortical Bone Thickness and Implant Placement Torque on Stability of Orthodontic Mini-Implants. *Int. J. Oral Maxillofac. Implants* **2007**, *22*, 779–784.
13. Wang, Z.; Zhao, Z.; Xue, J.; Song, J.; Deng, F.; Yang, P. Pullout Strength of Miniscrews Placed in Anterior Mandibles of Adult and Adolescent Dogs: A Microcomputed Tomographic Analysis. *Am. J. Orthod. Dentofac. Orthop.* **2010**, *137*, 100–107. [CrossRef]
14. Kim, J.W.; Ahn, S.J.; Chang, Y.I. Histomorphometric and Mechanical Analyses of the Drill-Free Screw as Orthodontic Anchorage. *Am. J. Orthod. Dentofac. Orthop.* **2005**, *128*, 190–194. [CrossRef]
15. Wilmes, B.; Su, Y.Y.; Drescher, D. Insertion Angle Impact on Primary Stability of Orthodontic Mini-Implants. *Angle Orthod.* **2008**, *78*, 1065–1070. [CrossRef]
16. Motoyoshi, M.; Hirabayashi, M.; Uemura, M.; Shimizu, N. Recommended Placement Torque When Tightening an Orthodontic Mini-Implant. *Clin. Oral Implants Res.* **2006**, *17*, 109–114. [CrossRef]
17. Stahl, E.; Keilig, L.; Abdelgader, I.; Jäger, A.; Bourauel, C. Numerical Analyses of Biomechanical Behavior of Various Orthodontic Anchorage Implants. *J. Orofac. Orthop.* **2009**, *70*, 115–127. [CrossRef]
18. Liu, T.C.; Chang, C.H.; Wong, T.Y.; Liu, J.K. Finite Element Analysis of Miniscrew Implants Used for Orthodontic Anchorage. *Am. J. Orthod. Dentofac. Orthop.* **2012**, *141*, 468–476. [CrossRef]
19. Miyawaki, S.; Koyama, I.; Inoue, M.; Mishima, K.; Sugahara, T.; Takano-Yamamoto, T. Factors Associated with the Stability of Titanium Screws Placed in the Posterior Region for Orthodontic Anchorage. *Am. J. Orthod. Dentofac. Orthop.* **2003**, *124*, 373–378. [CrossRef]
20. Cheng, S.J.; Tseng, I.Y.; Lee, J.J.; Kok, S.H. A Prospective Study of the Risk Factors Associated with Failure of Mini-Implants Used for Orthodontic Anchorage. *Int. J. Oral Maxillofac. Implants* **2004**, *19*, 100–106.
21. Papadopoulos, M.A.; Tarawneh, F. The Use of Miniscrew Implants for Temporary Skeletal Anchorage in Orthodontics: A Comprehensive Review. *Oral Surg. Oral Med. Oral Pathol. Oral Radiol. Endod.* **2007**, *103*, e6–e15. [CrossRef]
22. Justens, E.; De Bruyn, H. Clinical Outcome of Mini-Screws Used as Orthodontic Anchorage. *Clin. Implant Dent. Relat. Res.* **2008**, *10*, 174–180. [CrossRef] [PubMed]
23. Chen, Y.J.; Chang, H.H.; Huang, C.Y.; Hung, H.C.; Lai, E.H.; Yao, C.C. A Retrospective Analysis of the Failure Rate of Three Different Orthodontic Skeletal Anchorage Systems. *Clin. Oral Implants Res.* **2007**, *18*, 768–775. [CrossRef] [PubMed]
24. Crismani, A.G.; Bertl, M.H.; Celar, A.G.; Bantleon, H.P.; Burstone, C.J. Miniscrews in Orthodontic Treatment: Review and Analysis of Published Clinical Trials. *Am. J. Orthod. Dentofac. Orthop.* **2010**, *137*, 108–113. [CrossRef] [PubMed]
25. Alharbi, F.; Almuzian, M.; Bearn, D. Miniscrews Failure Rate in Orthodontics: Systematic Review and Meta-Analysis. *Eur. J. Orthod.* **2018**, *40*, 519–530. [CrossRef] [PubMed]
26. Deguchi, T.; Takano-Yamamoto, T.; Kanomi, R.; Hartsfield, J.K., Jr.; Roberts, W.E.; Garetto, L.P. The Use of Small Titanium Screws for Orthodontic Anchorage. *J. Dent. Res.* **2003**, *82*, 377–381. [CrossRef]
27. Park, H.S.; Kwon, T.G. Sliding Mechanics with Microscrew Implant Anchorage. *Angle Orthod.* **2004**, *74*, 703–710. [CrossRef]
28. Cope, J.B. Temporary Anchorage Devices in Orthodontics: A Paradigm Shift. *Semin. Orthod.* **2005**, *11*, 3–9. [CrossRef]
29. Motoyoshi, M.; Ueno, S.; Okazaki, K.; Shimizu, N. Bone Stress for a Mini-Implant Close to the Roots of Adjacent Teeth—3D Finite Element Analysis. *Int. J. Oral Maxillofac. Surg.* **2009**, *38*, 363–368. [CrossRef]
30. Park, H.S.; Lee, S.K.; Kwon, O.W. Group Distal Movement of Teeth Using Microscrew Implant Anchorage. *Angle Orthod.* **2005**, *75*, 602–609. [CrossRef]
31. Parmar, R.; Reddy, V.; Reddy, S.K.; Reddy, D. Determination of Soft Tissue Thickness at Orthodontic Miniscrew Placement Sites Using Ultrasonography for Customizing Screw Selection. *Am. J. Orthod. Dentofac. Orthop.* **2016**, *150*, 651–658. [CrossRef]
32. Luzi, C.; Verna, C.; Melsen, B. Guidelines for Success in Placement of Orthodontic Mini-Implants. *J. Clin. Orthod.* **2009**, *43*, 39–44.
33. Hong, S.B.; Kusnoto, B.; Kim, E.J.; BeGole, E.A.; Hwang, H.S.; Lim, H.J. Prognostic Factors Associated with the Success Rates of Posterior Orthodontic Miniscrew Implants: A Subgroup Meta-Analysis. *Korean J. Orthod.* **2016**, *46*, 111–126. [CrossRef]

Disclaimer/Publisher's Note: The statements, opinions and data contained in all publications are solely those of the individual author(s) and contributor(s) and not of MDPI and/or the editor(s). MDPI and/or the editor(s) disclaim responsibility for any injury to people or property resulting from any ideas, methods, instructions or products referred to in the content.

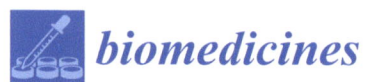
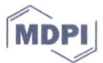

Systematic Review

A Systematic Review and Meta-Analysis on the Efficacy of Locally Delivered Adjunctive Curcumin (*Curcuma longa* L.) in the Treatment of Periodontitis

Louisa M. Wendorff-Tobolla [1,†], Michael Wolgin [1,*,†], Gernot Wagner [2], Irma Klerings [2], Anna Dvornyk [3] and Andrej M. Kielbassa [1]

1. Center for Operative Dentistry, Periodontology, and Endodontology, Department of Dentistry, Faculty of Medicine and Dentistry, Danube Private University (DPU), 3500 Krems, Austria
2. Department of Evidence-based Medicine and Evaluation, Danube University Krems, 3500 Krems, Austria
3. Department of Propaedeutics of Therapeutic Dentistry, Faculty of Dentistry, Poltava State Medical University (PSMU), 36011 Poltava, Ukraine
* Correspondence: michael.wolgin@dp-uni.ac.at
† These authors contributed equally to this work.

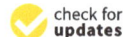

Citation: Wendorff-Tobolla, L.M.; Wolgin, M.; Wagner, G.; Klerings, I.; Dvornyk, A.; Kielbassa, A.M. A Systematic Review and Meta-Analysis on the Efficacy of Locally Delivered Adjunctive Curcumin (*Curcuma longa* L.) in the Treatment of Periodontitis. *Biomedicines* **2023**, *11*, 481. https://doi.org/10.3390/biomedicines11020481

Academic Editors: Giuseppe Minervini and Gianmarco Abbadessa

Received: 13 December 2022
Revised: 30 January 2023
Accepted: 1 February 2023
Published: 7 February 2023

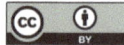

Copyright: © 2023 by the authors. Licensee MDPI, Basel, Switzerland. This article is an open access article distributed under the terms and conditions of the Creative Commons Attribution (CC BY) license (https://creativecommons.org/licenses/by/4.0/).

Abstract: This meta-analysis intended to assess evidence on the efficacy of locally delivered curcumin/turmeric as an adjunctive to scaling and root planing (SRP), on clinical attachment level (CAL) and probing pocket depth (PPD), compared to SRP alone or in combination with chlorhexidine (CHX). RCTs were identified from PubMed, Cochrane Library, BASE, LIVIVO, Dentistry Oral Sciences Source, MEDLINE Complete, Scopus, ClinicalTrials.gov, and eLibrary, until August 2022. The risk of bias (RoB) was assessed with the Cochrane Risk of Bias tool 2.0. A random-effects meta-analysis was performed by pooling mean differences with 95% confidence intervals. Out of 827 references yielded by the search, 23 trials meeting the eligibility criteria were included. The meta-analysis revealed that SRP and curcumin/turmeric application were statistically significantly different compared to SRP alone for CAL (-0.33 mm; $p = 0.03$; 95% CI -0.54 to -0.11; $I^2 = 62.3\%$), and for PPD (-0.47 mm; $p = 0.024$; 95% CI -0.88 to -0.06; $I^2 = 95.5\%$); however, this difference was considered clinically meaningless. No significant differences were obtained between patients treated with SRP and CHX, compared to SRP and curcumin/turmeric. The RoB assessment revealed numerous inaccuracies, thus raising concerns about previous overestimates of potential treatment effects.

Keywords: chlorhexidine; clinical attachment level; curcumin/turmeric; mechanical debridement; periodontitis; periodontal treatment; probing pocket depth

1. Introduction

Severe periodontal disease affected about 1.1 billion people globally in 2019 [1], with an overall prevalence of 67.4% (probing pocket depths between 4 and 5 mm), with 9.1% accounting for adolescents, 27.7% for adults, and 30.6% for elderly people [2]. Consequently, periodontitis can be considered a cross-generational, global public health problem with widely ranging effects such as bleeding gums, periodontal pockets, bone loss, and functional as well as aesthetic issues [3]. Furthermore, it is considered a risk factor for several systematic diseases, including cardiovascular disorders, rheumatoid arthritis, and chronic obstructive pulmonary diseases, as well as non-alcoholic liver diseases [3,4].

The primary goal of periodontal treatment is the removal of highly organized microorganisms embedded in an extracellular, polysaccharide matrix attached to the tooth's surface [5]. Biofilm management is usually achieved by sustainable biofilm disintegration consisting of instructions on effective oral hygiene, mechanical debridement of tooth surfaces, and removal of co-factors favoring re-accumulation, together with a regular recall system in which the current periodontal situation is evaluated [6]. Local therapeutical substances such as rinsing solutions, gels, and chips are administered to increase the success of the treatment and enable long-term clinical management of periodontitis [7].

One such therapeutical substance is chlorhexidine, which is bacteriostatic and bactericidal to gram-positive and gram-negative bacteria; additionally, chlorhexidine inhibits plaque formation by having a high affinity for binding spots of bacteria [8]. Application of chlorhexidine as a standard chemotherapeutic agent can, however, be associated with several undesirable side effects. Being exposed over a longer period of time, chlorhexidine can cause brown staining of the teeth, decreased taste sensation, oral mucosal lesions, and/or increased calculus formation [8].

Another common therapeutic substance is hydrogen peroxide, which operates as a disinfecting agent by releasing oxygen, thus creating an environment that is able to inhibit anerobic bacteria growth [9]. Notwithstanding, several adverse reactions to highly concentrated hydrogen peroxide may be observed; short durations can cause erythema or mucosal sloughing, whereas application for longer periods can lead to inflammation and/or hyperplasia [10].

Investigations have been initiated to examine the use of cytostatics, photodynamic therapy, metal ions, and natural compounds/oils in inflammatory-mediated conditions [11–16]. One of these alternatives is curcumin, which is a natural constituent found in the turmeric plant [17]. In contrast to conventional therapeutic substances, curcumin intervenes in the pathophysiological process of inflammation rather than working solely as an antibacterial [17]. It is extracted from the turmeric plant *Curcuma longa* L. (http://www.theplantlist.org; accessed on 29 July 2022) [17], and is thought to act anti-inflammatory by inhibiting the mRNA and protein expression of Cyclo-oxygenase-2 (COX-2) [18,19], through down-regulation of NF-kB activation [20]. Further proposed anti-inflammatory methods of action are that curcumin declines the activity of phospholipase A2, C and D [21,22] and inhibits lipoxygenase [23–25]. Additionally, an anti-bacterial mode of action is observed by curcumin; by inserting itself into the hydrophobic cellular membrane, thus disrupting membrane integrity, curcumin results in a leakage of cytoplasm [17]. A similar mode of action is executed by human beta-defensins (hBDs) [26] and artificially produced peptides, such as artilysine (an amphipathic structure that destabilizes bacteria's cell walls by hydrolysis) [27]. Furthermore, it has been demonstrated that curcumin is responsible for the down-regulation of 31 quorum-sensing genes required for biofilm production [28]. Additionally, a number of studies have postulated a correlation between curcumin and reduced adherence of *Streptococus mutans* to the tooth surfaces, thereby suppressing biofilm formation [29,30]. In the light of those respective results, these later trials have supported curcumin's ability to influence multiple signaling pathways and have paved the way for ongoing clinical trials. The respective literature search has proven that there are a remarkable number of clinical investigations focusing on the local application of curcumin administered either as an aqueous solution, gel, chip, or strip [31–53].

Although some meta-analyses have already addressed the issue of curcumin application during periodontal treatment, the present work is not a repetition of previously published results, since most published papers have not dealt with the evaluation of periodontal parameters such as CAL [54–56]. Therefore, the overall aim of this systematic review and meta-analysis was to compare the efficacy of scaling and root planing (SRP) alone or in combination with chlorhexidine (CHX) to SRP in combination with local curcumin with respect to key periodontal outcome indicators such as clinical attachment levels and probing pocket depths.

2. Materials and Methods

The authors focused on a researchable and answerable study question to the established PICO(ST) format [57]: For adult patients suffering from chronic generalized periodontitis (probing pocket depth of ≥ 4 mm) (P), will scaling and root planing (SRP), local *Curcuma longa* L. application (I) as compared to SRP or SRP, and local chlorhexidine (CHX) application (C) result in a change of clinical attachment levels (CAL: primary outcome) and probing pocket depths, (PPD: secondary outcome)(O) in a randomized split-mouth design and/or parallel group design studies (S) in a defined period of time (T)? The protocol of the present review was registered at the Prospero Register of Systematic Reviews (registration number: CRD42022290324,10/01/2022; registration name: Effect of locally delivered adjunctive Curcumin in the Treatment of Periodontitis—a Systematic Review and Meta-analysis). The current review was conducted in accordance with the "Preferred Reporting Items for Systematic Reviews and Meta-analyses" (PRISMA) statement checklist [58].

The following databases were searched until August 2022: PubMed, Cochrane Library (Wiley), BASE (base-search.net), LIVIVO, Dentistry Oral Sciences Source (Ebsco), MEDLINE Complete (Ebsco), Scopus, ClinicalTrials.gov, and eLibrary (https://www.elibrary.ru/defaultx.asp; accessed on 3 August 2022.). This combination of information sources retrieved both published journal articles and gray literature (e.g., dissertations, or study register entries). The search strategies were designed by an experienced information specialist (IK). In addition to the search in electronic databases, reference lists of included studies were checked manually. Search results were imported and deduplicated in Endnote 20 (Version 2013; The Endnote Team; Clarivate Analytics, Philadelphia, PA, USA). Additional data for individual search strategies are presented in the Supplementary Materials. The study selection process was performed stepwise. First, two reviewers (LWT and MW) independently screened the titles and abstracts of references found with the literature search. Second, the full texts of the studies included during the previous step were assessed for eligibility. Randomized controlled trials (RCTs) were included that compared SRP alone or in combination with chlorhexidine to SRP and local curcumin/turmeric regarding clinical attachment level and probing pocket depth. Table 1 presents details of the study eligibility criteria.

The quality of the included trials was methodically assessed by two authors (LWT and MW) using the revised Cochrane risk of bias tool 2.0 for randomized trials (RoB2). Any possible dissensions were resolved by discussion and mutual agreement. RoB2 is arranged into five different disciplines (randomization process, deviations from intended interventions, missing outcome data, measurement of the outcome, and selection of the reported results) that aim to evaluate all aspects of the study that are related to the risk of bias [59]. The five different disciplines were judged as having either low risk, some concerns, or high risk, and according to this judgment, an overall assessment of the risk of bias level in each individual study was made.

One author (LWT) collected the relevant data from the included articles. This was cross-checked for accuracy and completeness by another author (MW). The data of interest were methodology, number of participants, participants baseline characteristics, concentration of curcumin/turmeric and chlorhexidine, evaluation period, and results for primary and secondary outcomes. The authors of the Dave et al. (2018) study were contacted to gather missing information concerning initial PPD and curcumin concentration.

A random-effects meta-analysis was performed using an inverse-variance model with the DerSimonian–Laird estimate of squared tau (τ^2) by pooling mean differences with 95% confidence intervals, if the number of identified investigations that were similar in population and outcome was sufficient. The statistical heterogeneity was assessed across trials by visually inspecting the forest plots and calculating the I^2 statistics. STATA release 17.0 was used for all analyses (StataCorp LLC; College Station, TX, USA). Additional calculations had to be performed for the data published by Raghava et al. (2019) and Farhood et al. (2020); CAL was presented in variance (PPD in standard error), and CAL and PPD were presented in standard error, respectively. Conversions were made to the standard deviation.

3. Results

3.1. Literature Search and Screening

A total of 827 records were identified through the literature search. After deduplication, 222 studies were screened by title and abstract. Consecutively, 33 full-text articles were assessed for eligibility, and, finally, 23 investigations were included [31–53]. Details of the study selection process are presented in Figure 1.

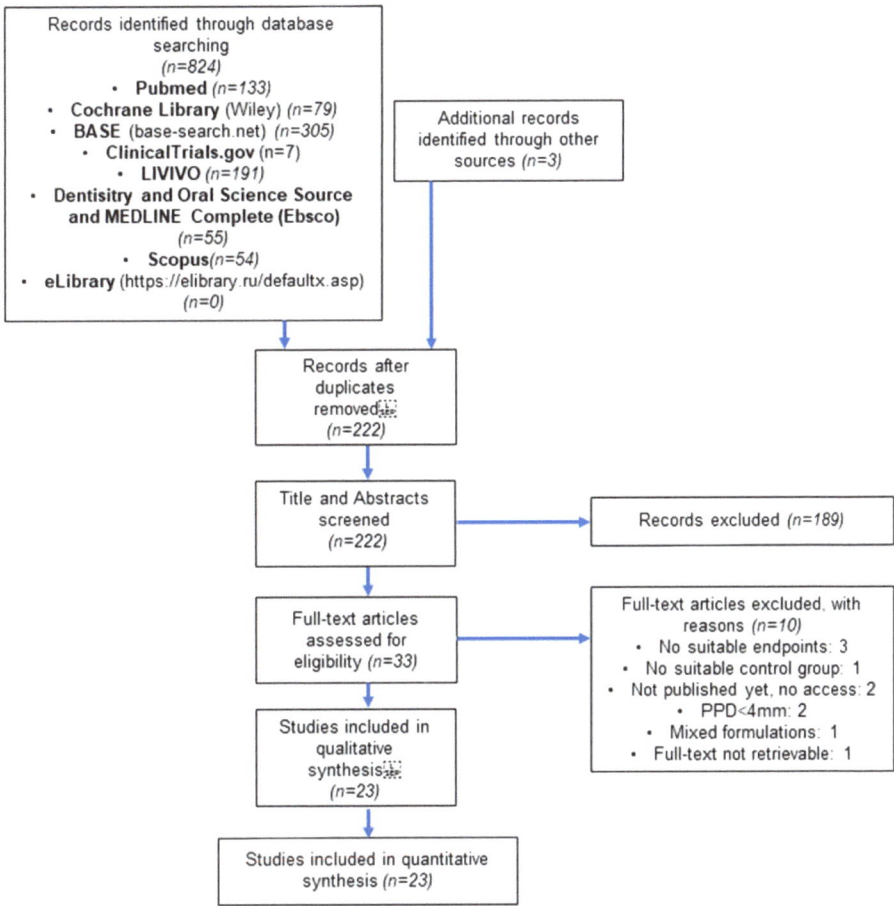

Figure 1. PRISMA Flow Diagram modified from Moher et al. (2009) [60], showing the number of studies identified, screened, assessed for eligibility, excluded, and included in the systematic research [31–53].

3.2. Study and Patient Characteristics

Sixteen studies compared SRP with SRP and local curcumin/turmeric application [31–46], three investigations compared SRP and chlorhexidine application with SRP and local curcumin/turmeric application [47–49], while another four studies evaluated SRP and SRP in combination with CHX compared to SRP and local curcumin/turmeric [50–53]. While a split-mouth design was applied in 18 investigations [31–35,38,40,41,43–51,53], five investigations employed a parallel group design [36,37,39,42,52]. The number of participants in the included studies ranged from 10 to 90. The age of participants ranged from 20 to 65 years; the mean age or gender ratio could not be calculated due to missing uniform data concerning these variables among certain studies.

Included were studies carried out at university hospitals in India, Iraq, Egypt, and Brazil, where participants were recruited from the departments of periodontology.

Study duration ranged from 21 days to 3 months. Thirteen studies used an acrylic stent to measure probing pocket depth and/or clinical attachment level [31–34,39,41,43,45–47,51–53]. Fourteen investigations used a COE pack to ensure the duration of the applied medicament [31–33,35,38,39,41–43,45,48–50,52]. The periodontal condition requiring treatment was defined as a probing pocket depth of ≥ 5 mm in ten studies [34,38–40,43,45–47,49,53], between 5 and 7 mm in seven [31,33,35,36,41,50,52], and between 4 and 6 mm in two investigations [37,48]. The following initial PPDs were observed once: between 5 and 8 mm [51], between 5 and 6 mm [44], >5 mm [32], and ≥ 4 mm [42]. Three studies were included that solely reported PPD [36,44,53]. Details of study characteristics are summarized and presented according to their controls and interventions in Table 1.

Table 1. Characteristics of included studies. SMD: split-mouth design, PGD: parallel-group design PPD: probing pocket depth, SBI: sulcus bleeding index, PI: plaque index, CAL: clinical attachment level, SRP: scaling and root planning, GI: gingival index, BOP: bleeding on probing, CHX: chlorhexidine [31–53].

Study	Sample Size	Study Design	Clinical Parameters	Intervention and Control		Stent	COE Pack	Follow-Up Periods
				Studies Comparing SRP alone to SRP and Curcumin				
Behal et al., 2011 [31]	n = 30 PPD 5–7 mm	SMD	PI (Turesky-Gilmore-Glickman), GI (Löe and Silness), SBI (Muhlemann), PPD (William probe), CAL	Group 1: SRP alone	Group 2: SRP was followed by local application 2% turmeric gel	yes	yes	0, 30, 45 d /0, 30 d
Bhatia et al., 2014 [32]	n = 25, (15♂, 10♀, 21–45 y.o.) PPD > 5 mm.	SMD	PI (Silness and Löe), SBI (Muhlemann), PPD, CAL	Group 1: SRP alone	Group 2: SRP was followed by local application of 1% curcumin gel	yes	yes	0, 1, 3, 6 m /0, 1 m
Anuradha et al., 2015 [33]	n = 30 (25–60 y.o.) PPD 5–7 mm	SMD	PI (Turesky-Gilmore-Glickman), GI (Löe and Silness), PPD, CAL (UNC-15)	Group 1: SRP alone	Group 2: SRP was followed by local application of curcumin gel (10 mg of *Curcuma longa* extract/g)	yes	yes	0, 30, 45 d /0, 30 d
Nagasri et al., 2015 [34]	n = 30 (12♂, 18♀, 35–60 y.o.) PPD ≥ 5 mm	SMD	PI (Silness and Löe), GI (Löe and Silness), PPD, CAL	Group 1: SRP alone	Group 2: SRP was followed by local application of curcumin gel (10 mg of *Curcuma longa* extract/g)	yes	no	0, 4 w /0, 4 w
Shivanand et al., 2016 [35]	n = 14 (6♂, 8♀, 35–50 y.o.) PPD 5–7 mm	SMD	PI (Silness and Löe), GI (Löe and Silness), BOP, PPD, CAL	Group 1: upper arch received SRP alone	Group 2: lower arch received SRP and application of curcumin gel (10 mg of *Curcuma longa* extract/g)	no	yes	0, 21, 30, 90 d /0, 30 d
Nasra et al., 2017 [36]	n = 10 (35–55 y.o.) PPD 5–7 mm	PGD	PPD (Glavind and Löe), SBI (Checchi), GI (Löe and Silness), PI (Silness and Löe)	Group 1: SRP alone	Group 2: SRP and curcumin gel 2%, the application was repeated once weekly over three weeks period	no	no	0, 1 m /0, 1 m
Dave et al., 2018 [37]	n = 20 (9♂, 11♀, 20–59 y.o.) PPD 4–6 mm	PGD	PI, BOP, SBI, PPD, CAL (UNC15)	Group1: SRP alone	Group 2: SRP and curcumin gel 10%, patients were instructed to apply gel for 2–3 min once daily	no	no	0, 2 m /0, 2 m
Raghava et al., 2019 [38]	n = 10 (5♂, 5♀, 25–40 y.o.) PPD ≥ 5 mm	SMD	PI (Silness and Löe), GI (Löe and Silness), PPD, CAL	Group 1: SRP alone	Group 2: SRP was followed by local application of curcumin gel (10 mg of *Curcuma longa* extract/g)	no	yes	0, 4 w /0, 4 w
Kaur et al., 2019 [39]	n = 29 (20♂, 9♀, 20–65 y.o.) PPD ≥ 5 mm	PGD	PI (Silness and Löe), SBI (Muhlemann), PPD, CAL (UNC-15)	Group 1: SRP alone	Group 2: SRP was followed by local application 1% curcumin gel (10 mg of *Curcuma longa* extract/g)	yes	yes	0, 1, 3 m /0, 1 m

Table 1. *Cont.*

Study	Sample Size	Study Design	Clinical Parameters	Intervention and Control			Stent	COE Pack	Follow-Up Periods
Perez-Pacheco et al., 2020 [40]	n = 20 (6♂, 14♀, 37–62 y.o., PPD ≥ 5 mm)	SMD	PI (O'Leary), GI (Ainamo and Bay), BOP, PPD, gingival recession, CAL (UNC-15)	Group 1: SRP and 0.05 mg/mL nano capsulated curcumin	Group 2: SRP and empty nanoparticles		no	no	0, 1, 2, 6 m / 0, 1 m
Farhood et al., 2020 [41]	n = 20 (9♂, 11♀, ≥21–45 y.o., PPD 5–7 mm)	SMD	PI, GI, BOP, PPD, CAL	Group 1: SRP alone	Group 2: SRP was followed by local application of curcumin gel (10 mg of *Curcuma longa* extract/g) Second application after 1 week		yes	yes	0, 1 m / 0, 1 m
Studies comparing SRP alone to SRP and Curcumin and a third or fourth control (not included in this meta-analysis)									
Mohammed et al., 2020 [42]	n = 90 (35♂, 55♀, 25–54 y.o., PPD ≥ 4 mm)	PGD	PPD, CAL, GI, BOP	Group 1: healthy periodontium (control group)	Group 2: for periodontitis patients SRP and curcumin gel (C. Longa extract, 10 mg)	Group 3: periodontitis patients receiving SRP alone	no	yes	0, 1 m / 0, 1 m
Rahalkar et al., 2021 [43]	n = 15 (5♂, 10♀, 37–57 y.o., PPD ≥ 5 mm)	SMD	PPD, CAL, GI (Löe and Silness), PI (Silness and Löe), SBI (Mombelli)	Group 1: SRP alone	Group 2: SRP and curcumin gel (C. Longa extract, 10 mg)	Group 3: SRP and tulsi extract	yes	yes	0, 30 d / 0, 30 d
Elavarasu et al., 2016 [44]	n = 15 (35–50 y.o., PPD 5–6 mm)	SMD	PI, GI, SBI, PPD	Group 1: Healthy periodontium (control)	Group 2: SRP alone	Group 3: SRP and curcumin strip placement 0.2% loaded on to guided tissue membrane (GTR)	no	no	0, 21 d / 0, 21 d
Saini et al., 2021 [45]	n = 30 (30–65 y.o., PPD ≥ 5 mm)	SMD	PI, GI, PPD, CAL (UNC-15)	Group 1: SRP and 5% neem chip	Group 2: SRP and 5% turmeric chip	Group 3: SRP and placebo chip	yes	yes	0, 1, 3 m / 0, 1 m
Sreedhar et al., 2015 [46]	n = 15 (15♀, 7♂, 8♀, 35–55 y.o., PPD ≥ 5 mm)	SMD	PI, SBI, PPD, CAL	Group 1: SRP alone.	Group 2: SRP anfd curcumin gel (10 mg of *Curcuma longa* extract/g) application for 5 min	Group 3: SRP and curcumin application for 5 min and irradiation with blue light emitting diode	Group 4: SRP and curcumin PDT	yes	no	0, 1, 3 m / 0, 3 m

Table 1. Cont.

Study	Sample Size	Study Design	Clinical Parameters	Intervention and Control		Stent	COE Pack	Follow-Up Periods
\multicolumn{9}{c}{Studies comparing SRP and CHX to SRP and Curcumin}								
Gottumukkala et al., 2014 [47]	$n = 60$ (25–55 y.o.), PPD $\geq$ 5 mm	SMD	PPD, CAL, GI (Löe and Silness), PI (Silness and Löe)	Group 1: SRP alone along with CHX chip (2.5 mg)	Group 2: received SRP along with curcumin chip (CU extract concentration of 50 mg/cm)	yes	no	0, 1, 3, 6 m /0, 1 m
Anitha et al., 2015 [48]	$n = 30$ (20♂, 10♀, 20–50 y.o.), PPD 4–6 mm	SMD	PPD, CAL, GI (Löe and Silness), PI (Turesky-Gillmore)	Group 1: receiving SRP and curcumin gel (250 g of the powdered rhizome of Curcuma longa in 5 mL ethanol) Repeated application at day 15	Group 2: SRP and CHX gel 0.1% Repeated application at day 15	no	yes	0, 15, 30 d /0, 30 d
Siddarth et al., 2020 [49]	$n = 25$ (20♂, 5♀, $\geq$30 y.o.), PPD $\geq$ 5 mm	SMD	GI (Löe and Silness), PI (Silness and Löe), SBI (Muhlemann), PPD, CAL	Group 1: SRP and application of 2% curcumin gel	Group 2: SRP and application of 0.2% CHX gel	no	yes	0, 1, 3 m /0, 1 m
\multicolumn{9}{c}{Studies comparing SRP alone to SRP and Curcumin and SRP and CHX}								
Jaswal et al., 2014 [50]	$n = 15$ (12♂, 3♀, 21–55 y.o.), PPD 5–7 mm	SMD	PI (Silness and Löe), GI (Löe and Silness), PPD, CAL (UNC-15)	Group 1: received SRP and 2% turmeric gel	Group 2: receiving SRP and 1% CHX	Group 3: SRP alone	yes	0, 30, 45 d /0, 30 d
Singh et al., 2018 [51]	$n = 40$ (22♂, 18♀, 30–50 y.o.), PPD 5–8 mm	SMD	PI, GI, PPD, CAL (UNC-15)	Group 1: SRP and sites treated with CHX chip (2.5 mg)	Group 2: SRP and sites treated with 5% turmeric chip	Group 3: SRP alone	yes	no	0, 1, 3 m /0, 1 m
Guru et al., 2020 [52]	$n = 45$ (36♂, 9♀, 25–50 y.o.), PPD 5–7 mm	PGD	PI, GI, PPD, CAL (UNC-15)	Group 1: SRP alone	Group 2: SRP, 2%curcumin with nanogel	Group 3: SRP, 1% CHX gel	yes	yes	0, 21, 45 d /0, 21 d
Gottumukkala et al., 2013 [53]	$n = 26$ (12♂, 14♀, 30–55 y.o.), PPD $\geq$ 5 mm	SMD	PI (Silness and Löe), BOP, redness, PPD (UNC15)	Group 1: SRP and saline irrigation Repeated gingival irrigation at 7, 14 and 21 d	Group 2: SRP and 1% curcumin solution, repeated gingival irrigation at 7, 14 and 21 d	Group 3: SRP and 0.2% CHX Repeated gingival irrigation at 7, 14 and 21 d	yes	no	0, 1, 3, 6 m /0, 1 m

3.3. Quality Assessment

The possibility of bias in design and analysis was evaluated by the Cochrane Risk of Bias tool 2.0 [59] (this tool was designed for randomized parallel group design investigations, and, consequently, this should be carefully considered when interpreting the following results). In total, 23 studies were rated with a moderate risk of bias. The most common source of potential bias was domain four ("measurement of the outcome"). In all included studies, investigators probed manually, which was judged to have a poor validity. The second most common source of bias was domain three ("missing outcome data"); many investigations [31–35,38,41–51,53] failed to comment on the loss of follow-up, which led to the present judgment. The third most common source of bias was the "randomization process", which certain investigations could have described it in greater detail [31,32,35,36,41–44,50,53]. The remaining domains, "effect of assigning to intervention", as well as "selection to reported results", performed acceptably throughout the included investigations. Details of the RoB Assessment are provided in Figure 2.

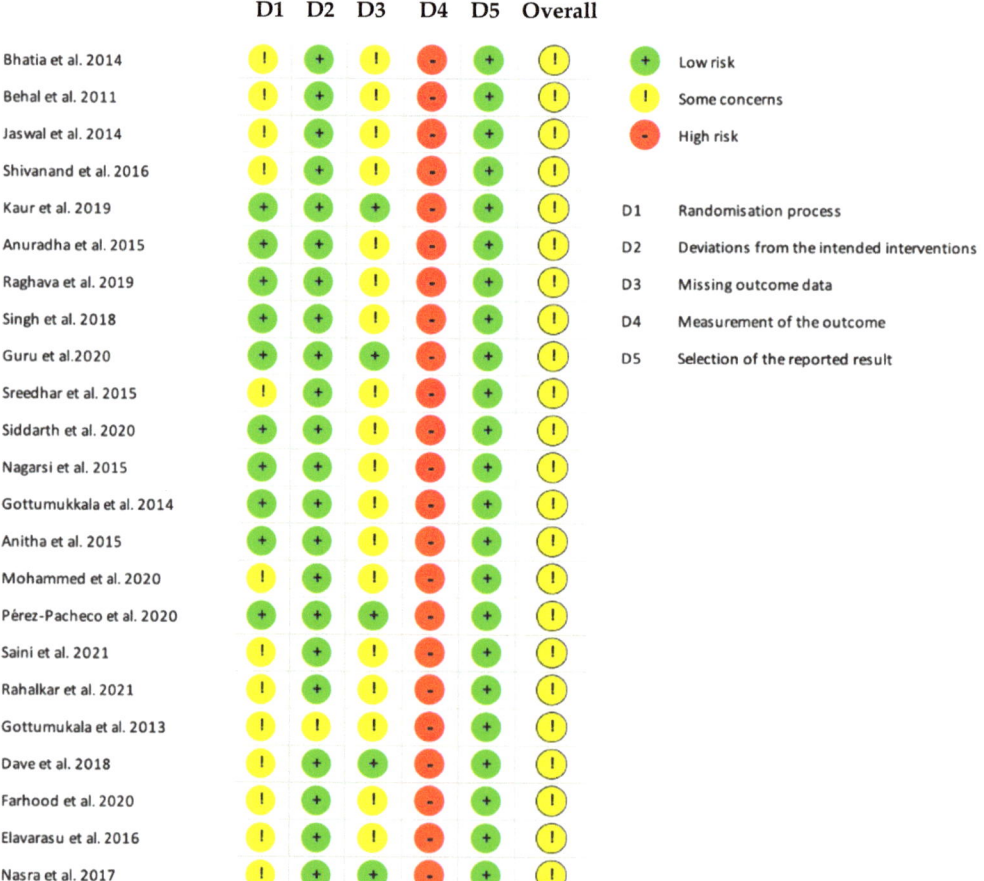

Figure 2. Diagram showing the bias detected in the different domains and overall bias of studies included [31–53]. Based on Sterne et al. (2019) [59].

3.4. Clinical Attachment Level Loss

3.4.1. SRP Alone Compared to SRP and Local Curcumin

Seventeen investigations [31–35,37–43,45,46,50–52] evaluated the effects of SRP and curcumin/turmeric on the loss of CAL. In random effects meta-analysis, a statistically significant mean difference of −0.33 mm (95% CI −0.54 to −0.11; $p = 0.03$, $I^2 = 62.3\%$; 453 sites; see Figure 3) was favoring SRP and curcumin/turmeric was observed.

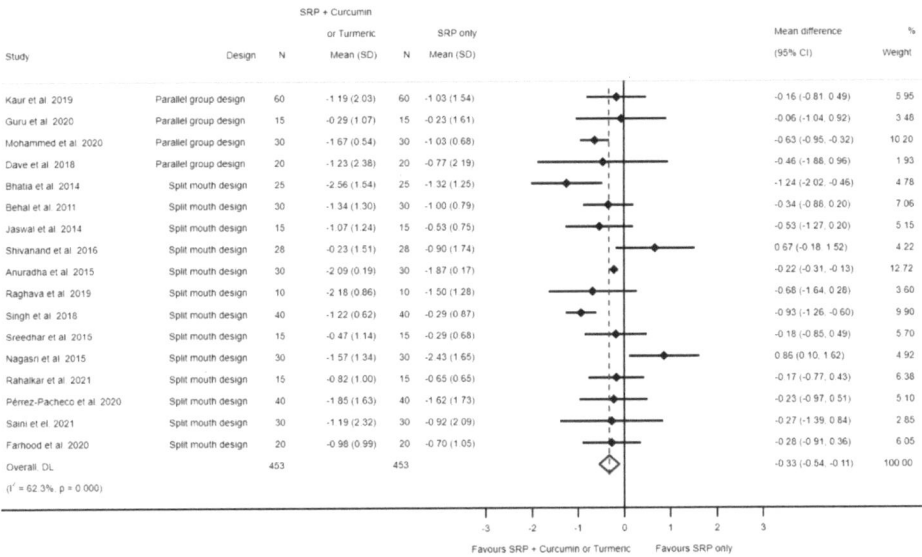

Figure 3. Forest plot for the comparison of SRP to SRP and local curcumin/turmeric application related to clinical attachment level loss [31–35,37–43,45,46,50–52].

3.4.2. SRP and Chlorhexidine Compared to SRP and Local Curcumin

The effect of SRP and chlorhexidine application, in comparison to SRP and local curcumin/turmeric application, on the loss of CAL was evaluated by six investigations [47–52]. Random effects meta-analysis showed a statistically non-significant mean difference of −0.42 mm (95% CI −1.15 to 0.31; $p = 0.258$, $I^2 = 93.6\%$; 185 sites; see Figure 4) in favor of SRP and curcumin/turmeric.

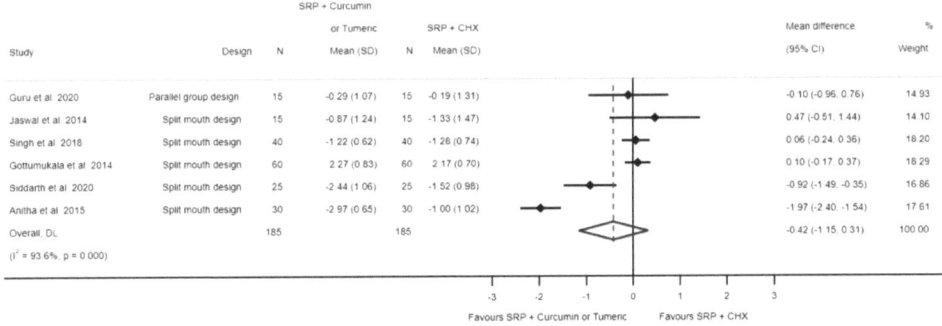

Figure 4. Forest plot for the comparison of SRP and chlorhexidine to SRP and local curcumin/turmeric related to clinical attachment level loss [47–52].

3.5. Probing Pocket Depth Reduction

3.5.1. SRP Alone Compared to SRP and Local Curcumin

Twenty studies with a moderate risk of bias [31–46,50–53] reported on the difference in probing pocket depth reduction between SRP alone and SRP with local curcumin/turmeric application. Random effects meta-analysis showed a statistically significant difference of -0.47 mm (95% CI -0.88 to -0.06; $p = 0.024$; $I^2 = 95.5\%$; 501 sites; see Figure 5).

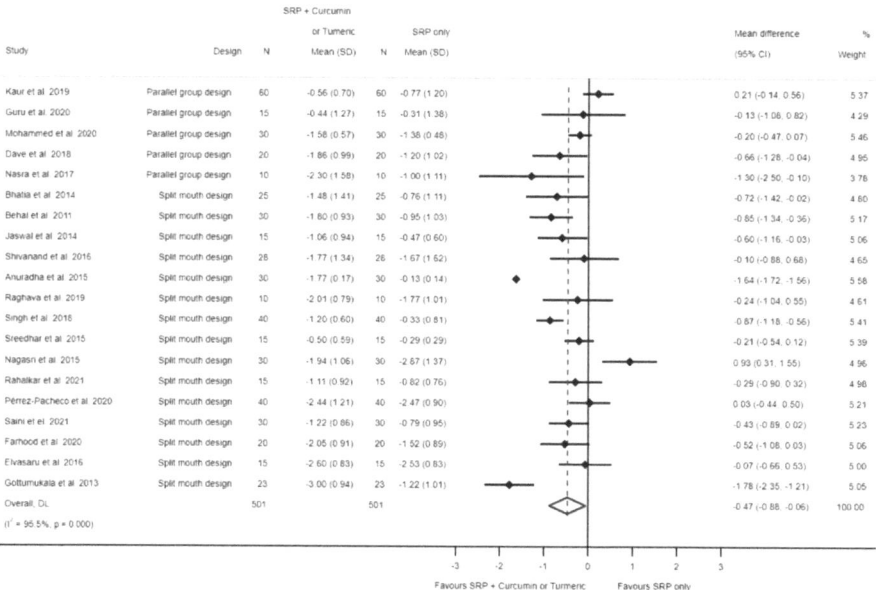

Figure 5. Forest plot for the comparison of SRP to SRP and local curcumin/turmeric application related to probing pocket depth reduction [31–46,50–53].

3.5.2. SRP and Chlorhexidine Compared to SRP and Local Curcumin

Figure 6 presents the effects of seven investigations [47–53] comparing SRP and chlorhexidine application, in contrast to SRP and curcumin/turmeric application on probing pocket depth reduction. Random effects meta-analysis exhibited a pooled mean difference of -0.54 mm (95% CI -1.19 to 0.12; $p = 0.108$, $I^2 = 93.4\%$, 208 sites; see Figure 6), which was statistically non-significant.

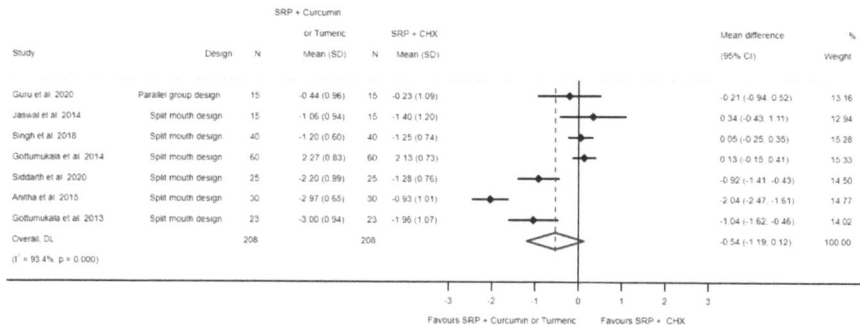

Figure 6. Forest plot for the comparison of SRP and chlorhexidine to SRP and local curcumin/turmeric application related to probing pocket depth reduction [47–53].

4. Discussion

This systematic review and meta-analysis revealed a statistically significant difference between SRP alone, compared to SRP and curcumin/turmeric application for CAL and PPD. However, these significant decreases (CAL −0.33 mm; PPD −0.47 mm) are not considered clinically relevant. Included studies showed a notable degree of heterogeneity, which is probably due to different application methods, varying concentrations of curcumin/CHX, and the unreliability of outcome measurements.

All periodontal pockets were probed manually by all investigators, even though one investigation used a pressure-sensitive manual probe [53] and two investigations measured six sites around each tooth [40,43]. It is well accepted that probing manually might be unreliable, and can result in certain inaccuracies [61,62], at least to some extent. A standardized measuring method using electronic periodontal probes, thus controlling probing force and measuring to the closest tenth of a millimeter and, therefore, generating reproducible results, even with different examiners, would seem generally preferable [63,64]. Furthermore, factors like the design of the probe, probing position, visual observational error, and tissue inflammation could influence the reproducibility of readings, thus leading to detection bias [65,66]. Nevertheless, the assessors of the present investigation decided to override the suggested overall judgment for the risk of bias assessment. This is justified by the fact that all treatment groups measured the outcomes manually, in most cases uniformly using a UNC 15 periodontal probe [33,37,39,40,45,50–53]. Additionally, studies have shown that there is a tendency to have similar reliability between manual and electronic probes [67,68]. Furthermore, many investigations [31–35,38,41–51,53] failed to comment on the loss of follow-up, and this sort of attrition bias led to the present judgment.

A further plausible explanation for the observed heterogeneity might be the varying application methods. To a certain extent, gels have several advantages over other application methods. They are biocompatible and bioadhesive, allowing them to attach to periodontal pockets and, furthermore, enabling a controlled drug release and minimum dose frequency [69]. While most studies applied a conventional gel [32–37,39–45,48,50,51], two used a nanoparticle gel system, which is expected to have several advantages. Due to their nanoparticle size, these gel systems are able to penetrate into the most apical regions of periodontal pockets, thus ensuring a homogenous disposal of the drug over a long interval, along with a reduction in drug quantity and high bioavailability [69]. Matrix delivery systems such as chips and strips, as used in four trials [46,47,49,52], have the benefit of sustained drug release patterns. In contrast, solutions, as used in one investigation [54], provide high concentrations initially and will be diluted promptly by liquids, for example, by gingival crevicular fluid [69].

There are numerous issues to be discussed about the stated concentrations in the included investigations. Certain studies used different degrees of purity as starting products. The majority of selected studies, nine in total, used the product "Curenext oral gel" (Abbott Healthcare Limited, Mumbai, India), which contains 10 mg of *Curcuma longa* extract/g [34–37,39,42–45]. The company (Abbott Healthcare) was contacted, and they stated that "*Curcuma longa* extract" contains 72.77% curcumin. Turmeric contains, apart from curcumin and curcumin's analogs, several other substances and phytochemicals, such as zingiberene, eugenol, turmerin, turmerones, and turmeronols [70]. Additionally, different manufacturing processes were used to yield curcumin products. One study used a 95% pure curcumin powder to create a 2% curcumin gel [36], while another investigation purified curcumin by the method of evaporation, thus generating 99% curcumin powder [49]. A further investigation used a >65% curcumin powder to create curcumin nanoparticles [40,71], whereas another investigation estimated the curcumin content by measuring the absorbance of curcumin spectrophotometrically [32]. The starting product of one study (using >10% curcumin) might have contained a range of other substances [52,72]. The remaining investigations did not describe the initial product used in sufficient detail, and the amount of curcumin was not specified [31,37,44,45,48,50,51,53]. Additionally, varying CHX concentrations were noted: 0.1% [48], 0.2% [49,53], 1% [50,52], and 2.5 mg [47,51].

Although the studies under investigation all revealed varying curcumin concentrations, it can be assumed that the latter was effective, since an inhibitory effect on 61.01% of the MMP-9 activity has been determined at a curcumin concentration of 1500 µg/mL [73]. Additionally, a few investigations repeated the curcumin application. Patients were either instructed to apply the gel daily [37], or the application was repeated once weekly (over a three-week period) [36], with a second application of gel after one week [41], repeated application at day 15 [48], or repeated applications after 7, 14, and 21 days [53]. Furthermore, the use of a COE pack after drug application, aiming to ensure the persistence of the applied drug and prevent site contamination, could be a positive influencing factor for the concentration of the drug applied; however, this has not been proven clinically up to now.

Previous trials have commented on curcumin's poor bioavailability, and this was probably due to low absorption, rapid metabolism, and quick systemic elimination [74,75]. To date, a number of investigations have begun to examine the use of synthetic, structural analogues and various nanoforms of curcumin, as they have improved plasma and tissue levels [74–76]. The effect of oral application of curcumin and modified curcumin on bone resorption, inflammation, and apoptosis in rats, was compared by a previous study. It was concluded that administration of chemically modified curcumin significantly reduced the inflammatory infiltrate in comparison to natural curcumin [77]. This should encourage interest in planning and conducting trials to explore the qualities of chemically modified curcumin.

Limitations of this work are that the risk of bias assessment used was based on a study design used in general medicine. There seems to be a lack of risk of bias in assessments designed for split-mouth trials, which is a common design in oral health. It is worth noting that, even though a split-mouth design can be considered powerful, this latter methodology may result in considerable variability, which is a result of characteristic differences between examiners. No doubt, and this cannot be ruled out, there was a potential risk of contamination of the control site, as it could be possible for the drugs to diffuse to the other site (carry-across effects) [78]. In comparison to the protocol registration, a few amendments would seem worth mentioning. No subgroup analysis was conducted; more data bases were searched; the search was updated in April 2022, and a slight alteration was made to the title; the STATA release 17.0 was used for all analyses (StataCorp LLC; College Station, TX, USA).

The search for new anti-microbial and anti-inflammatory substances as potential agents in the treatment of oral diseases, especially those that cannot develop antibiotic resistance, has gained much importance in recent years. Curcumin appears to possess these valuable properties and has reached the clinical testing phase. At first glance, the results of these clinical studies appear very promising. On a closer inspection, however, it must be stated that several issues in relation to the risk of bias, as discussed in detail, must be elucidated. Uniform study designs and methods with accurate and reproducible measurements of endpoints and homogenous concentrations would be desirable. Interestingly, a recently published meta-analysis of the effect of adjuvant curcumin in the treatment of periodontitis, came to the conclusion that curcumin can be successfully used in periodontal therapy [57]. Another meta-analysis concerning this topic, evaluating gingival index, sulcus bleeding index, and bleeding on probing as primary outcomes, concluded that curcumin is a "good candidate as an adjunct treatment for periodontal disease" [56]. Another meta-analysis concludes that locally applied curcumins "were found to be equally effective compared to the routinely used agents for reduction of plaque and gingival inflammation" [55]. Undoubtedly, such statements should be carefully but critically weighed; when reflecting on several aspects, like the lack of sufficient details concerning study quality, this would seem more than justified. Moreover, to recommend curcumin for periodontal therapy would call for clear endpoints assessing the effectiveness of curcumin in periodontal treatment, and any possible effects of the oral hygiene of participants must be clearly distinguished.

When pondering on the treatment of periodontal disease with adjuvant curcumin, the data available from this present meta-analysis would suggest that there is obviously no reason for any further investigations, and this would refer both to large-scale and high-quality studies. At the end of the day, the available data base could reveal that the proven (and noteworthy, no doubt) biochemical properties of curcumin would justify the previous research projects in the first instance, but, notwithstanding, no clinically significant improvements could be proven with the current systematic review. Consequently, a clinical implementation of adjuvant curcumin for periodontal treatment is not recommended.

5. Conclusions

In conclusion, with reference to clinical attachment level and probing pocket depth, the present results cannot indicate that curcumin's/turmeric's anti-bacterial and anti-inflammatory properties result in an additionally beneficial clinical outcome, when combining this adjunct to scaling and root planing. Therefore, our findings do not support the application of curcumin-/turmeric-based products in non-surgical periodontal treatment scenarios.

Supplementary Materials: The following supporting information can be downloaded at: https://www.mdpi.com/article/10.3390/biomedicines11020481/s1, Table S1: Search strategies.

Author Contributions: Conceptualization, L.M.W.-T., M.W. and A.M.K.; methodology, L.M.W.-T., M.W., I.K., A.D. and A.M.K.; validation, L.M.W.-T., M.W. and A.M.K.; formal analysis, L.M.W.-T. and G.W.; investigation, L.M.W.-T. and M.W.; resources, L.M.W.-T. and M.W.; data curation, G.W.; writing—original draft preparation, L.M.W.-T.; writing—review and editing, L.M.W.-T., M.W., G.W. and A.M.K.; visualization, G.W.; supervision, M.W. and A.M.K.; project administration, M.W. and A.M.K. All authors have read and agreed to the published version of the manuscript.

Funding: This research did not receive any specific grant from funding agencies in the public, commercial, or not-for-profit sectors.

Institutional Review Board Statement: Not applicable.

Informed Consent Statement: Patient consent was waived as specific patient details were not mentioned or anonymized.

Data Availability Statement: Datasets generated in this study can be found in the Supplementary Materials.

Conflicts of Interest: The authors declare no conflict of interest.

References

1. Chen, M.X.; Zhong, Y.J.; Dong, Q.Q.; Wong, H.M.; Wen, Y.F. Global, Regional, and National Burden of Severe Periodontitis, 1990–2019: An Analysis of the Global Burden of Disease Study 2019. *J. Clin. Periodontol.* **2021**, *48*, 1165–1188. [CrossRef] [PubMed]
2. Nazir, M.; Al-Ansari, A.; Al-Khalifa, K.; Alhareky, M.; Gaffar, B.; Almas, K. Global Prevalence of Periodontal Disease and Lack of Its Surveillance. *Sci. World J.* **2020**, *2020*, 2146160. [CrossRef] [PubMed]
3. Arigbede, A.; Babatope, B.; Bamidele, M. Periodontitis and Systemic Diseases: A Literature Review. *J. Indian Soc. Periodontol.* **2012**, *16*, 487–491. [CrossRef]
4. Kuraji, R.; Sekino, S.; Kapila, Y.; Numabe, Y. Periodontal Disease–Related Nonalcoholic Fatty Liver Disease and Nonalcoholic Steatohepatitis: An Emerging Concept of Oral-liver Axis. *Periodontol. 2000* **2021**, *87*, 204–240. [CrossRef] [PubMed]
5. Jakubovics, N.S.; Goodman, S.D.; Mashburn-Warren, L.; Stafford, G.P.; Cieplik, F. The Dental Plaque Biofilm Matrix. *Periodontol. 2000* **2021**, *86*, 32–56. [CrossRef]
6. Kwon, T.; Lamster, I.B.; Levin, L. Current Concepts in the Management of Periodontitis. *Int. Dent. J.* **2021**, *71*, 462–476. [CrossRef]
7. Isola, G.; Polizzi, A.; Santonocito, S.; Dalessandri, D.; Migliorati, M.; Indelicato, F. New Frontiers on Adjuvants Drug Strategies and Treatments in Periodontitis. *Sci. Pharm.* **2021**, *89*, 46. [CrossRef]
8. James, P.; Worthington, H.V.; Parnell, C.; Harding, M.; Lamont, T.; Cheung, A.; Whelton, H.; Riley, P. Chlorhexidine Mouthrinse as an Adjunctive Treatment for Gingival Health. *Cochrane Database Syst. Rev.* **2017**, *2021*, CD008676. [CrossRef]
9. Marshall, M.V.; Cancro, L.P.; Fischman, S.L. Hydrogen Peroxide: A Review of Its Use in Dentistry. *J. Periodontol.* **1995**, *66*, 786–796. [CrossRef]
10. Walsh, L.J. Safety Issues Relating to the Use of Hydrogen Peroxide in Dentistry. *Aust. Dent. J.* **2000**, *45*, 257–269. [CrossRef]
11. Karygianni, L.; Al-Ahmad, A.; Argyropoulou, A.; Hellwig, E.; Anderson, A.C.; Skaltsounis, A.L. Natural Antimicrobials and Oral Microorganisms: A Systematic Review on Herbal Interventions for the Eradication of Multispecies Oral Biofilms. *Front. Microbiol.* **2016**, *6*, 1529. [CrossRef]
12. Goudouri, O.-M.; Kontonasaki, E.; Lohbauer, U.; Boccaccini, A.R. Antibacterial Properties of Metal and Metalloid Ions in Chronic Periodontitis and Peri-Implantitis Therapy. *Acta Biomater.* **2014**, *10*, 3795–3810. [CrossRef]

13. Sgolastra, F.; Petrucci, A.; Gatto, R.; Marzo, G.; Monaco, A. Photodynamic Therapy in the Treatment of Chronic Periodontitis: A Systematic Review and Meta-Analysis. *Lasers Med. Sci.* **2013**, *28*, 669–682. [CrossRef]
14. Novaes, V.C.N.; Ervolino, E.; Fernandes, G.L.; Cunha, C.P.; Theodoro, L.H.; Garcia, V.G.; de Almeida, J.M. Influence of the Treatment with the Antineoplastic Agents 5-Fluorouracil and Cisplatin on the Severity of Experimental Periodontitis in Rats. *Support. Care Cancer* **2021**, *30*, 1967–1980. [CrossRef]
15. Engel Naves Freire, A.; Macedo Iunes Carrera, T.; de Oliveira, G.J.P.L.; Pigossi, S.C.; Vital Ribeiro Júnior, N. Comparison between Antimicrobial Photodynamic Therapy and Low-Level Laser Therapy on Non-Surgical Periodontal Treatment: A Clinical Study. *Photodiagnosis Photodyn. Ther.* **2020**, *31*, 101756. [CrossRef]
16. Zielińska, A.; Kubasiewicz, K.; Wójcicki, K.; Silva, A.M.; Nunes, F.M.; Szalata, M.; Słomski, R.; Eder, P.; Souto, E.B. Two- and Three-Dimensional Spectrofluorimetric Qualitative Analysis of Selected Vegetable Oils for Biomedical Applications. *Molecules* **2020**, *25*, 5608. [CrossRef]
17. Livada, R.; Shiloah, J.; Tipton, D.A.; Dabbous, M. The Potential Role of Curcumin in Periodontal Therapy: A Review of the Literature. *J. Int. Acad. Periodontol.* **2017**, *19*, 70–79.
18. Goel, A.; Boland, C.R.; Chauhan, D.P. Specific Inhibition of Cyclooxygenase-2 (COX-2) Expression by Dietary Curcumin in HT-29 Human Colon Cancer Cells. *Cancer Lett.* **2001**, *172*, 111–118. [CrossRef]
19. Zhang, F.; Altorki, N.K.; Mestre, J.R.; Subbaramaiah, K.; Dannenberg, A.J. Curcumin Inhibits Cyclooxygenase-2 Transcription in Bile Acid- and Phorbol Ester-Treated Human Gastrointestinal Epithelial Cells. *Carcinogenesis* **1999**, *20*, 445–451. [CrossRef]
20. Plummer, S.M.; Holloway, K.A.; Manson, M.M.; Munks, R.J.; Kaptein, A.; Farrow, S.; Howells, L. Inhibition of Cyclo-Oxygenase 2 Expression in Colon Cells by the Chemopreventive Agent Curcumin Involves Inhibition of NF-KB Activation via the NIK/IKK Signalling Complex. *Oncogene* **1999**, *18*, 6013–6020. [CrossRef]
21. Rao, C.V.; Rivenson, A.; Simi, B. Chemoprevention of Colon Carcinogenesis by Dietary Curcumin, a Naturally Occurring Plant Phenolic Compound. *Cancer Res.* **1995**, *55*, 259–266. [PubMed]
22. Yamamoto, H.; Hanada, K.; Kawasaki, K.; Nishijima, M. Inhibitory Effect of Curcumin on Mammalian Phospholipase D Activity. *FEBS Lett.* **1997**, *417*, 196–198. [CrossRef] [PubMed]
23. Ammon, H.P.T.; Safayhi, H.; Mack, T.; Sabieraj, J. Mechanism of Antiinflammatory Actions of Curcumine and Boswellic Acids. *J. Ethnopharmacol.* **1993**, *38*, 105–112. [CrossRef] [PubMed]
24. Began, G.; Sudharshan, E.; Rao, A.G.A. Inhibition of Lipoxygenase 1 by Phosphatidylcholine Micelles-Bound Curcumin. *Lipids* **1998**, *33*, 1223–1228. [CrossRef] [PubMed]
25. Skrzypczak-Jankun, E.; McCabe, N.P.; Selman, S.H.; Jankun, J. Curcumin Inhibits Lipoxygenase by Binding to Its Central Cavity: Theoretical and X-Ray Evidence. *Int. J. Mol. Med.* **2000**, *6*, 521–527. [CrossRef]
26. Paris, S.; Wolgin, M.; Kielbassa, A.M.; Pries, A.; Zakrzewicz, A. Gene Expression of Human Beta-Defensins in Healthy and Inflamed Human Dental Pulps. *J. Endod.* **2009**, *35*, 520–523. [CrossRef]
27. Briers, Y.; Walmagh, M.; Van Puyenbroeck, V.; Cornelissen, A.; Cenens, W.; Aertsen, A.; Oliveira, H.; Azeredo, J.; Verween, G.; Pirnay, J.-P.; et al. Engineered Endolysin-Based "Artilysins" To Combat Multidrug-Resistant Gram-Negative Pathogens. *mBio* **2014**, *5*, e01379-14. [CrossRef]
28. Rudrappa, T.; Bais, H.P. Curcumin, a Known Phenolic from *Curcuma Longa*, Attenuates the Virulence of Pseudomonas Aeruginosa PAO1 in Whole Plant and Animal Pathogenicity Models. *J. Agric. Food Chem.* **2008**, *56*, 1955–1962. [CrossRef]
29. Helalat, L.; Zarejavid, A.; Ekrami, A. The Effect of Curcumin on Growth and Adherence of Major Microorganisms Causing Tooth Decay. *Middle East J. Fam. Med.* **2017**, *15*, 214–220. [CrossRef]
30. Song, J.; Choi, B.; Jin, E.-J.; Yoon, Y.; Choi, K.-H. Curcumin Suppresses Streptococcus Mutans Adherence to Human Tooth Surfaces and Extracellular Matrix Proteins. *Eur. J. Clin. Microbiol. Infect. Dis.* **2012**, *31*, 1347–1352. [CrossRef]
31. Behal, R.; Gilda, S.; Paradkar, A.; Mali, A. Evaluation of Local Drug-Delivery System Containing 2% Whole Turmeric Gel Used as an Adjunct to Scaling and Root Planing in Chronic Periodontitis: A Clinical and Microbiological Study. *J. Indian Soc. Periodontol.* **2011**, *15*, 35. [CrossRef]
32. Bhatia, M.; Urolagin, S.S.; Pentyala, K.B.; Urolagin, S.B.; Menaka, K.B.; Bhoi, S. Novel Therapeutic Approach for the Treatment of Periodontitis by Curcumin. *J. Clin. Diagn. Res.* **2014**, *8*, ZC65–ZC69. [CrossRef]
33. Anuradha, B.R.; Bai, Y.D.; Sailaja, S.; Sudhakar, J.; Priyanka, M.; Deepika, V. Evaluation of Anti-Inflammatory Effects of Curcumin Gel as an Adjunct to Scaling and Root Planing: A Clinical Study. *J. Int. Oral Health* **2015**, *7*, 93.
34. Nagasri, M.; Madhulatha, M.; Musalaiah, S.V.V.S.; Kumar, P.M.; Krishna, C.M. Efficacy of Curcumin as an Adjunct to Scaling and Root Planning in Chronic Periodontitis Patients: A Clinical and Microbiological Study. *J. Pharm. Bioallied Sci.* **2015**, *7*, 554. [CrossRef]
35. Shivanand, P.; Vandana, K.V.; Vandana, K.L.; Praksh, S. Evaluation of Curcumin 10 Mg (Curenext ®) as Local Drug Delivery Adjunct in the Treatment of Chronic Periodontitis: A Clinical Trial. *CODS J. Dent.* **2016**, *8*, 59–63. [CrossRef]
36. Nasra, M.M.A.; Khiri, H.M.; Hazzah, H.A.; Abdallah, O.Y. Formulation, in-Vitro Characterization and Clinical Evaluation of Curcumin in-Situ Gel for Treatment of Periodontitis. *Drug Deliv.* **2017**, *24*, 133–142. [CrossRef]
37. Dave, D.; Patel, P.; Shah, M.; Dadawala, S.; Saraiya, K.; Sant, A. Comparative Evaluation of Efficacy of Oral Curcumin Gel as an Adjunct to Scaling and Root Planing in the Treatment of Chronic Periodontitis. *Adv. Hum. Biol.* **2018**, *8*, 79. [CrossRef]

38. Raghava, K.V.; Sistla, K.P.; Narayan, S.J.; Yadalam, U.; Bose, A.; Mitra, K. Efficacy of Curcumin as an Adjunct to Scaling and Root Planing in Chronic Periodontitis Patients: A Randomized Controlled Clinical Trial. *J. Contemp. Dent. Pract.* **2019**, *20*, 842–846. [CrossRef]
39. Kaur, H.; Malhotra, R.; Gupta, M.; Grover, D.V. Evaluation_of_Curcumin_Gel_as_Adjunct_to_Scaling_Root Planning in the Mangement of Periodontitis- Randomized Clinical & Biochemical Investigation. *Infect. Disord. Drug Targets* **2019**, *18*, 1. [CrossRef]
40. Pérez-Pacheco, C.G.; Fernandes, N.A.R.; Primo, F.L.; Tedesco, A.C.; Bellile, E.; Retamal-Valdes, B.; Feres, M.; Guimarães-Stabili, M.R.; Rossa, C. Local Application of Curcumin-Loaded Nanoparticles as an Adjunct to Scaling and Root Planing in Periodontitis: Randomized, Placebo-Controlled, Double-Blind Split-Mouth Clinical Trial. *Clin. Oral Investig.* **2020**, *25*, 3217–3227. [CrossRef]
41. Farhood, H.T.; Ali, B.G. Clinical and Anti-Inflammatory Effect of Curcumin Oral Gel as Adjuncts in Treatment of Periodontal Pocket. *J. Res. Med. Dent. Sci.* **2020**, *8*, 83–90.
42. Mohammad, C.A. Efficacy of Curcumin Gel on Zinc, Magnesium, Copper, IL-1β, and TNF-α in Chronic Periodontitis Patients. *BioMed Res. Int.* **2020**, *2020*, 1–11. [CrossRef] [PubMed]
43. Rahalkar, A.; Kumathalli, K.; Kumar, R. Determination of Efficacy of Curcumin and Tulsi Extracts as Local Drugs in Periodontal Pocket Reduction: A Clinical and Microbiological Study. *J. Indian Soc. Periodontol.* **2021**, *25*, 197. [CrossRef] [PubMed]
44. Elavarasu, S.; Suthanthiran, T.; Kumar, S. Evaluation of Superoxide Dismutase Levels in Local Drug Delivery System Containing 0.2% Curcumin Strip as an Adjunct to Scaling and Root Planing in Chronic Periodontitis: A Clinical and Biochemical Study. *Pharm. Bioallied Sci.* **2016**, *8*, S48–S52. [CrossRef]
45. Saini, K.; Yadav, M.; Bhardway, A.; Chopra, P.; Saini, S. Comparative Clinical Evaluation of Two Local Drug Delivery Agents (Neem Chip and Turmeric Chip) in Chronic Periodontitis: An Experimental Study. *World J. Dent.* **2021**, *12*, 138–143. [CrossRef]
46. Sreedhar, A.; Sarkar, I.; Rajan, P.; Pai, J.; Malagi, S.; Kamath, V.; Barmappa, R. Comparative Evaluation of the Efficacy of Curcumin Gel with and without Photo Activation as an Adjunct to Scaling and Root Planing in the Treatment of Chronic Periodontitis: A Split Mouth Clinical and Microbiological Study. *J. Nat. Sci. Biol. Med.* **2015**, *6*, 102. [CrossRef]
47. Gottumukkala, S.N.V.S.; Sudarshan, S.; Mantena, S.R. Comparative Evaluation of the Efficacy of Two Controlled Release Devices: Chlorhexidine Chips and Indigenous Curcumin Based Collagen as Local Drug Delivery Systems. *Contemp. Clin. Dent.* **2014**, *5*, 175. [CrossRef]
48. Anitha, V.; Rajesh, P.; Shanmugam, M.; Priya, B.M.; Prabhu, S.; Shivakumar, V. Comparative Evaluation of Natural Curcumin and Synthetic Chlorhexidine in the Management of Chronic Periodontitis as a Local Drug Delivery: A Clinical and Microbiological Study. *Indian J. Dent. Res.* **2015**, *26*, 53–56. [CrossRef]
49. Siddharth, M.; Gupta, R.; Singh, P.; Sinha, A.; Shree, S.; Sharma, K. Comparative Evaluation of Subgingivally Delivered 2% Curcumin and 0.2% Chlorhexidine Gel Adjunctive to Scaling and Root Planing in Chronic Periodontitis. *J. Contemp. Dent. Pract.* **2020**, *21*, 494–499. [CrossRef]
50. Jaswal, R.; Dhawan, S.; Grover, V.; Malhotra, R. Comparative Evaluation of Single Application of 2% Whole Turmeric Gel versus 1% Chlorhexidine Gel in Chronic Periodontitis Patients: A Pilot Study. *J. Indian Soc. Periodontol.* **2014**, *18*, 575–580. [CrossRef]
51. Singh, A.; Sridhar, R.; Shrihatti, R.; Mandloy, A. Evaluation of Turmeric Chip Compared with Chlorhexidine Chip as a Local Drug Delivery Agent in the Treatment of Chronic Periodontitis: A Split Mouth Randomized Controlled Clinical Trial. *J. Altern. Complement. Med.* **2018**, *24*, 76–84. [CrossRef]
52. Guru, S.R.; Reddy, K.A.; Rao, R.J.; Padmanabhan, S.; Guru, R.; Srinivasa, T. Comparative Evaluation of 2% Turmeric Extract with Nanocarrier and 1% Chlorhexidine Gel as an Adjunct to Scaling and Root Planing in Patients with Chronic Periodontitis: A Pilot Randomized Controlled Clinical Trial. *J. Ind. Soc Periodontol.* **2020**, *24*, 224. [CrossRef]
53. Gottumukkala, S.; Koneru, S.; Mannem, S.; Mandalapu, N. Effectiveness of Sub Gingival Irrigation of an Indigenous 1% Curcumin Solution on Clinical and Microbiological Parameters in Chronic Periodontitis Patients: A Pilot Randomized Clinical Trial. *Contemp. Clin. Dent.* **2013**, *4*, 186–191. [CrossRef]
54. De Oliveira, R.C.G.; Costa, C.A.; Costa, N.L.; Silva, G.C.; de Souza, J.A.C. Effects of Curcuma as an Adjunct Therapy on Periodontal Disease: A Systematic Review and Meta-Analysis. *Complement. Ther. Clin. Pract.* **2021**, *45*, 101493. [CrossRef]
55. Terby, S.; Shereef, M.; Ramanarayanan, V.; Balakrishnan, B. The Effect of Curcumin as an Adjunct in the Treatment of Chronic Periodontitis: A Systematic Review and Meta-Analysis. *Saudi Dent. J.* **2021**, *33*, 375–385. [CrossRef]
56. Zhang, Y.; Huang, L.; Zhang, J.; De Souza Rastelli, A.N.; Yang, J.; Deng, D. Anti-Inflammatory Efficacy of Curcumin as an Adjunct to Non-Surgical Periodontal Treatment: A Systematic Review and Meta-Analysis. *Front. Pharmacol.* **2022**, *13*, 808460. [CrossRef]
57. Higgins, J.; Thomas, J. *Cochrane Handbook for Systematic Reviews of Interventions*; Cochrane: London, UK, 2022.
58. Page, M.J.; McKenzie, J.E.; Bossuyt, P.M.; Boutron, I.; Hoffmann, T.C.; Mulrow, C.D.; Shamseer, L.; Tetzlaff, J.M.; Akl, E.A.; Brennan, S.E.; et al. The PRISMA 2020 Statement: An Updated Guideline for Reporting Systematic Reviews. *BMJ* **2021**, *372*, n71. [CrossRef]
59. Sterne, J.A.C.; Savović, J.; Page, M.J.; Elbers, R.G.; Lasserson, T.; McAleenan, A.; Reeves, B.C.; Shepperd, S.; Shrier, I.; Tilling, K.; et al. RoB 2: A Revised Tool for Assessing Risk of Bias in Randomised Trials. *BMJ* **2019**, *366*, l4898. [CrossRef]
60. Moher, D.; Liberati, A.; Tetzlaff, J.; Altman, D.G. Preferred Reporting Items for Systematic Reviews and Meta-analyses: The Prisma Statement. *PLoS Med.* **2019**, *6*, e1000097. [CrossRef]
61. Gupta, N.; Rath, S.K.; Lohra, P. Comparative Evaluation of Accuracy of Periodontal Probing Depth and Attachment Levels Using a Florida Probe versus Traditional Probes. *Med. J. Armed Forces India* **2015**, *71*, 352–358. [CrossRef]

62. Oringer, R.J.; Fiorellini, J.P.; Koch, G.G.; Sharp, T.J.; Nevins, M.L.; Davis, G.H.; Howell, T.H. Comparison of Manual and Automated Probing in an Untreated Periodontitis Population. *J. Periodontol.* **1997**, *68*, 1156–1162. [CrossRef] [PubMed]
63. Araujo, M.W.B.; Hovey, K.M.; Benedek, J.R.; Grossi, S.G.; Dorn, J.; Wactawski-Wende, J.; Genco, R.J.; Trevisan, M. Reproducibility of Probing Depth Measurement Using a Constant-Force Electronic Probe: Analysis of Inter- and Intraexaminer Variability. *J. Periodontol.* **2003**, *74*, 1736–1740. [CrossRef] [PubMed]
64. Hefti, A.F. Periodontal Probing. *Crit. Rev. Oral Biol. Med.* **1997**, *8*, 336–356. [CrossRef] [PubMed]
65. Watts, T. Constant Force Probing with and without a Stent in Untreated Periodontal Disease: The Clinical Reproducibility Problem and Possible Sources of Error. *J. Clin. Periodontol.* **1987**, *14*, 407–411. [CrossRef] [PubMed]
66. Larsen, C.; Barendregt, D.S.; Slot, D.E.; Van der Velden, U.; Van der Weijden, F. Probing Pressure, a Highly Undervalued Unit of Measure in Periodontal Probing: A Systematic Review on Its Effect on Probing Pocket Depth. *J. Clin. Periodontol.* **2009**, *36*, 315–322. [CrossRef]
67. Niederman, R. Manual and Electronic Probes Have Similar Reliability in the Measurement of Untreated Periodontitis: Question: Do Manual or Electronic Probes Produce the Most Reproducible Measurements of Clinical Attachment Level in Periodontitis Patients? *Evid. Based Dent.* **2009**, *10*, 39. [CrossRef]
68. Silva-Boghossian, C.M.; Amaral, C.S.F.; Maia, L.C.; Luiz, R.R.; Colombo, A.P.V. Manual and Electronic Probing of the Periodontal Attachment Level in Untreated Periodontitis: A Systematic Review. *J. Dent.* **2008**, *36*, 651–657. [CrossRef]
69. Sholapurkar, A.; Sharma, D.; Glass, B.; Miller, C.; Nimmo, A.; Jennings, E. Professionally Delivered Local Antimicrobials in the Treatment of Patients with Periodontitis—A Narrative Review. *Dent. J.* **2021**, *9*, 2. [CrossRef]
70. Aggarwal, B.B.; Sundaram, C.; Malani, N.; Ichikawa, H. Curcumin: The Indian Solid Gold. In *The Molecular Targets and Therapeutic Uses of Curcumin in Health and Disease*; Aggarwal, B.B., Surh, Y.-J., Shishodia, S., Eds.; Springer: Boston, MA, USA, 2007; Volume 595, pp. 1–75. ISBN 978-0-387-46400-8.
71. Sigma-Aldrich. Curcumin. Available online: https://www.sigmaaldrich.com/AT/de/product/sigma/c1386?gclid=EAIaIQobChMI_ff86b_i9wIVBZ53Ch3R5gqrEAAYASAAEgK1YPD_BwE (accessed on 10 April 2022).
72. Konark Herbals & Health Care Curcuma Longa-Haldi. Available online: https://www.kherbalhealthcare.com/commiphora-mukul-guggal.html#curcuma-longa-haldi (accessed on 10 April 2022).
73. Guru, S.; Kothiwale, S.; Saroch, N.; Guru, R. Comparative Evaluation of Inhibitory Effect of Curcumin and Doxycycline on Matrix Metalloproteinase-9 Activity in Chronic Periodontitis. *Indian J. Dent. Res.* **2017**, *28*, 560. [CrossRef]
74. Anand, P.; Kunnumakkara, A.B.; Newman, R.A.; Aggarwal, B.B. Bioavailability of Curcumin: Problems and Promises. *Mol. Pharm.* **2007**, *4*, 807–818. [CrossRef]
75. Sohn, S.-I.; Priya, A.; Balasubramaniam, B.; Muthuramalingam, P.; Sivasankar, C.; Selvaraj, A.; Valliammai, A.; Jothi, R.; Pandian, S. Biomedical Applications and Bioavailability of Curcumin—An Updated Overview. *Pharmaceutics* **2021**, *13*, 2102. [CrossRef]
76. Karthikeyan, A.; Senthil, N.; Min, T. Nanocurcumin: A Promising Candidate for Therapeutic Applications. *Front. Pharmacol.* **2020**, *11*, 487. [CrossRef]
77. Curylofo-Zotti, F.A.; Elburki, M.S.; Oliveira, P.A.; Cerri, P.S.; Santos, L.A.; Lee, H.-M.; Johnson, F.; Golub, L.M.; Rossa, C.; Guimarães-Stabili, M.R. Differential Effects of Natural Curcumin and Chemically Modified Curcumin on Inflammation and Bone Resorption in Model of Experimental Periodontitis. *Arch. Oral Biol.* **2018**, *91*, 42–50. [CrossRef]
78. Smaïl-Faugeron, V.; Fron-Chabouis, H.; Courson, F.; Durieux, P. Comparison of Intervention Effects in Split-Mouth and Parallel-Arm Randomized Controlled Trials: A Meta-Epidemiological Study. *BMC Med. Res. Methodol.* **2014**, *14*, 64. [CrossRef]

Disclaimer/Publisher's Note: The statements, opinions and data contained in all publications are solely those of the individual author(s) and contributor(s) and not of MDPI and/or the editor(s). MDPI and/or the editor(s) disclaim responsibility for any injury to people or property resulting from any ideas, methods, instructions or products referred to in the content.

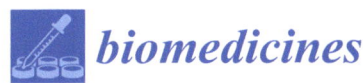

Article

Heat Accumulation in Implant Inter-Osteotomy Areas—An Experimental In Vitro Study

Shanlin Li [1], Adam Tanner [1], Georgios Romanos [2] and Rafael Delgado-Ruiz [3,*]

- [1] School of Dental Medicine, Stony Brook University, Stony Brook, New York, NY 11794, USA
- [2] Department of Periodontology, School of Dental Medicine, Stony Brook University, Stony Brook, New York, NY 11794, USA
- [3] Department of Prosthodontics and Digital Technology, School of Dental Medicine, Stony Brook University, Stony Brook, New York, NY 11794, USA
- * Correspondence: rafael.delgado-ruiz@stonybrookmedicine.edu

Abstract: To examine the influence of the distance between adjacent implant osteotomies on heat accumulation in the inter-osteotomy area, two experimental groups with 15 pairs of osteotomies in Type II polyurethane blocks were compared: 7 mm inter-osteotomy separations (Group A, $n = 15$) and 14 mm inter-osteotomy separations (Group B, $n = 15$). An infrared thermographic analysis of thermal changes in the inter-osteotomy area was completed. A one-way analysis of variance (ANOVA) and Fisher post-test were used to determine group differences. Higher temperatures were recorded in Group A at the coronal and middle levels compared to the apical level in both groups. The temperature reached max temperatures at T80s and T100s. In Group A, the threshold for thermal necrosis was exceeded. Meanwhile, Group B did not reach the threshold for thermal necrosis. Preparing adjacent implant osteotomies in dense bone with a 7 mm separation between their centers increases the temperature in the inter-osteotomy area, exceeding the threshold for bone thermal necrosis; meanwhile, increasing the distance between osteotomies reduces the thermal accumulation and the risk for thermal necrosis.

Keywords: bone drilling; implant osteotomy; implant site preparation; infrared thermographic analysis

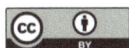

Citation: Li, S.; Tanner, A.; Romanos, G.; Delgado-Ruiz, R. Heat Accumulation in Implant Inter-Osteotomy Areas—An Experimental In Vitro Study. *Biomedicines* **2023**, *11*, 9. https://doi.org/10.3390/biomedicines11010009

Academic Editors: Gianmarco Abbadessa, Giuseppe Minervini and Gianluca Gambarini

Received: 5 October 2022
Revised: 26 November 2022
Accepted: 14 December 2022
Published: 21 December 2022

Copyright: © 2022 by the authors. Licensee MDPI, Basel, Switzerland. This article is an open access article distributed under the terms and conditions of the Creative Commons Attribution (CC BY) license (https://creativecommons.org/licenses/by/4.0/).

1. Introduction

Dental implants are an excellent treatment option for partially or fully edentulous patients, given their high survival (94.6% ± 5.97%) and success rates (89.7% ± 10.2%) after ten years in function [1]. In general, dental implant beds are prepared through a series of drilling steps prior to implant insertion; these procedures are also called implant bed or implant site preparation [2–4]. The implant bed preparation traditionally requires one or more rotating drills to complete the osteotomy, which also produces local microfractures and temperature elevation [5]. If the levels of local trauma and temperature cannot be controlled, the risk for bone thermomechanical damage might increase [5].

Exposure time and temperature elevation are determinants of the degree of bone damage. If the bone temperature reaches the limit of 47 °C for one minute or more, irreversible thermal necrosis occurs [4,6]. In addition, alkaline phosphatase degrades at temperatures above 56 °C; necrosis of the surrounding tissues can occur when the bone reaches temperatures over 60 °C; and temperatures over 70 °C can produce fulminant bone necrosis [7].

The temperature elevation produced during bone drilling is related to a combination of various parameters, with bone density and the drilling technique being the most relevant [8]. Bone density influences how heat is produced and how temperature dissipates [9,10]. Higher temperatures are produced in dense (cortical) bone compared to softer (trabecular) bone [10] because higher frictional forces are produced when drilling in dense bone. Meanwhile, drilling in soft bone will result in lower frictional forces and less heat generation. Furthermore, the low dissipation rates of the temperature produced in dense bone can explain why it is at a higher risk for osteonecrosis than is soft bone [11].

Considering the drilling technique for the implant bed preparation, parameters such as thrust force, feed rate, irrigation, drilling speed, and operator experience have been investigated [12–18]. Thrust force and feed rate are influenced by the operator, and it seems that novices produce higher forces and feed rates compared to experts, resulting in higher temperatures during bone drilling [12,13]. Irrigation is essential for controlling the temperature during high-speed drilling. Specifically, external irrigation is more efficient for cooling than internal irrigation; high volumes of irrigation reduce the temperature more than low volumes of irrigation [14]; and reduced coolant temperature controls the thermal increase better than higher coolant temperatures [15,16]. If the coolant cannot reach the targets (drill surface and bone), the temperature elevation is not controlled. This occurs when irrigation lines are obstructed or in guided surgery, when the surgical guide and metallic sleeves impede the contact of the coolant with the drill and the bone [17].

Finally, when comparing conventional drilling speeds (1200 rpm–2000 rpm) with slow drilling speeds (50 rpm, 150 rpm, or 300 rpm), it was observed that slow drilling speeds resulted in minimal temperature elevation in soft and dense bone [18]. This was confirmed by a recent systematic review that showed that slow-speed drilling produced minimal temperature increases and similar osseointegration and crestal bone loss compared to what was observed in conventional drilling with irrigation [19].

In relation to sequential osteotomies (one osteotomy adjacent to another) there are not reports in the dental field, and there is only one study by Palmisano et al. [20] that evaluated the heat accumulation phenomenon in orthopedic surgery when multiple adjacent osteotomies are prepared. In their study, it was observed that drilling nine adjacent osteotomies in sequence increased the temperature in the inter-osteotomy space after the fifth osteotomy, and the highest temperatures were measured during the ninth osteotomy [20].

In implant dentistry, the thermal effects of bone drilling are commonly evaluated at the site of the implant osteotomy, but a significant lack of knowledge remains concerning the cumulative thermal effect of drilling adjacent implant osteotomies in Type II bone, where the risk of thermal damage is increased. Specifically, what is the impact of the distance between osteotomies on the heat generated in the inter-osteotomy area of sequentially prepared dental implant osteotomies?

This study aimed to test the null hypothesis, stating there is no difference in temperature accumulation between adjacent implant osteotomies separated by 7 or 14 mm, against the alternative hypothesis that there are differences in temperature accumulation between adjacent implant osteotomies separated by 7 or 14 mm.

2. Materials and Methods

2.1. Sample Size and Calibration

Sample size for this in vitro study was determined as fifteen pairs of osteotomies per group A and B ($n = 15$). The sample size was estimated for a confidence level of 95% and a confidence interval of 25% using the sample size application from StatPlus: Mac, (Analyst Soft Inc., Walnut, CA, USA)- statistical analysis program for macOS. Version v8.

The osteotomies were prepared by two calibrated operators using an implant motor Frios® S/I connected to a contra-angle WS-75 (Friadent, Dentsply Sirona, Bürmoos, Austria). Tapered implant drills Ref. HIKELT-5-3810 (Bioner Sistemas Implantologicos, Barcelona, Spain; Ref. HIKELT-5-3810) with 3.8 mm diameter and 10 mm length were used. Solid close-cell polyurethane blocks (Sawbones, Pacific Research Labs, Vashon, WA, USA) with a density of 0.64 g/cm^3 and 40 PCF (pounds per cubic foot) were used for this experiment. The thermal conductivity of this type of block (0.47 W/mK) is comparable to Type II dense bone [21–23].

2.2. Experimental Setup

Sixty simulated osteotomies, divided into fifteen pairs with 7 mm separation in Type II blocks (Test A, $n = 15$), and fifteen pairs of simulated osteotomies with 14 mm separation in Type II blocks (Test B, $n = 15$) were created. Polyurethane blocks were fixed in a vise oriented with their major diameter parallel to the floor and the border of the surface for evaluation facing upwards. The top side of the blocks that was facing the camera served as reference for marking a line parallel to the edge of the block. The line was traced with a pencil at a 4 mm distance from the edge of the blocks. The centers of the future osteotomies were marked on the line, maintaining 7 mm or 14 mm inter-osteotomy distance depending on the experimental group.

2.3. Thermal Analysis

One infrared thermographic camera FLIR A325sc (FLIR Systems Inc, Nashua, NH, USA) equipped with macro lenses FLIR T97215 (FLIR Systems Inc, Nashua, NH, USA) was oriented to the inter-osteotomy area of the future osteotomies (aligned with the osteotomy marks completed previously). This allowed for the recording of the inter-osteotomy area temperatures and produced thermal maps at the surface of the blocks. The camera orientation was adjusted to include in the recordings the top of the block and an additional 15 mm above the block (Figure 1).

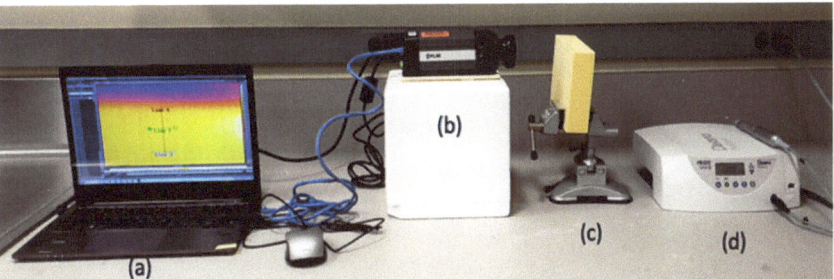

Figure 1. (**a**) Laptop with thermography camera software, (**b**) thermographic camera, (**c**) polyurethane bone block mounted in a vise, and (**d**) implant motor and contra angle.

The recording parameters were room temperature at 21 degrees Celsius, relative humidity of 50%, and focal distance of 7 cm. The blocks were used in dry conditions, and no irrigation was used during the simulated drilling. Each recording of the thermographic camera started before initializing any implant osteotomy preparation. Before the drills contacted the blocks, a calibration recording of the block's temperature was documented as a baseline. The temperature was recorded in degrees Celsius. Afterwards, using the software FLIR Research Studio Professional Edition, a vertical line of 10 mm was placed in the inter-osteotomy area. Then, three equidistant lines perpendicular to the first vertical line were drawn at the coronal, middle, and apical levels. Thus, each intersection between the vertical and the horizontal lines evaluated the inter-osteotomy area temperature at the coronal, middle, and apical levels (Figure 2).

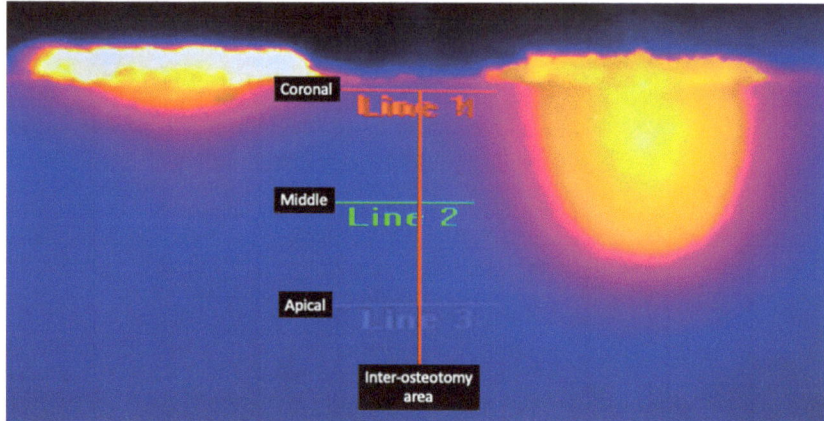

Figure 2. Image demonstrating the setup of measurement recording. The vertical red line in the middle signifies the inter-osteotomy center where the measurements were taken. Lines 1, 2, and 3 indicate the coronal, middle, and apical levels of the inter-osteotomy area, respectively.

The infrared thermographic camera was set in continuous video-capture mode to register the temperature changes at the unit sample (each unit sample comprised a pair of adjacent osteotomies evaluated during a period of ±120 s). The changes produced during drilling at the first and second implant sites and temperature accumulation in the inter-osteotomy area were analyzed in standardized measurements at 20 s, 40 s, 60 s, 80 s, and 100 s.

2.4. Statistical Analysis

Statistical analysis was completed using the statistical software Minitab web app. The normality of the data was evaluated using the Kolmogorov–Smirnoff test. ANOVA test was completed. Fisher post-test was used to evaluate the temperature differences in the coronal, middle, and apical areas at 7 mm and 14 mm and at 20 s, 40 s, 60 s, 80 s, and 100 s. Significance was set as $p < 0.05$.

3. Results

The temperature increased gradually during and after the preparation of the first and second osteotomies and reached peaks between 60 s and 100 s. The temperature accumulation toward the centers of the inter-osteotomy areas was higher at 80 and 100 s (Figure 3).

3.1. Coronal Temperature for 7 mm and 14 mm Inter-Osteotomy Separations

Higher temperatures were observed at the coronal level in 7 mm inter-osteotomy separations compared to 14 mm inter-osteotomy separations. Specifically, at 7 mm, the temperature reached peak values at 60 s (58.86 °C ± SD 19.32 °C). Meanwhile, at 14 mm, peak values were reached at 100 s (28.307 °C ± SD 1.52 °C), as shown in Table 1. Figure 4 illustrates mean temperatures and standard deviations recorded in the coronal region at different time points and different inter-osteotomy distances (Table 1 and Figure 4).

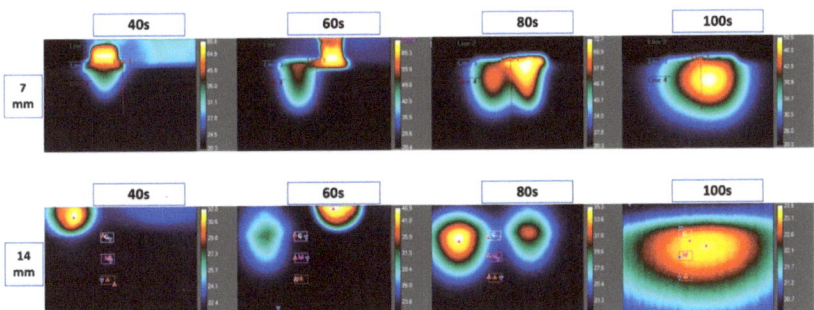

Figure 3. Thermal camera recordings from 7 mm and 14 mm inter-osteotomy distances at 40 s, 60 s, 80 s, and 100 s. This figure illustrates the live recording of the thermal behavior during the preparation of the osteotomies. The red line represents the center between osteotomies. Along the red line, three zones: coronal, middle, and apical. Higher temperatures were recorded at the 7 mm distance compared to 14 mm. Each of the screenshots in the 14 mm recordings shows three letters: C, M, A (coronal, middle, and apical). Each of the screenshots in the 14 mm recordings shows three letters: C, M, A (coronal, middle, and apical). There are also red solid arrows illustrating the hottest region and blue solid arrows illustrating the coldest regions within the zone of evaluation.

Table 1. Descriptive statistics of inter-implant bed temperature at distances of 7 mm and 14 mm in the coronal area of the dense bone. D = distance, C = coronal, T = time (T1 = 20 s, T2 = 40 s, T3 = 60 s, T4 = 80 s, T5 = 100 s).

Inter-Osteotomy Distance and Time. Coronal Area	Sample Size	Mean	Standard Deviation	95% CI
D7CT0	15	21.133	0.713	(15.976, 26.290)
D7CT20	15	26.03	4.97	(20.87, 31.19)
D7CT40	15	39.08	11.90	(33.92, 44.23)
D7CT60	15	58.86	19.32	(53.70, 64.01)
D7CT80	15	59.74	18.51	(54.59, 64.90)
D7CT100	15	54.07	18.19	(48.91, 59.22)
D14CT0	15	22.040	1.679	(16.883, 27.197)
D14CT20	15	22.597	1.084	(17.440, 27.754)
D14CT40	15	22.655	0.835	(17.498, 27.812)
D14CT60	15	25.195	1.837	(20.038, 30.352)
D14CT80	15	25.692	2.034	(20.535, 30.849)
D14CT100	15	28.307	1.520	(23.150, 33.464)

3.2. Middle Temperature for 7 mm and 14 mm Inter-Osteotomy Separations

Higher temperatures were observed at the middle level for 7 mm compared to 14 mm inter-osteotomy separations. Specifically, at 7 mm, the temperature reached the higher peak values at 100 s (52.60 °C ± SD 17.39 °C) compared to the peak values for 14 mm distances at 100 s (28.252 °C ± SD 1.972 °C), as shown in Table 2. Figure 5 demonstrates the mean temperatures and standard deviations recorded at the middle region of the inter-osteotomy area at each time point and distance (Table 2 and Figure 5).

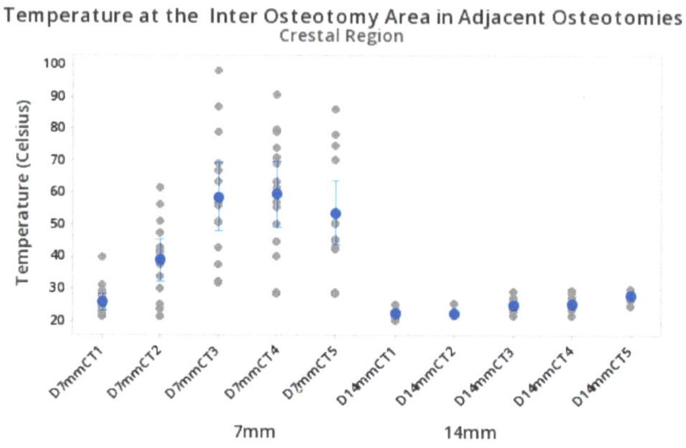

Temperature at the Inter Osteotomy Area in Adjacent Osteotomies
Crestal Region

Figure 4. Temperature in the inter-osteotomy area. Measurements at the coronal level. The y axis shows the temperature reached during the preparation of the osteotomies. The x axis indicates the different test groups at 7 mm and 14 mm inter-osteotomy separations at the coronal level. Ascending temperatures were observed in both groups and were influenced by the time and separation between osteotomies. D = distance, C = crestal, T = time (T1 = 20 s, T2 = 40 s, T3 = 60 s, T4 = 80 s, T5 = 100 s). The blue dots represent the central mean value. The grey dots represent the distribution of upper and lower temperatures (sometimes overlapping). The blue lines if present, represent standard deviations.

Table 2. Descriptive statistics of inter-implant bed temperature at distances of 7 mm and 14 mm in the middle area of the dense bone. D = distance, M = middle, T = time (T1 = 20 s, T2 = 40 s, T3 = 60 s, T4 = 80 s, T5 = 100 s).

Inter-Osteotomy Distance and Time. Middle Area	Sample Size	Mean	Standard Deviation	95% CI
D7MT0	15	20.816	0.484	(17.158, 24.475)
D7M20	15	20.980	0.496	(17.322, 24.638)
D7MT40	15	26.90	4.91	(23.24, 30.55)
D7MT60	15	40.74	10.61	(37.08, 44.40)
D7MT80	15	43.42	13.13	(39.77, 47.08)
D7MT100	15	52.60	17.39	(48.94, 56.26)
D14MT0	15	21.223	0.450	(17.565, 24.881)
D14MT20	15	21.344	0.609	(17.686, 25.002)
D14MT40	15	21.376	0.452	(17.718, 25.034)
D14MT60	15	22.284	0.732	(18.626, 25.943)
D14MT80	15	22.524	0.707	(18.866, 26.182)
D14MT100	15	28.252	1.972	(24.594, 31.910)

3.3. Apical Temperatures for 7 mm and 14 mm Inter-Osteotomy Separations

Higher temperatures were observed at the apical level of the inter-osteotomy zone for 7 mm compared to 14 mm separations. Specifically, at 7 mm, the temperature reached the higher peak values at 100 s (28.89 °C ± SD 5.34 °C). At the 14 mm inter-osteotomy distance, peak values were lower at 100 s (23.025 °C ± SD 0.79 °C) (Table 3). Figure 5 demonstrates the peak values of the 15 measurements recorded at each time point and distance (Table 3 and Figure 6).

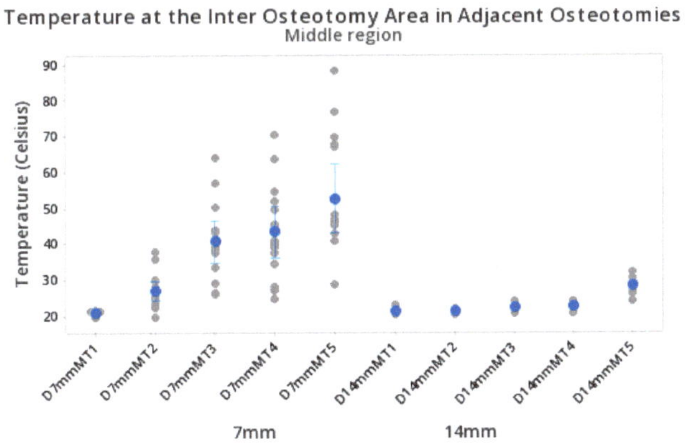

Temperature at the Inter Osteotomy Area in Adjacent Osteotomies
Middle region

Figure 5. Temperature in the inter-osteotomy area. Measurements at the middle level. The y axis shows the temperature reached during the preparation of the osteotomies. The x axis indicates the different test groups at 7 mm and 14 mm inter-osteotomy separations at the middle level. Ascending temperatures were observed in both groups and influenced by the time and separation between osteotomies. D = distance, M = middle, T = time (T1 = 20 s, T2 = 40 s, T3 = 60 s, T4 = 80 s, T5 = 100 s). The blue dots represent the central mean value. The grey dots represent the distribution of upper and lower temperatures (sometimes overlapping). The blue lines if present, represent standard deviations.

Table 3. Descriptive statistics of inter-implant bed temperature at distances of 7 mm and 14 mm in the apical area of the dense bone. D = distance, A = apical, T = time (T1 = 20 s, T2 = 40 s, T3 = 60 s, T4 = 80 s, T5 = 100 s).

Inter-Osteotomy Distance and Time. Apical Area	Sample Size	Mean	Standard Deviation	95% CI
D7AT0	15	20.740	0.523	(19.757, 21.723)
D7AT20	15	20.843	0.529	(19.860, 21.826)
D7AT40	15	21.132	0.658	(20.148, 22.115)
D7AT60	15	23.194	1.820	(22.211, 24.177)
D7AT80	15	24.131	3.247	(23.148, 25.114)
D7AT100	15	28.89	5.34	(27.91, 29.88)
D14AT0	15	21.092	0.387	(20.109, 22.075)
D14AT20	15	21.112	0.387	(20.128, 22.095)
D14AT40	15	21.148	0.392	(20.165, 22.131)
D14AT60	15	21.2436	0.3480	(20.2604, 22.2268)
D14AT80	15	21.2933	0.3576	(20.3101, 22.2765)
D14AT100	15	23.025	0.790	(22.041, 24.008)

3.4. Statistical Comparisons

Fisher tests showed higher temperatures in the inter-osteotomy area for 7 mm compared to 14 mm separation at 40, 60, 80, and 100 s. (Table 4).

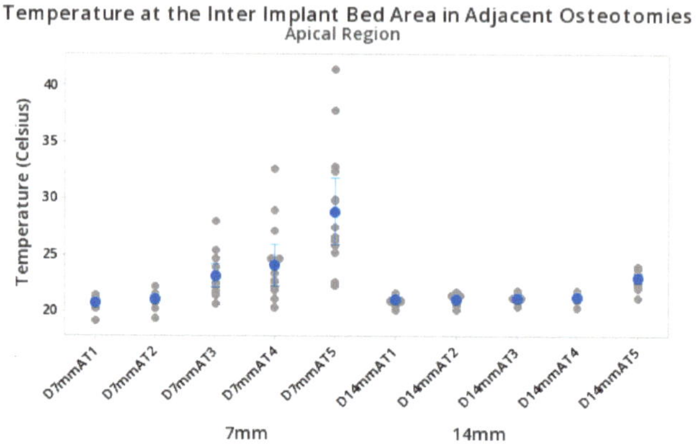

Temperature at the Inter Implant Bed Area in Adjacent Osteotomies
Apical Region

Figure 6. Temperature in the inter-osteotomy area in adjacent osteotomies. Measurements at the apical level. The y axis shows the temperature reached during the preparation of the osteotomies. The x axis indicates the different test groups at 7 mm and 14 mm inter-osteotomy area separations at the apical level. Ascending temperatures were observed in both groups, influenced by the time. D = distance, A = apical, T = time (T1 = 20 s, T2 = 40 s, T3 = 60 s, T4 = 80 s, T5 = 100 s). The blue dots represent the central mean value. The grey dots represent the distribution of upper and lower temperatures (sometimes overlapping). The blue lines if present, represent standard deviations.

Table 4. Fisher test for 14 mm vs. 7 mm in the coronal area. * $p < 0.05$.

Coronal Groups Comparison	Difference of Means	SE of Difference	95% CI	T-Value	Adjusted p Value
D14CT0–D7CT0	0.91	3.69	(−6.39, 8.20)	0.25	0.806
D14CT20–D7CT20	−3.43	3.69	(−10.72, 3.86)	−0.93	0.354
D14CT40–D7CT40	−16.42	3.69	(−23.72, −9.13)	−4.45	0.000 *
D14CT60–D7CT60	−33.66	3.69	(−40.95, −26.37)	−9.11	0.000 *
D14CT80–D7CT80	−34.05	3.69	(−41.34, −26.76)	−9.22	0.000 *
D14CT100–D7CT100	−25.76	3.69	(−33.05, −18.47)	−6.97	0.000 *

Similarly, the Fisher test showed higher temperatures in the middle region of the inter-osteotomy zones for 7 mm compared to 14 mm separations (Table 5).

Table 5. Fisher test for 14 mm vs. 7 mm in the middle area. * $p < 0.05$.

Middle Groups Comparison	Difference of Means	SE of Difference	95% CI	T-Value	Adjusted p Value
D14MT0–D7MT0	0.41	2.62	(−4.77, 5.58)	0.16	0.877
D14MT20–D7M20	0.36	2.62	(−4.81, 5.54)	0.14	0.890
D14MT40–D7MT40	−5.52	2.62	(−10.69, −0.35)	−2.11	0.037 *
D14MT40–D7MT60	−19.36	2.62	(−24.54, −14.19)	−7.39	0.000 *
D14MT80–D7MT80	−20.90	2.62	(−26.07, −15.73)	−7.98	0.000 *
D14MT100–D7MT100	−24.35	2.62	(−29.52, −19.17)	−9.29	0.000 *

In the apical region of the inter-osteotomy zone, statistical differences between 7mm and 14mm were observed at 60, 80, and 100 s (Table 6).

Table 6. Fisher test for 14 mm vs. 7 mm in the apical area. * $p < 0.05$.

Apical Groups Comparison	Difference of Means	SE of Difference	95% CI	T-Value	Adjusted p Value
D14AT0–D7AT0	0.352	0.704	(−1.038, 1.743)	0.50	0.618
D14AT20–D7AT20	0.268	0.704	(−1.122, 1.659)	0.38	0.704
D14AT40–D7AT40	0.017	0.704	(−1.374, 1.407)	0.02	0.981
D14AT60–D7AT60	−1.950	0.704	(−3.341, −0.560)	−2.77	0.006 *
D14AT80–D7AT80	−2.838	0.704	(−4.228, −1.447)	−4.03	0.00 *
D14AT100–D7AT100	−5.869	0.704	(−7.260, −4.479)	−8.33	0.00 *

4. Discussion

This study aimed to test the null hypothesis, stating there is no difference in temperature accumulation between adjacent implant osteotomies separated by 7 or 14 mm, against the alternative hypothesis that there are differences in temperature accumulation between adjacent implant osteotomies separated by 7 or 14 mm. The null hypothesis was rejected. Higher temperature accumulation was observed in shorter separations (7 mm between osteotomies), surpassing the threshold for thermal necrosis in the coronal and middle zones. In implant dentistry, the thermal analysis of bone drilling is centered in the evaluation of the temperature changes at the osteotomy sites, and existing evidence indicates that frictional forces, drilling forces, drilling speed, and bone density all contribute to thermal changes during implant osteotomy [24–26].

The direct consequences of the bone overheating are either bone necrosis, increased bone resorption, or implant failure [27–29]. In addition, the effects of increased temperature on bone can be influenced by the phenomena of temperature dissipation and temperature accumulation [20,30–33]. Temperature dissipation in bone can be observed as the heat transfer from one area to another, and temperature accumulation can be observed as the summation of heat dissipated from more than one heat source [21,26]. When multiple adjacent implant osteotomies are required, the risk for thermal necrosis of the inter-osteotomy area should be evaluated because this parameter could explain interproximal bone resorption. The results of the present study showed that 7 mm of separation produced higher temperatures in the inter-osteotomy area than did a 14 mm separation.

This agrees with the studies in orthopedic surgery completed by Gholampour et al., 2019 [34], who prepared adjacent osteotomies at 6 mm, 12 mm, and 16 mm separations in femoral bone. Thermocouples and an infrared camera were used to evaluate the effects of a coolant and separation on the temperature at the first osteotomy site. The results showed that 6 mm separation resulted in higher temperatures, and increasing the time between drilling and the use of coolant limited the temperature increase.

The results of the present study are also in agreement with Palmisano et al., 2015 [20], who investigated the heat-accumulation phenomenon in sequential orthopedic drilling. In their study, nine sequential osteotomies were prepared in a 3 × 3 array on cadaver tibia, using three different drill types. Temperature changes were recorded at the center of four adjacent osteotomies using thermocouples. Their findings demonstrated that the temperatures were higher after the last osteotomy compared to the temperatures after the first osteotomy, and they demonstrated that the heat accumulation and heat dispersion increased when adjacent preparations were completed in dense bone.

In the present study, the results showed that the coronal and middle levels of the inter-osteotomy area presented the highest temperatures at times T4 and T5. Meanwhile, a minimal thermal increment was detected at the apical levels at all the evaluated times.

These findings can be explained by three factors. The first factor is the continued contact of the drills with the cortical compared to the middle and apical. The second factor is the tapered drill design toward the apex, and the third factor is the larger distance between adjacent osteotomies at the apical. This agrees with the study by Heydari et al., [35], who observed higher temperatures during drilling in dense bone due to increased fiction and heat accumulation from the increased time that the drills were in contact with the bone.

In the present study, the distances of 7 mm or 14 mm between the centers of the osteotomies were used, assuming that either adjacent implants with regular diameters (3.8 mm–4 mm) are inserted or adjacent implants are inserted but include a space for a pontic for the fabrication of a bridge. It has been recommended to maintain a distance of 3 mm between adjacent implants because it can preserve the bone and gingival papilla height. When the distance between adjacent implants is reduced to 2 mm or 1 mm, the bone remodeling between implants increases, resulting in bone loss. In addition, when the distance between adjacent implants is less than 3 mm, angiogenesis is reduced. Additionally, the number of blood vessels decreases, and the bone formation is impaired [36–39]. Within the limitations of this study, it seems also reasonable to think that distances smaller than 3 mm can also produce increased temperature accumulation and increased risk of osteonecrosis in adjacent osteotomies.

Limitations of this study include: only one type of polyurethane block was used, and given the homogeneous characteristic of the blocks, the results can be extrapolated only to bone with similar conditions (dense bone); only one type of drill was used, and the effect of other drill designs remains unknown; only two inter-osteotomy distances were evaluated, and therefore, the information related to the thermal behavior when drilling adjacent osteotomies with shorter or larger separations is missing.

The strengths of this study include: the use of a controlled experimental setup, calibrated operators, and the utilization of bone blocks with a well-known thermal coefficient comparable to human dense bone. This study alerts clinicians to the thermal risks of drilling adjacent dental implant osteotomies. In addition, potential methods for reducing thermal accumulation in the inter-osteotomy zone require further investigation.

5. Conclusions

Preparing adjacent implant osteotomies in dense bone with a 7 mm separation between their centers increases the temperature in the inter-osteotomy area, exceeding the threshold for bone thermal necrosis; meanwhile, increasing the distance between osteotomies reduces the thermal accumulation and the risk for thermal necrosis.

Author Contributions: Conceptualization, R.D.-R.; methodology, R.D.-R. and G.R.; formal analysis, R.D.-R., G.R., S.L. and A.T.; investigation, R.D.-R., S.L. and A.T.; resources, R.D.-R. and G.R.; data curation, S.L. and A.T.; writing—original draft preparation, S.L., A.T. and R.D.-R.; writing—review and editing, S.L., A.T., R.D.-R. and G.R. All authors have read and agreed to the published version of the manuscript.

Funding: This work was self-funded by resources and materials from the Department of Prosthodontics and Digital Technology of the School of Dental Medicine at Stony Brook University.

Institutional Review Board Statement: Not applicable.

Informed Consent Statement: Not applicable.

Data Availability Statement: The data from this experiment will be provided after request to the authors.

Acknowledgments: The authors acknowledge the support of the Digital Implant Prosthodontics Research Laboratory (DIPRESLAB) and the Laboratory for Periodontal Implant and Phototherapy (LA-PIP) of the School of Dental Medicine at Stony Brook University.

Conflicts of Interest: The authors declare no conflict of interest.

References

1. Moraschini, V.; Poubel, L.; Ferreira, V.; Barboza Edos, S. Evaluation of survival and success rates of dental implants reported in longitudinal studies with a follow-up period of at least 10 years: A systematic review. *Int. J. Oral. Maxillofac. Surg.* **2015**, *44*, 377–388. [CrossRef] [PubMed]
2. Benington, I.; Biagioni, P.; Briggs, J.; Sheridan, S.; Lamey, P. Thermal changes observed at implant sites during internal and external irrigation. *Clin. Oral. Implants Res.* **2002**, *13*, 293–297. [CrossRef] [PubMed]

3. Gehrke, S.; Bettach, R.; Taschieri, S.; Boukhris, G.; Corbella, S.; Del Fabbro, M. Temperature Changes in Cortical Bone after Implant Site Preparation Using a Single Bur versus Multiple Drilling Steps: An In Vitro Investigation. *Clin. Implant Dent. Relat. Res.* **2015**, *17*, 700–707. [CrossRef] [PubMed]
4. Kotsakis, G.; Romanos, G. Biological mechanisms underlying complications related to implant site preparation. *Periodontol. 2000* **2022**, *88*, 52–63. [CrossRef]
5. Akhbar, M.; Sulong, A. Surgical Drill Bit Design and Thermomechanical Damage in Bone Drilling: A Review. *Ann. Biomed. Eng.* **2021**, *49*, 29–56. [CrossRef]
6. Hochscheidt, C.; Shimizu, R.; Andrighetto, A.; Moura, L.; Golin, A.; Hochscheidt, R. Thermal variation during osteotomy with different dental implant drills: A standardized study in bovine ribs. *Implant Dent.* **2017**, *26*, 73–79. [CrossRef]
7. Gungormus, M.; Neda, G.; Erbasar, H. Transient Heat Transfer in Dental Implants for Thermal Necrosis-Aided Implant Removal: A 3D Finite Element Analysis. *J. Oral. Implantol.* **2019**, *45*, 196–201. [CrossRef]
8. Palmisano, A.; Tai, B.; Belmont, B.; Irwin, T.; Shih, A.; Holmes, J. Comparison of cortical bone drilling induced heat production among common drilling tools. *J. Orthop. Trauma.* **2015**, *29*, e188–e193. [CrossRef]
9. Liu, Y.; Wu, J.; Zhang, J.; Peng, W.; Liao, W. Numerical and Experimental Analyses on the Temperature Distribution in the Dental Implant Preparation Area when Using a Surgical Guide. *J. Prosthodont.* **2018**, *27*, 42–51. [CrossRef]
10. Augustin, G.; Davila, S.; Udiljak, T.; Vedrina, D.; Bagatin, D. Determination of spatial distribution of increase in bone temperature during drilling by infrared thermography: Preliminary report. *Arch. Orthop. Trauma Surg.* **2009**, *129*, 703–709. [CrossRef]
11. Gehrke, S.; Aramburú, J.; Pérez-Albacete, C.; Ramirez-Fernandez, M.; Sánchez de Val, J.M.; Calvo-Guirado, J. The influence of drill length and irrigation system on heat production during osteotomy preparation for dental implants: An ex vivo study. *Clin. Oral. Implants Res.* **2018**, *29*, 772–778. [CrossRef] [PubMed]
12. Lee, J.; Chavez, C.; Park, J. Parameters affecting mechanical and thermal responses in bone drilling: A review. *J. Biomech.* **2018**, *71*, 4–21. [CrossRef] [PubMed]
13. Golahmadi, A.; Khan, D.; Mylonas, G.; Marcus, H. Tool-tissue forces in surgery: A systematic review. *Ann. Med. Surg.* **2021**, *65*, 102268. [CrossRef] [PubMed]
14. Timon, C.; Keady, C. Thermal Osteonecrosis Caused by Bone Drilling in Orthopedic Surgery: A Literature Review. *Cureus* **2019**, *11*, e5226. [CrossRef]
15. Sindel, A.; Dereci, Ö.; Hatipoğlu, M.; Altay, M.; Özalp, Ö.; Öztürk, A. The effects of irrigation volume to the heat generation during implant surgery. *Med. Oral. Patol. Oral. Cir. Bucal* **2017**, *22*, e506–e511. [CrossRef]
16. Ashry, A.; Elattar, M.; Elsamni, O.; Soliman, I. Effect of Guiding Sleeve Design on Intraosseous Heat Generation During Implant Site Preparation (In Vitro Study). *J. Prosthodont.* **2022**, *31*, 147–154. [CrossRef]
17. Alhroob, K.; Alsabbagh, M.; Alsabbagh, A. Effect of the use of a surgical guide on heat generation during implant placement: A comparative in vitro study. *Dent. Med. Probl.* **2021**, *58*, 55–59. [CrossRef]
18. Delgado-Ruiz, R.; Velasco Ortega, E.; Romanosm, G.; Gerhkem, S.; Newen, I.; Calvo-Guirado, J. Slow drilling speeds for single-drill implant bed preparation. Experimental in vitro study. *Clin. Oral. Investig.* **2018**, *22*, 349–359. [CrossRef]
19. Di Stefano, D.; Arosio, P. Correlation Between Bone Density and Instantaneous Torque at Implant Site Preparation: A Validation on Polyurethane Foam Blocks of a Device Assessing Density of Jawbones. *Int. J. Oral. Maxillofac. Implants* **2016**, *31*, e128–e135. [CrossRef]
20. Palmisano, A.; Tai, B.; Belmont, B.; Irwin, T.; Shih, A.; Holmes, J. Heat accumulation during sequential cortical bone drilling. *J. Orthop. Res.* **2016**, *34*, 463–470. [CrossRef]
21. Cseke, A.; Heinemann, R. The effects of cutting parameters on cutting forces and heat generation when drilling animal bone and biomechanical test materials. *Med. Eng. Phys.* **2018**, *51*, 24–30. [CrossRef] [PubMed]
22. Horak, Z.; Dvorak, K.; Zarybnicka, H.; Vojackova, H.; Dvorakova, J.; Vilimek, M. Experimental Measurements of Mechanical Properties of PUR Foam Used for Testing Medical Devices and Instruments Depending on Temperature, Density and Strain Rate. *Materials* **2020**, *13*, 4560. [CrossRef] [PubMed]
23. Zhang, H.; Fang, W.; Li, Y.; Tao, W. Experimental study of the thermal conductivity of polyurethane foams. *Appl. Thermal. Eng.* **2017**, *115*, 528–538. [CrossRef]
24. Szalma, J.; Lovász, B.; Vajta, L.; Soós, B.; Lempel, E.; Möhlhenrich, S. The influence of the chosen in vitro bone simulation model on intraosseous temperatures and drilling times. *Sci. Rep.* **2019**, *9*, 11817. [CrossRef] [PubMed]
25. Bernabeu-Mira, J.; Soto-Peñaloza, D.; Peñarrocha-Diago, M.; Camacho-Alonso, F.; Rivas-Ballester, R.; Peñarrocha-Oltra, D. Low-speed drilling without irrigation versus conventional drilling for dental implant osteotomy preparation: A systematic review. *Clin. Oral. Investig.* **2021**, *25*, 4251–4267. [CrossRef]
26. Lee, J.; Gozen, B.; Ozdoganlar, O. Modeling and experimentation of bone drilling forces. *J. Biomech.* **2012**, *45*, 1076–1083. [CrossRef]
27. Lughmani, W.; Bouazza-Marouf, K.; Ashcroft, I. Drilling in cortical bone: A finite element model and experimental investigations. *J. Mech. Behav. Biomed. Mater.* **2015**, *42*, 32–42. [CrossRef]
28. Shakouri, E.; Sadeghi, M.; Maerefat, M.; Shajari, S. Experimental and analytical investigation of the thermal necrosis in high-speed drilling of bone. *Proc. Inst. Mech. Eng. H* **2014**, *228*, 330–341. [CrossRef]
29. Trisi, P.; Berardini, M.; Falco, A.; Podaliri Vulpiani, M.; Perfetti, G. Insufficient irrigation induces peri-implant bone resorption: An in vivo histologic analysis in sheep. *Clin. Oral. Implants Res.* **2014**, *25*, 696–701. [CrossRef]

30. Yoshida, K.; Uoshima, K.; Oda, K.; Maeda, T. Influence of heat stress to matrix on bone formation. *Clin. Oral. Implants Res.* **2009**, *20*, 782–790. [CrossRef]
31. Piattelli, A.; Piattelli, M.; Mangano, C.; Scarano, A. A histologic evaluation of eight cases of failed dental implants: Is bone overheating the most probable cause? *Biomaterials* **1998**, *19*, 683–690. [CrossRef]
32. Reingewirtz, Y.; Szmukler-Moncler, S.; Senger, B. Influence of different parameters on bone heating and drilling time in implantology. *Clin. Oral. Implants Res.* **1997**, *8*, 189–197. [CrossRef]
33. Islam, M.; Wang, X. Effect of coring conditions on temperature rise in bone. *Biomed. Mater. Eng.* **2017**, *28*, 201–211. [CrossRef]
34. Gholampour, S.; Deh, H. The effect of spatial distances between holes and time delays between bone drillings based on examination of heat accumulation and risk of bone thermal necrosis. *Biomed. Eng. Online* **2019**, *18*, 65. [CrossRef]
35. Heydari, H.; Kazerooni, N.C.; Zolfaghari, M.; Ghoreishi, M.; Tahmasbi, V. Analytical and experimental study of effective parameters on process temperature during cortical bone drilling. *Proc. Inst. Mech. Eng. H.* **2018**, *232*, 871–883. [CrossRef]
36. Tarnow, D.; Cho, S.; Wallace, S. The effect of inter-implant distance on the height of inter-implant bone crest. *J. Periodontol.* **2000**, *71*, 546–549. [CrossRef] [PubMed]
37. Ramanauskaite, A.; Sader, R. Esthetic complications in implant dentistry. *Periodontol. 2000* **2022**, *88*, 73–85. [CrossRef] [PubMed]
38. Gastaldo, J.; Cury, P.; Sendyk, W. Effect of the vertical and horizontal distances between adjacent implants and between a tooth and an implant on the incidence of interproximal papilla. *J. Periodontol.* **2004**, *75*, 1242–1246. [CrossRef]
39. Traini, T.; Novaes, A.; Piattelli, A.; Papalexiou, V.; Muglia, V. The relationship between interimplant distances and vascularization of the interimplant bone. *Clin. Oral. Implants Res.* **2010**, *21*, 822–829. [CrossRef] [PubMed]

Disclaimer/Publisher's Note: The statements, opinions and data contained in all publications are solely those of the individual author(s) and contributor(s) and not of MDPI and/or the editor(s). MDPI and/or the editor(s) disclaim responsibility for any injury to people or property resulting from any ideas, methods, instructions or products referred to in the content.

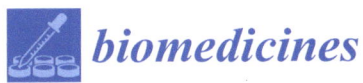 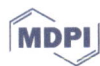

Article

Evaluation of the Efficacy of CPP-ACP Remineralizing Mousse in Molar-Incisor Hypomineralized Teeth Using Polarized Raman and Scanning Electron Microscopy—An *In Vitro* Study

Inês Cardoso-Martins [1,*], Sofia Pessanha [2], Ana Coelho [1], Sofia Arantes-Oliveira [1] and Paula F. Marques [1]

1. Faculdade de Medicina Dentária da Universidade de Lisboa, Rua Professora Teresa Ambrósio, 1600-277 Lisbon, Portugal
2. NOVA School of Science and Technology, Campus Caparica, 2829-516 Caparica, Portugal
* Correspondence: inescardosomartins@yahoo.com; Tel.: +351-919-638-288

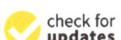

Citation: Cardoso-Martins, I.; Pessanha, S.; Coelho, A.; Arantes-Oliveira, S.; Marques, P.F. Evaluation of the Efficacy of CPP-ACP Remineralizing Mousse in Molar-Incisor Hypomineralized Teeth Using Polarized Raman and Scanning Electron Microscopy—An *In Vitro* Study. *Biomedicines* **2022**, *10*, 3086. https://doi.org/10.3390/biomedicines10123086

Academic Editors: Gianmarco Abbadessa and Giuseppe Minervini

Received: 10 November 2022
Accepted: 27 November 2022
Published: 1 December 2022

Publisher's Note: MDPI stays neutral with regard to jurisdictional claims in published maps and institutional affiliations.

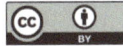

Copyright: © 2022 by the authors. Licensee MDPI, Basel, Switzerland. This article is an open access article distributed under the terms and conditions of the Creative Commons Attribution (CC BY) license (https://creativecommons.org/licenses/by/4.0/).

Abstract: Remineralization of tooth enamel can be achieved by applying a complex of casein phosphopeptides and amorphous calcium phosphate (CPP-ACP). However, the efficacy and optimization of this agent in molar–incisor hypomineralization (MIH) lacks evidence. The purpose of this study is to evaluate the efficacy of CPP-ACP tooth mousse in remineralizing MIH-affected enamel in an optimized 28-day protocol using polarized Raman microscopy and scanning electron microscopy. The protocol was applied to two types of MIH opacities, white and yellow, and compared against sound enamel specimens before and after treatment. Data was analyzed using a one-way ANOVA and LSD post hoc multiple comparisons test ($p < 0.05$) for the Raman analysis. Hypomineralized enamel showed an improvement of its structure after CPP-ACP supplementation. In addition, Raman spectroscopy results showed a decrease in the depolarization ratio of the symmetric stretching band of phosphate ($p < 0.05$ for both groups). In conclusion, there was an improvement in mineral density and organization of the hypomineralized enamel after treatment with CPP-ACP tooth mousse.

Keywords: Raman spectroscopy; electron scanning microscopy; molar–incisor hypomineralization; tooth remineralization; dental enamel; enamel; pediatric dentistry

1. Introduction

Molar–incisor hypomineralization (MIH) is described as the hypomineralization of one to four permanent first molars frequently in combination with affected incisors [1]. This hypomineralization occurs when systemic factors affect the ameloblastic function during the maturation phase of amelogenesis [2]. The global and European prevalence of MIH ranges from 13.1% to 14.2% [3] and 3.6 to 25% [1,4], respectively. Enamel from the MIH-affected surface is characterized by a lower mineral concentration, lower organization of the crystalline structure, and higher porosity, making those teeth more vulnerable to abrasion and carious lesions [5]. The presence of chronic pulpal inflammation in MIH teeth may be due to their increased enamel porosity and possible bacterial penetration through the large dentinal tubules, making them extremely sensitive, arduous to hygiene, and difficult to anesthetize [1,6]. In more severe cases, the porous enamel may even fracture after eruption or under masticatory forces, creating post-eruptive enamel breakdowns (PEB) [1].

Clinically, MIH teeth present clearly demarcated opacities that vary in size, shape, and color, from white to yellow/brownish [1,2]. Several studies showed that these defects have increased carbon and carbonate concentrations and higher protein content when compared to normal enamel [2,5,7–9]. To enhance the mechanical properties of MIH teeth, remineralization is a good treatment option that can increase the mineral content of enamel and prevent its post-eruptive enamel breakdowns [10]. The literature shows that fluoride varnish can be effective in remineralizing MIH teeth [2]. Furthermore, in a recent study, a novel remineralizing agent, a biomimetic hydroxyapatite, was successfully used in the improvement of the MIH condition [11]. The remineralization of tooth enamel can also be achieved by applying a complex of casein phosphopeptides and amorphous calcium phosphate (CPP-ACP), that acts as a reservoir of calcium and phosphate, stabilizing high concentrations of these ions [12–14]. There is evidence that the application of CPP-ACP cream decreases the loss of minerals, and the depth and width of lesions [14]. Several studies demonstrated that the consistent use of CPP-ACP promotes an increase in mineral density and inhibits demineralization [15,16]. In 2011, Baroni and Marchionni observed an improvement in mineralization, morphology, and porosities of MIH-affected enamel following a continued use of a cream containing 10% CPP-ACP [17]. However, there is still a limited number of studies in the literature regarding the remineralizing efficacy of this agent in MIH-affected teeth [7,13].

Raman spectroscopy has been used to evaluate the symmetric stretching mode of the tetrahedral phosphate group (PO43-, with a Raman shift of ~959 cm^{-1}) and infer upon the mineral phase of enamel [18]. Fraser et al. evaluated changes in the intensity and peak shape of this Raman band, together with the ratios to the amide I and carbonate, to study teeth affected with MIH [5]. Raman spectroscopy was also used in combination with SEM to evaluate MIH-affected permanent molars through the phosphate-to-carbonate ratio [19]. Recent advances in Raman microscopy also showed the suitability, sensitivity, and specificity of polarized Raman spectroscopy for the evaluation of demineralized enamel [20]. Studies have also showed an increase in the depolarization ratio of this band in demineralized enamel, prompting the use of this methodology for carious lesion diagnosis [21,22]. Franco et al. used Raman microscopy to evaluate the effectiveness of CPP-ACP tooth mousse on the remineralization of MIH opacities after a single application [23].

According to the recent literature, there is no study that has used polarized Raman microscopy combined with SEM to evaluate the efficacy of remineralization protocols in different MIH opacities.

The aim of the present study is to understand, through polarized Raman spectroscopy analysis and SEM observation, if a 28-day protocol of application of CPP-ACP is effective in remineralizing hypomineralized enamel in two types of MIH lesions (white and yellow). The tested hypothesis was that the application of CPP-ACP did not increase the organization of the enamel apatite crystals of MIH molars in vitro.

2. Materials and Methods

The sample size consisted of 20 severely hypomineralized maxillary and mandibular molar teeth extracted due the presence of severe painful symptoms conditioning the patient's quality of life. The selection of severe hypomineralized teeth was based on the EAPD diagnostic criteria of MIH [2]. An orthodontic consultation was performed, and the extractions were adapted to the patient's orthodontic treatment plan. Upon extraction and verbal consent of the guardian of the patient, each tooth was stored and preserved in accordance with ISO conditions (ISO/TS 11405) in a refrigerated 1% chloramine solution for 1 week, and then in Hank's solution (BioWhittaker™, Lonza, MD, USA). A control group was created using 12 sound molar teeth extracted mainly for orthodontic reasons. The control teeth were sound teeth that presented no enamel defects, cracks, caries, or fractures.

2.1. Sample Description and Preparation

All teeth went through a prophylactic protocol using a polishing brush with pumice paste in a low rotation handpiece (0.04 mg of pumice; 0.8 mL of water) for 60 s, before being washed with distilled water for 60 s and submitted to an ultrasound bath in ethanol 100% for 60 s using the Bransonic® M2800-E, Emerson, Danbury, CT, USA, electronic cleaning device. Each tooth was encased in an acrylic block using a hot glue pistol and sectioned parallel to the occlusal surface to split the root from the crown using a water-cooled diamond-impregnated circular saw (Isomet, Buehler Ltd., Lake Bluff, IL, USA).

The SEM analysis requires metallization that makes a before–after approach unfeasible; however, Raman analyses are non-invasive and do not require specific sample preparation, so a before–after approach was undertaken. Twenty hypomineralized teeth were then sectioned perpendicular to the occlusal surface to obtain the following: one enamel opacity in sixteen teeth and two enamel opacities in four teeth. The 12 sound teeth were also sectioned perpendicular to the occlusal surface.

2.1.1. Raman Spectroscopy

The 12 opacities from the MIH teeth and the 6 surfaces of the sound teeth were allocated to one of the three groups: Group A—6 white hypomineralized opacities; Group B—6 yellow hypomineralized opacities; Group C—6 sound teeth. Once prepared and whilst awaiting testing, the samples were stored fully hydrated in Hank's solution BioWhittaker ™ (Lonza, MD, USA).

2.1.2. Scanning Electron Microscopy (SEM)

The 12 opacities from the MIH teeth and the 6 surfaces of the sound teeth were allocated to one of the following 6 groups: Group D—3 white hypomineralized opacities; Group E—3 yellow hypomineralized opacities; Group F—3 sound teeth; Group G—3 white hypomineralized opacities for CPP-ACP treatment protocol; Group H—3 yellow hypomineralized opacities for CPP-ACP treatment protocol; Group I—3 sound teeth for CPP-ACP treatment protocol. Once prepared and whilst awaiting testing, the samples were stored fully hydrated in Hank's solution (BioWhittaker™, Lonza, MD, USA). Figure 1 represents a flowchart of the study design.

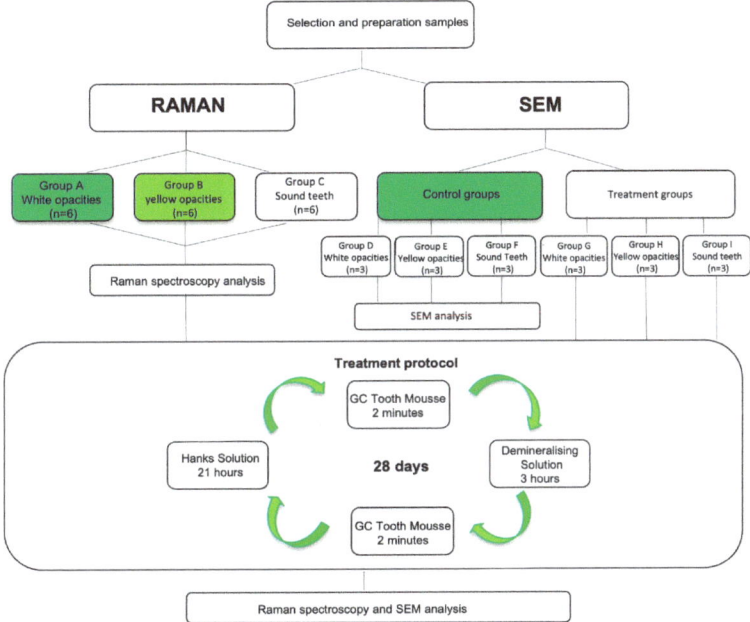

Figure 1. Scheme of the study design.

2.2. Analysis and Treatment Protocol

2.2.1. Raman Spectroscopy Analysis

Each sample from groups A, B and C was removed from the Hanks' solution (BioWhittaker™, Lonza, MD, USA), washed with distilled water for 5 s, dried with absorbent paper, placed on a holder, and analyzed with Raman microscopy to determine the depolarization ratio before and after the CPP-ACP treatment protocol.

Polarized Raman spectra of samples were obtained using an XploRA Confocal Microscope (Horiba, Palaiseau, France) with a 785 nm laser. Using an entrance slit of 200 µm, and a confocal hole of 300 µm, the scattered light collected by the objective was dispersed onto the air-cooled CCD array of an Andor iDus detector (Oxford instruments, Bristol, UK) with a 1200 lines/mm grating. This way, the spectral range investigated was from 200 cm^{-1} to 1300 cm^{-1} with a spectral resolution of 4 cm^{-1}. A 100× objective (N.A. = 0.9) was used to focus on the surface of enamel, as well as a 50% neutral density filter rendering an incident power on the sample of 4.8 ± 0.4 mW (Lasercheck®, Edmund Optics, Mainz, Germany). Each spectrum was obtained by 3 accumulations of 20 s each and an average of 10 spot analyses were performed for each sample. In order to determine the depolarization ratio (ρ959) of the symmetric stretching band of phosphate ions (ν1~959 cm^{-1}), in each spot, spectra were recorded with cross and parallel polarization to the polarization of the incident laser. The depolarization ratio was then determined as follows:

$$\rho_{959} = \frac{I_{959} \perp}{I_{959} \parallel}$$

where I_{959} II is the intensity of the Raman band at ~959 cm^{-1} using parallel polarization, and $I_{959}\perp$ is the intensity of the Raman band at ~959 cm^{-1} using perpendicular polarization.

2.2.2. SEM Analysis

Regarding the treatment groups (G, H, and I), the samples were removed from the Hank's solution and the treatment protocol with CPP-ACP was performed daily for a period of 28 consecutive days. The samples of the control groups (D, E, and F) were kept in a balanced Hanks solution for 28 days. On day 29, all specimens from all groups were prepared according to the following protocol for debris removal and enamel prism revealing (Figure 2):

(1) Conditioning with 2 mL of 5.25% sodium hypochlorite for 60 s;
(2) Washing with distilled water for 10 s;
(3) Ultrasound cleaning with 100% ethanol for 60 s;
(4) Washing with distilled water for 5 s;
(5) Drying with air syringe for 10 s;
(6) Conditioning with 2 mL of 10% phosphoric acid for 20 s;
(7) Washing with distilled water for 10 s;
(8) Ultrasound cleaning with 100% ethanol for 60 s;
(9) Washing with distilled water for 5 s;
(10) Drying with air syringe for 10 s.

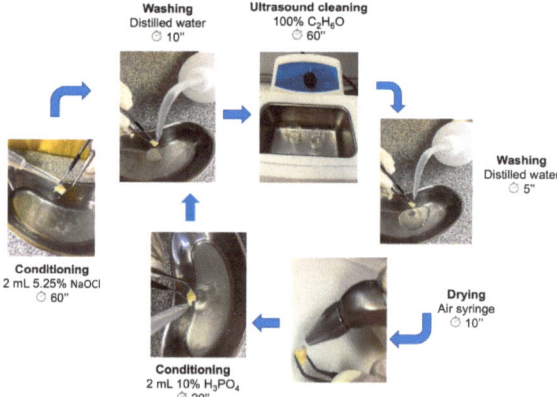

Figure 2. Protocol for debris removal and enamel prism revealing.

After debris removal protocol application, specimens were attached to metallic supports with double sided carbon tape (NemTape, Nisshin, Japan) and sputter-coated with 200 nm gold/palladium in an argon atmosphere (Jeol, Tokyo, Japan). Specimens' surfaces were examined using a Hitachi, SU3800 (Tokyo, Japan) scanning electron microscope. Microphotographs of representative areas at 1000×, 2000×, 5000×, and 10,000× magnifications were obtained for each specimen using Esprit software (v1.8.2.2167, Bruker, MA, EUA).

2.2.3. CPP-ACP Treatment Protocol

The treatment procedure was adapted from the protocol used by Cardoso-Martins et al. and Shetty et al. for in vitro studies with CPP-ACP [24,25]. The binding of ACP to CPP is pH-dependent and decreases as the pH decreases [26]. Enamel remineralization by CPP-ACP can occur over a range of pH values from 4.5 to 7 [27]. In this protocol, the decrease in the pH by a demineralizing agent enables this remineralization process. Through the local release of calcium and phosphate ions, this nanoaggregate allows the maintenance of a supersaturated mineral state that suppresses demineralization and promotes mineralization. The treatment procedure was carried out daily for a period of 28 days [24,25]. Each of the enamel samples were treated with the remineralizing agent—10% CPP-ACP (GC Tooth mousse™, GC, Leuven, Belgium)—for a period of 2 min, following which the samples were individually immersed in 2 mL of a demineralizing solution (2.0 mMol/L calcium, 2.0 mMol/L phosphate, 75 mMol/L acetic acid, pH 4.4) for a period of 3 h. Afterwards, samples were re-treated with the remineralizing agent for 2 min. To finalize, the enamel samples were individually immersed in 2 mL of Hank's balanced salt solution (BioWhittaker™, Lonza, MD, USA) for a period of 21 h.

The demineralizing agent was replaced every 5 days, and the Hank's solution every 48 h.

2.3. Statistical Analysis

The sample size was calculated according to $n = 1 + 2C (S/D)^2$ [28], which resulted in $n = 6$. The sample size calculation was based on results of a pilot study and used the following assumptions: the mean of differences (D = 0.0117), standard deviation (S = 0.0057), and considering the degree of significance, a = 0.05 and 90% power.

Statistical analysis was performed with SPSS v26.0, (IBM, New York, NY, USA). A Shapiro–Wilk test for normal distribution evaluation was performed. Levene's test showed that the values obtained have equal variances. Since data distribution was normal, a one-way ANOVA and an LSD post hoc multiple comparisons test were performed. A significance level of 0.05 was considered.

3. Results

The Raman band of interest corresponding to the symmetric stretching of phosphate (v1 PO_4^{3-} ~959 cm^{-1}) was identified. The spectra recorded for a sample presenting a hypomineralized white opacity before (Figure 3) and after (Figure 4) treatment with GC Tooth Mousse containing CPP-ACP is shown, before baseline correction.

There was an increase in the main band in the parallel mode concomitant with a decrease in the same band in the perpendicular mode, after treatment. The results for the mean depolarization ratio of the symmetric stretching band of phosphate for the three studied groups (A, B, C) are presented in Table 1.

Table 1. Mean depolarization ratio and standard deviations (SD) of the symmetric stretching band of phosphate values for the three groups.

Study Group	Depolarization Ratio Pre-Treatment (Mean ± SD)	Depolarization Ratio Post-Treatment (Mean ± SD)	Significance Level (p)
A—White opacity teeth	0.029 ± 0.004	0.021 ± 0.003	0.004
B—Yellow opacity teeth	0.044 ± 0.004	0.037 ± 0.008	0.015
C—Sound teeth	0.019 ± 0.002	0.017 ± 0.003	0.5

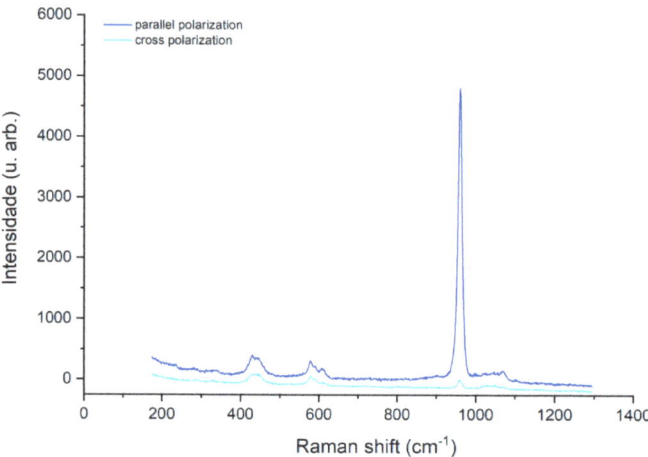

Figure 3. Spectra of a hypomineralized white opacity before treatment with GC Tooth Mousse.

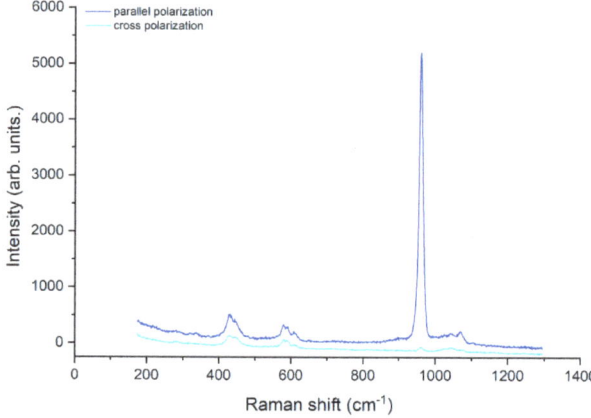

Figure 4. Spectra of a hypomineralized white opacity after treatment with GC Tooth Mousse.

For group A, the hypomineralized teeth with white opacities, the mean values obtained for the depolarization ratio before and after treatment were 0.029 ± 0.004 and 0.021 ± 0.003, respectively. There was a statistically significant decrease ($p < 0.05$) in the mean values of the depolarization ratio, which suggests an improvement in the enamel mineralization after treatment.

Furthermore, in group B, comprising the teeth presenting yellow hypomineralized opacities, there was a statistically significant decrease ($p < 0.05$) in the mean values of the depolarization ratio after treatment, with values ranging from 0.044 ± 0.004 before to 0.037 ± 0.008 after treatment. Therefore, there was also an improvement in the enamel mineralization with treatment in this group.

The mean values for the depolarization ratio for the sound teeth (C group) before treatment was 0.019 ± 0.002, and after treatment it was 0.017 ± 0.003. There was no statistically significant difference ($p > 0.05$) in the enamel mineralization of the sound teeth group before and after treatment. The sound teeth enamel surface presents apatite crystals methodically organized perpendicular to the surface, revealing a high anisotropy of the symmetric stretching band of phosphate. Candido et al. and Ko et al., using Raman spectroscopy, showed that the arrangement of apatite crystals is altered in demineralized enamel, since they present a more disordered structure. Accordingly, in demineralized enamel, the depolarization ratio value is higher [18,20].

The SEM images of the white and yellow opacities (D and E groups) revealed deficient or hollow rod cores. The crystals building up the enamel rods were disorganized, rock-shaped, without a uniform orientation, and difficult to distinguish. In the white opacities group, the borders of the enamel rods were dissolved with prominent inter-rod spaces, and a structureless layer was partially covering the enamel prisms (Figure 5a). In the yellow opacities group, the borders of the enamel rods were indistinct, with fewer visible inter-rod areas (Figure 6a). White and yellow opacities submitted to CPP-ACP treatment (G and H groups) showed filled rod cores with tighter packed and more well-organized crystals when compared with hypomineralized teeth not submitted to the remineralization CPP-ACP protocol, where wider inter-rod spaces were present (Figures 5b and 6b)

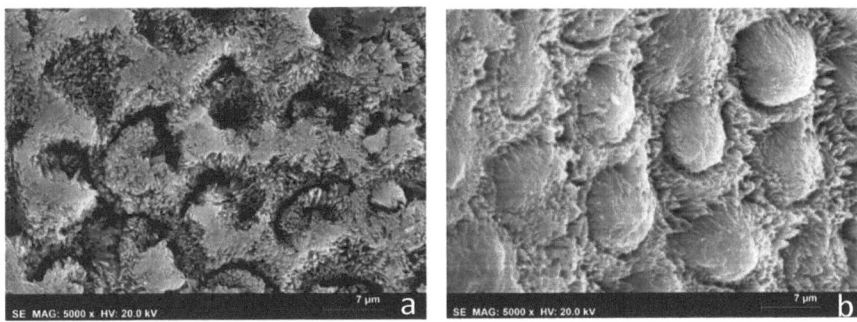

Figure 5. MIH specimens' SEM photograph (5000×). (**a**) Group D—white hypomineralized opacities; (**b**) Group G—white hypomineralized opacities after CPP-ACP protocol.

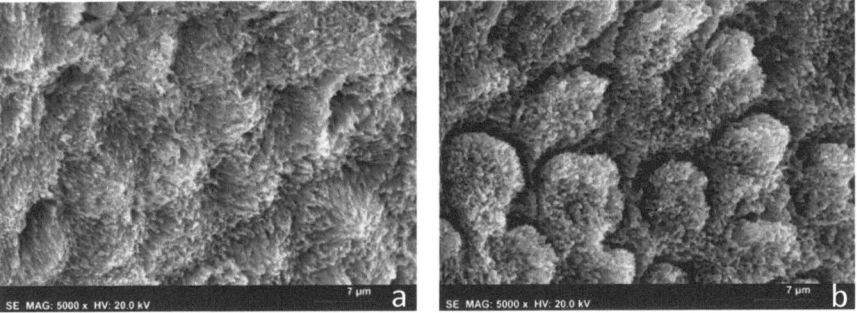

Figure 6. MIHs specimens' SEM photographs (5000×). (**a**) Group E—yellow hypomineralized opacities; (**b**) Group H—yellow hypomineralized opacities after CPP-ACP protocol.

A normal prismatic surface without structural alterations was present for both sound teeth groups. There were well-defined enamel rods with distinct borders and narrow inter-rod areas. The crystals in the enamel rods were densely packed, well organized, and presented a uniform orientation (F and I groups) (Figure 7).

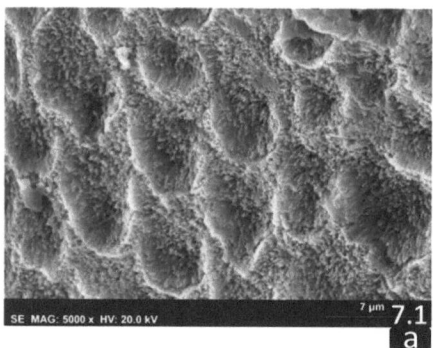 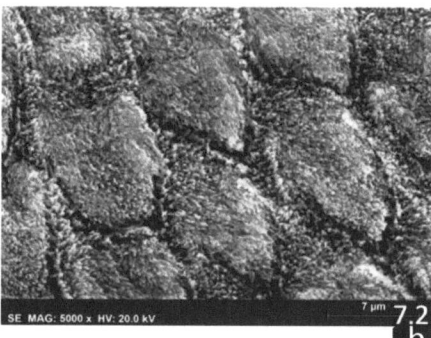

Figure 7. Sound specimens' SEM photographs (5000×). (**a**) Group F—sound tooth; (**b**) Group I—sound tooth after CPP-ACP protocol.

4. Discussion

The Raman spectroscopy analysis of this study demonstrated that the treatment protocol used for CPP-ACP application had a positive and a statistically significant effect in reducing the depolarization ratio on enamel surfaces with either white or yellow hypomineralized opacities.

The SEM study showed that hypomineralized enamel of white and yellow opacities after CPP-ACP treatment protocol had an improvement on the enamel structure, that exhibited filled rod cores with tighter packed and more well-organized crystals when compared with hypomineralized teeth not submitted to remineralization protocol. The SEM images of the sound teeth enamel opacities non-submitted and submitted to CPP-ACP treatment (F and I groups) showed a normal prismatic surface.

Results from this study demonstrated that MIH opacities' enamel structure in the white and yellow opacities (D and E groups) is characterized by having hydroxyapatite crystals more loosely and irregularly packed than in sound teeth (Figures 5a and 6a). This is consistent with Raman results with a higher value of depolarization ratio for groups A and B when compared with Group C. The literature also shows that hypomineralized areas have a disordered, structureless configuration of hydroxyapatite crystals compared with sound enamel [29]. Lygidakis et al., showed that the unorganized microstructure of MIH teeth led to a reduction in mechanical properties, such as hardness and modules of elasticity [2].

White and yellow opacities (G and H groups) showed an improvement in the enamel structure after CPP-ACP treatment. Rods evolved a more mature and geometric structure, showing filled cores with tighter packed and more well-organized crystals (Figures 5b and 6b). This is corroborated by Raman spectroscopy results comparing the before and after in groups A and B, which showed a decrease in depolarization ratio values and, therefore, an increase in the organization of the enamel apatite crystals after CPP-ACP treatment. Cevc et al. observed that there was a larger proportion of well-oriented microcrystals in caries-resistant teeth, indicating that the degree of hydroxyapatite microcrystal alignment is a property that may help determine their mechanical resistance [30]. The results obtained in this study are suggestive of an increased mineralization of MIH teeth after CPP-ACP treatment that could reflect an increased mechanical resistance. Baroni et al. also observed a marked improvement in enamel morphology after the application of CPP-ACP on MIH molars [17]. Franco et al. also showed an improvement in the degree of crystallite orientation in both white and yellow enamel opacities after treatment with CPP-ACP tooth mousse [23].

According to the Raman data obtained, there was a greater improvement in the organization of the enamel apatite crystals of MIH teeth after CPP-ACP treatment in the white opacities group compared to the yellow group. This difference might be explained due to the higher porosity and larger prismatic cracks of the yellow lesions when compared to the white ones [5].

The protocol with the CPP-ACP treatment was adapted from the protocol used by Cardoso-Martins et al. in an in vitro study with the same remineralizing agent assessed over 28 days in MIH teeth [24]. As a result, it was possible to decrease the samples depolarization ratio, which represents an improvement in the degree of crystallite orientation. The white opacities' depolarization ratio mean values reached the corresponding level of the healthy teeth mean values before treatment.

A potential limitation of this study rests on the fact that it was based on an in vitro environment. Moreover, a single remineralizing agent was used and, therefore, a control group with another agent was lacking. Furthermore, a SEM–EDS (energy-dispersive X-ray spectroscopy) could have been used, but in this study Raman spectroscopy was preferred instead. There is extensive evidence that Raman spectroscopy is a very sensitive tool for the evaluation of the demineralization of enamel and that it can be used to study slight changes in the enamel structure, so we used this methodology for the evaluation of the opposite process [23]. Furthermore, due to the metallization process, a direct comparison of the Ca and P content and the depolarization ratio of phosphate would not be possible, as the sample groups were different. The small sample size must also be considered, which was due to the challenges in obtaining the specimens, since they relate to the extraction of hypomineralized permanent molars in children.

The results of the present study support the rejection of the tested hypothesis, warranting in vivo studies in MIH teeth with this remineralizing agent where administration protocols can be adjusted. In future studies, this protocol should evolve, either by increasing the number of applications or extending the duration, in order to improve the yellow opacities' depolarization ratio, mean values and to achieve values close to the healthy teeth.

This study highlights the importance of more research using this type of remineralization protocols to improve MIH teeth properties, as well as the need for further clinical trials to support the recommendation for the use of CPP-ACP to increase the mineral content of hypomineralized teeth. In the future, it would be of interest to study new remineralizing agents, such as a biomimetic nano-hydroxyapatite based on the integration of calcium and phosphate, at the level of demineralized dental surfaces of MIH teeth [11]. Hence, managing this condition appropriately could prevent its associated negative impacts on the patient's quality of life [2,7].

5. Conclusions

In this in vitro study, as determined through Raman spectroscopy analysis and SEM evaluation, there were significant improvements in the organization of MIH enamel apatite crystals after CPP-ACP treatment. In conclusion, there was a significant remineralization of enamel after a consecutive daily application of CPP-ACP tooth mousse over 28 days.

Author Contributions: Conceptualization, I.C.-M., S.P., S.A.-O. and P.F.M.; methodology, I.C.-M., S.P., S.A.-O. and P.F.M.; validation, I.C.-M., S.P., S.A.-O. and P.F.M.; formal analysis, I.C.-M.; investigation, I.C.-M.; resources, I.C.-M., S.P., S.A.-O. and P.F.M.; writing—original draft preparation, I.C.-M., S.A.-O., S.P., A.C. and P.F.M.; visualization, I.C.-M., S.A.-O., S.P., A.C. and P.F.M.; supervision, S.A.-O. and P.F.M. All authors have read and agreed to the published version of the manuscript.

Funding: This research was funded by Fundação para a Ciência e Tecnologia (FCT) (Portugal) by the research center grant UID/FIS/04559/2021 to LIBPhys from the FCT/MCTES/PIDDAC, Portugal.

Institutional Review Board Statement: The study was conducted in accordance with the Declaration of Helsinki and approved by the Institutional Review Board (or Ethics Committee) of Faculdade de Medicina Dentária da Universidade de Lisboa (protocol code CE-FMDUL201701 and date of approval: January 2017).

Informed Consent Statement: Informed consent was obtained from all subjects involved in the study.

Data Availability Statement: Not applicable.

Acknowledgments: Inês Cardoso-Martins acknowledges Cuf, SA for the PhD scholarship.

Conflicts of Interest: The authors declare no conflict of interest.

References

1. Weerheijm, K.L. Molar incisor hypomineralisation (MIH). *Eur. J. Paediatr. Dent.* **2003**, *4*, 114–120. [PubMed]
2. Lygidakis, N.A.; Garot, E.; Somani, C.; Taylor, G.D.; Rouas, P.; Wong, F.S.L. Best clinical practice guidance for clinicians dealing with children presenting with molar-incisor-hypomineralisation (MIH): An updated European Academy of Paediatric Dentistry policy document. *Eur. Arch. Paediatr. Dent.* **2022**, *23*, 3–21. [CrossRef] [PubMed]
3. Zhao, D.; Dong, B.; Yu, D.; Ren, Q.; Sun, Y. The prevalence of molar incisor hypomineralization: Evidence from 70 studies. *Int. J. Paediatr. Dent.* **2018**, *28*, 170–179. [CrossRef]
4. Abdelaziz, M.; Krejci, I.; Banon, J. Prevalence of Molar Incisor Hypomineralization in over 30,000 Schoolchildren in Switzerland. *J. Clin. Pediatr. Dent.* **2022**, *46*, 1–5. [CrossRef]
5. Fraser, S.J.; Natarajan, A.K.; Clark, A.S.S.; Drummond, B.K.; Gordon, K.C. A Raman spectroscopic study of teeth affected with molar–incisor hypomineralisation. *J. Raman Spectrosc.* **2015**, *46*, 202–210. [CrossRef]
6. Özgül, B.M.; Sakaryalı, D.; Tirali, R.E.; Çehreli, S.B. Does MIH Affects Preoperative and Intraoperative Hypersensitivity? *J. Clin. Pediatr. Dent.* **2022**, *46*, 204–210. [CrossRef]
7. Somani, C.; Taylor, G.D.; Garot, E.; Rouas, P.; Lygidakis, N.A.; Wong, F.S.L. An update of treatment modalities in children and adolescents with teeth affected by molar incisor hypomineralisation (MIH): A systematic review. *Eur. Arch. Paediatr. Dent.* **2022**, *23*, 39–64. [CrossRef]
8. Farah, R.A.; Swain, M.V.; Drummond, B.K.; Cook, R.; Atieh, M. Mineral density of hypomineralised enamel. *J. Dent.* **2010**, *38*, 50–58. [CrossRef]
9. Crombie, F.A.; Cochrane, N.J.; Manton, D.J.; Palamara, J.E.; Reynolds, E.C. Mineralisation of developmentally hypomineralised human enamel in vitro. *Caries Res.* **2013**, *47*, 259–263. [CrossRef]
10. Kumar, A.; Goyal, A.; Gauba, K.; Kapur, A.; Singh, S.K.; Mehta, S.K. An evaluation of remineralised MIH using CPP-ACP and fluoride varnish: An in-situ and in-vitro study. *Eur. Arch. Paediatr. Dent.* **2022**, *23*, 79–87. [CrossRef]
11. Butera, A.; Pascadopoli, M.; Pellegrini, M.; Trapani, B.; Gallo, S.; Radu, M.; Scribante, A. Biomimetic hydroxyapatite paste for molar–incisor hypomineralization: A randomized clinical trial. *Oral Dis.* **2022**. [CrossRef]
12. Reynolds, E.C. Calcium phosphate-based remineralization systems: Scientific evidence? *Aust. Dent. J.* **2008**, *53*, 268–273. [CrossRef] [PubMed]
13. Bakkal, M.; Abbasoglu, Z.; Kargul, B. The Effect of Casein Phosphopeptide-Amorphous Calcium Phosphate on Molar-Incisor Hypomineralisation: A Pilot Study. *Oral Health Prev. Dent.* **2017**, *15*, 163–167. [PubMed]
14. Garry, A.P.; Flannigan, N.L.; Cooper, L.; Komarov, G.; Burnside, G.; Higham, S.M. A randomised controlled trial to investigate the remineralising potential of Tooth MousseTM in orthodontic patients. *J. Orthod.* **2017**, *44*, 147–156. [CrossRef] [PubMed]
15. Miyahira, K.; Coutinho, T.C.L.; da Silva, E.M.; Pereira, A.M.B.; Tostes, M.A. Evaluation of CPP-ACP and fluoride on inhibition of human enamel demineralisation: Cross-sectional hardness and MicroCT studies. *Oral Health Prev. Dent.* **2018**, *15*, 549–555.
16. Thierens, L.A.M.; Moerman, S.; Van Elst, C.; Vercruysse, C.; Maes, P.; Temmerman, L.; De Roo, N.M.C.; Verbeeck, R.M.H.; De Pauw, G.A.M. The in vitro remineralising effect of CPP-ACP and CPP-ACPF after 6 and 12 weeks on initial caries lesion. *J. Appl. Oral Sci.* **2019**, *27*, e20180589. [CrossRef]
17. Baroni, C.; Marchionni, S. MIH supplementation strategies: Prospective clinical and laboratory trial. *J. Dent. Res.* **2011**, *90*, 371–376. [CrossRef]
18. Cândido, M.; Silveira, J.M.; Mata, A.; Carvalho, M.L.; Pessanha, S. In vitro study of the demineralization induced in human enamel by an acidic beverage using X-ray fluorescence spectroscopy and Raman microscopy. *X-ray Spectrom.* **2019**, *48*, 61–69. [CrossRef]
19. Taube, F.; Marczewski, M.; Norén, J.G. Deviations of inorganic and organic carbon content in hypomineralised enamel. *J. Dent.* **2015**, *43*, 269–278. [CrossRef]
20. Ko, A.C.-T.; Choo-Smith, L.-P.; Hewko, M.; Sowa, M.G.; Dong, C.C.S.; Cleghorn, B. Detection of early dental caries using polarized Raman spectroscopy. *Opt. Express* **2006**, *14*, 203–215. [CrossRef]
21. Buchwald, T.; Okulus, Z.; Szybowicz, M. Raman spectroscopy as a tool of early dental caries detection–new insights. *J. Raman Spectrosc.* **2017**, *48*, 1094–1102. [CrossRef]
22. Monteiro, M.; Chasqueira, F.; Pessanha, S. Raman spectroscopy in the characterisation of carious dental tissues. *Spectrosc. Eur.* **2018**, *30*, 11–14.
23. Franco, S.; Cardoso-Martins, I.; Arantes-Oliveira, S.; Pessanha, S.; Marques, P.F. In vitro polarized Raman analysis for the evaluation of the efficacy of CPP-ACP remineralizing mousse in tooth hypomineralization. *Results Chem.* **2021**, *3*, 100232. [CrossRef]
24. Cardoso-Martins, I.; Arantes-Oliveira, S.; Coelho, A.; Pessanha, S.; Marques, P.F. Evaluation of the Efficacy of CPP-ACP Remineralizing Mousse in MIH White and Yellow Opacities—In Vitro Vickers Microhardness Analysis. *Dent. J.* **2022**, *10*, 186. [CrossRef]

25. Shetty, S.; Hegde, M.N.; Bopanna, T.P. Enamel remineralization assessment after treatment with three different remineralizing agents using surface microhardness: An in vitro study. *J. Conserv. Dent.* **2014**, *17*, 49–52. [CrossRef]
26. Reynolds, E.C. Anticariogenic complexes of amorphous calcium phosphate stabilized by casein phosphopeptides: A review. *Spec. Care Dent.* **1998**, *18*, 8–16. [CrossRef]
27. Nidhi, G.; Kunwarjeet, S. Try it to Believe it: Amazing Remineralization Technologies. *J. Pharm. Biomed. Sci.* **2012**, *24*, 79–82.
28. Dell, R.B.; Holleran, S.; Ramakrishnan, R. Sample size determination. *ILAR J.* **2002**, *43*, 207–213. [CrossRef]
29. Fagrell, T.G.; Dietz, W.; Jälevik, B.; Norén, J.G. Chemical, mechanical and morphological properties of hypomineralized enamel of permanent first molars. *Acta. Odontol. Scand.* **2010**, *68*, 215–222. [CrossRef]
30. Cevc, G.; Cevc, P.; Schara, M.; Skaleric, U. The caries resistance of human teeth is determined by the spatial arrangement of hydroxyapatite microcrystals in the enamel. *Nature* **1980**, *286*, 425–426. [CrossRef]

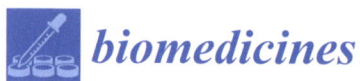 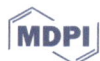

Article

Application of Two-Dimensional Entropy Measures to Detect the Radiographic Signs of Tooth Resorption and Hypercementosis in an Equine Model

Kamil Górski [1,*], Marta Borowska [2], Elżbieta Stefanik [1], Izabela Polkowska [3], Bernard Turek [1], Andrzej Bereznowski [4] and Małgorzata Domino [1,*]

1. Department of Large Animal Diseases and Clinic, Institute of Veterinary Medicine, Warsaw University of Life Sciences, 02-787 Warsaw, Poland
2. Institute of Biomedical Engineering, Faculty of Mechanical Engineering, Białystok University of Technology, 15-351 Białystok, Poland
3. Department and Clinic of Animal Surgery, Faculty of Veterinary Medicine, University of Life Sciences, 20-950 Lublin, Poland
4. Division of Veterinary Epidemiology and Economics, Institute of Veterinary Medicine, Warsaw University of Life Sciences, Nowoursynowska 159c, 02-776 Warsaw, Poland
* Correspondence: kamil_gorski@sggw.edu.pl (K.G.); malgorzata_domino@sggw.edu.pl (M.D.)

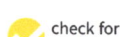

Citation: Górski, K.; Borowska, M.; Stefanik, E.; Polkowska, I.; Turek, B.; Bereznowski, A.; Domino, M. Application of Two-Dimensional Entropy Measures to Detect the Radiographic Signs of Tooth Resorption and Hypercementosis in an Equine Model. *Biomedicines* 2022, 10, 2914. https://doi.org/10.3390/biomedicines10112914

Academic Editors: Gianluca Gambarini; Giuseppe Minervini and Gianmarco Abbadessa

Received: 1 October 2022
Accepted: 11 November 2022
Published: 13 November 2022
Corrected: 29 June 2023

Publisher's Note: MDPI stays neutral with regard to jurisdictional claims in published maps and institutional affiliations.

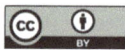

Copyright: © 2022 by the authors. Licensee MDPI, Basel, Switzerland. This article is an open access article distributed under the terms and conditions of the Creative Commons Attribution (CC BY) license (https://creativecommons.org/licenses/by/4.0/).

Abstract: Dental disorders are a serious health problem in equine medicine, their early recognition benefits the long-term general health of the horse. Most of the initial signs of Equine Odontoclastic Tooth Resorption and Hypercementosis (EOTRH) syndrome concern the alveolar aspect of the teeth, thus, the need for early recognition radiographic imaging. This study is aimed to evaluate the applicability of entropy measures to quantify the radiological signs of tooth resorption and hypercementosis as well as to enhance radiographic image quality in order to facilitate the identification of the signs of EOTRH syndrome. A detailed examination of the oral cavity was performed in eighty horses. Each evaluated incisor tooth was assigned to one of four grade–related EOTRH groups (0–3). Radiographs of the incisor teeth were taken and digitally processed. For each radiograph, two–dimensional sample (SampEn2D), fuzzy (FuzzEn2D), permutation (PermEn2D), dispersion (DispEn2D), and distribution (DistEn2D) entropies were measured after image filtering was performed using Normalize, Median, and LaplacianSharpening filters. Moreover, the similarities between entropy measures and selected Gray–Level Co–occurrence Matrix (GLCM) texture features were investigated. Among the 15 returned measures, DistEn2D was EOTRH grade–related. Moreover, DistEn2D extracted after Normalize filtering was the most informative. The EOTRH grade–related similarity between DistEn2D and Difference Entropy (GLCM) confirms the higher irregularity and complexity of incisor teeth radiographs in advanced EOTRH syndrome, demonstrating the greatest sensitivity (0.50) and specificity (0.95) of EOTRH 3 group detection. An application of DistEn2D to Normalize filtered incisor teeth radiographs enables the identification of the radiological signs of advanced EOTRH with higher accuracy than the previously used entropy–related GLCM texture features.

Keywords: radiographs; texture analysis; entropy–based approaches; equine odontoclastic tooth resorption and hypercementosis; dental care

1. Introduction

Dental disorders, including complications related to cases of oral cavity disease, constitute a serious health problem in equine medicine [1]. As equine hypsodont teeth slowly erupt over most of the horse's life [2], simple dental rasping is able to improve the welfare and possibly food digestion as well as biting behaviour of more than 70% of horses presenting dental disorders [3]. Thus, dental disorders are of major importance in equine veterinary practice, with up to 10% of practice time involving dental–related work [1].

The current standard of care in equine dentistry includes performing a complete visual oral examination, including general and dental history taking, observation and general physical examination, as well as comprehensive oral and dental examination [4]. However, radiography and possibly other imaging of dental apices and reserve crowns is essential in the evaluation of primary incisor and canine teeth disease affected by resorption and hypercementosis of the reserve crown [5,6], secondary periodontal disease with remodelling and lysis of the alveolar bone [1,7,8], traumatic disorders of teeth [1,9,10], as well as apical infections such as cheek teeth apical abscessation [1,9]. The welfare of the horse depends on skilled and knowledgeable veterinarians who can characterize normal and abnormal findings relative to the oral cavity [4], including frequently occurring dental disorders [1]. Therefore, the digital processing of dental radiographs is proposed here to enhance the quality of the image so that the veterinarians can more easily identify the radiographic signs of disease. As radiography is useful in the diagnosis of tooth resorption and hypercementosis [5,6], bone remodelling and lysis [1,7,8], as well as tooth fractures [1,9,10] and infections [1,9], these preliminary studies focus on the example of Equine Odontoclastic Tooth Resorption and Hypercementosis (EOTRH) syndrome. EOTRH requires radiographic imaging in the early stages to visualize the alveolar aspect of the teeth, where the signs are typically more advanced than is suggestive by the external appearance of the teeth [5,11]. Moreover, the radiographic signs of EOTRH appear earlier than the clinical signs [12–14], as 88% of horses with no apparent clinical signs demonstrated radiographic signs of incisor teeth resorption and 20% of horses demonstrated signs of incisor teeth hypercementosis [5]. Resorption and hypercementosis are two ongoing processes that progressively affect the structure of the tooth starting from the alveolar aspect (root and the reserve crown) [15]. Both processes are radiographically well–defined, as teeth demonstrate high radiodensity [16], where low radiopaque signs of resorption and high radiopaque signs of hypercementosis are alternately visible, thus, presenting the high irregularity and complexity of the image texture of radiographs [17].

The complete visual examination of the oral cavity allows the veterinarian to identify and manage dental problems and diagnose early stages of disease, benefiting the long–term general health of the horse and improving its quality of life [4], whereas the main aim of using digital processing of digital radiographs is to enhance the automated detection of early signs of EOTRH disease that might be missed by solely visual evaluation. Thus, the introduction of digital processing to the equine dental radiographs aims to improve the detection of specific signs of dental diseases which are not recognizable during the preliminary visual examination. It has been shown that raw radiographs collected directly from the X–ray scanner, which have not been digitally processed, are less effective in incisor teeth radiographic texture quantification than those that have been digitally processed. Due to the presence of noise, the radiographic filtering by filters improves the edge delimitation, such as Normalize or Bilateral filters, which increases the recognition of the radiographic signs of EOTRH syndrome [17]. However, the specific detection of grade 1, grade 2, and grade 3 EOTRH radiological signs remains challenging.

With the rapid advances in diagnostic imaging in equine dentistry [17–19], high–resolution detailed digital images [20] as well as a vast and ever–growing amount of data [17] are more readily available. Digital image processing is increasingly used to select and provide diagnostically important data [21] to avoid information noise that is difficult to evaluate. As the development of the computer–aided detection of image differences is a multi–stage process [22,23], the first two steps towards achieving the main goal have already been attained. The first step, concerning the preliminary demonstration of the possibility of quantifying the texture features of horses' incisor radiographs, has been previously published [17]. The second step is presented in this study. This second step concerns the advancement in image regularity evaluation, comparison of the novel and recent image regularity indicators, and demonstration of the detection accuracy of radiographic signs of teeth resorption and hypercementosis in both novel and recent experiments. To achieve this intermediate goal, the two–dimensional entropy measures [24], which are relatively recent methods of image irregularity and complexity quantification, have been proposed to obtain relevant and insightful data from equine dental radiographs, which could be applied in early EOTRH diagnosis. As entropy–based measurements represent a new class of easy–to–implement methods [25], their evaluation in different types of clinical applications [26] is advisable. In equine medicine, the entropy–based measurements have been successfully applied for the analysis of the texture of equine thermal images in pregnancy determination [27] and the rider:horse body weight ratio detection in horseback riding [28]. In the study examining the pregnancy model, four entropy–based measurements were used [27], however, in the horses' back load assessment model, a fifth measurement was added [28]. These five entropy–based measurements included: two–dimensional sample entropy (SampEn2D) [29], two–dimensional fuzzy entropy (FuzzEn2D) [30], two–dimensional permutation entropy (PermEn2D) [31], two–dimensional dispersion entropy (DispEn2D) [32], and two–dimensional distribution entropy (DistEn2D) [33]. These five aforementioned entropy–based measurements have been implemented in the current study. We hypothesize that the quantitative description of incisor tooth radiographs, by using filtrations and entropy measurement extraction, imply the specific detection of the radiological signs of grade 1, grade 2, and grade 3 EOTRH syndrome, which could be used in the future development of the automated detector of early signs of the disease.

Therefore, the study aimed to evaluate the applicability of entropy measures to quantify the radiological signs of tooth resorption and hypercementosis and to enhance the quality of the radiograph to improve the identification of the radiographic signs of EOTRH syndrome. To achieve this goal, the measures of five entropy–based measurements were extracted from radiographs of equine incisor teeth. Then, combinations of measures and filters were used to identify changes associated with the EOTRH grades. Next, the selected entropy measures and filters were compared with recently reported features of gray–level matrices texture analysis approaches to find similarities. Finally, for the selected measures and features, the detection accuracy of the radiographic signs of EOTRH syndrome was calculated.

2. Materials and Methods

2.1. Horses

Eighty privately owned horses ($n = 80$) (age mean $\pm$ SD: 16.9 ± 7.0; 37 geldings, 43 mares; 30 Polish Halfbred horses, 13 Arabian horses, 10 Schlesisches Warmblood horses, 8 Wielkopolska breed horses, 7 Dutch Warmblood horses, 5 Thoroughbred horses, 4 Polish coldblooded horses, and 3 Malopolska breed horses) were enrolled in the current study. The owners presented their horses for the standard veterinary diagnostic procedure including a basic clinical examination [34], a detailed examination of the oral cavity [35], and an additional examination [5]. In the current study, examination data collected from July 2021 to December 2021 were used.

A basic clinical examination was conducted following standard protocol [34], which allowed for the collection of the internal temperature, heart rate, respiratory rate, mucous membranes, capillary refill time, and lymph node evaluation. After a basic clinical examination–based qualification prior to the sedation procedure, the horses received a dose of detomidine hydrochloride (Domosedan; Orion Corporation, Espoo, Finland; 0.01 mg/kg bwt i.v.), xylazine hydrochloride (Xylapan; Vetoquinol Biowet Sp. z o.o., Gorzów Wielkopolski, Poland; 0.4 mg/kg bwt i.v.), or a combination of both. In some cases, the additional dose of butorphanol tartrate (Torbugesic; Zoetis Polska Sp. z o.o., Warsaw, Poland.; 0.01 mg/kg bwt i.v.) was required. No clinical contraindication to the sedation procedure was found in any of the examined horses.

A detailed examination of the oral cavity was conducted following standard protocol and included a visual examination and digital palpation of the teeth [35]. The Haussmann's mouth speculum was used to ensure the safety of the horse and veterinarian during a detailed examination. A 400 mL syringe was used to flush the oral cavity in order to remove any food which remained on, around, and between teeth. The periodontal probe was used for the evaluation of the interdental spaces. All clinical signs, including the condition of teeth, interdental spaces, gums, and mucosa of the cheeks and tongue, were documented on the equine dental chart [15] (Figure 1A).

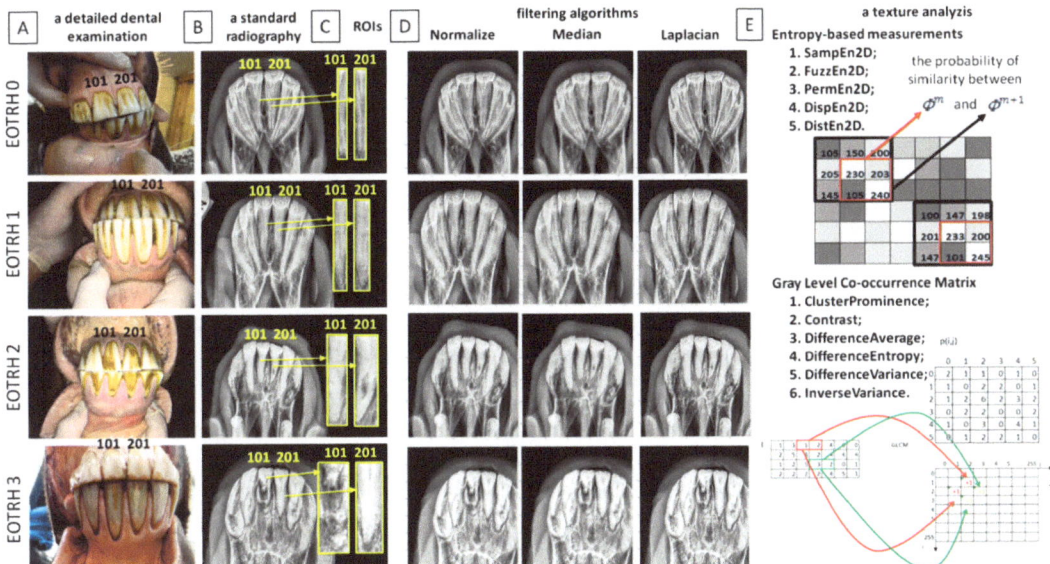

Figure 1. Scheme of radiographic–based detection of the signs of the Equine Odontoclastic Tooth Resorption and Hypercementosis (EOTRH) syndrome. A detailed dental examination (**A**); a standard radiography (**B**); segmentation of input radiographs with regions of interest (ROIs) of the first upper right incisor tooth (101) and the first upper left incisor tooth (201) marked with yellow lines (**C**); filtering of input radiographs by three filters—Normalize, Median, and Laplacian Sharpening (**D**); a texture analysis of output radiographs after filtering using entropy–based measures (five measures: SampEn2D—two-dimensional sample entropy, FuzzEn2D—two-dimensional fuzzy entropy, PermEn2D—two-dimensional permutation entropy, DispEn2D—two-dimensional dispersion entropy, DistEn2D—two-dimensional distribution entropy) and Gray–Level Co–occurrence Matrix (six selected features: Cluster Prominence, Contrast, Difference Average, Difference Entropy, Difference Variance, Inverse Variance) (**E**).

An additional examination allowed for radiography of the incisor teeth [5]. The radiographs were obtained by intraoral presentation, which required insertion of the protected radiographic cassette into the opened oral cavity of the horse, following the guidelines of the bisecting angle technique [13]. The dorsoventral projection for the maxillary teeth [15] was achieved by using the following settings: 2.5 mAs; 65 kV; of the x–ray tube (Orange 9020HF, Ecoray Co., Ltd.; 3F, Urbanlight B/D, 630, Eonju–ro, Gangnam–gu, Seoul, Korea) and the same distance (80 cm) to the radiographic cassette (Saturn 8000, Vievorks Co., Ltd., 41–3, Burim–ro, 170beon–gil, Dongan–gu, Anyang–si, Gyeonggi–do, 14055 Korea. The radiographs were acquired on HP portable computer (HP Inc UK Ltd., Earley West, 300 Thames Valley Park Drive, UK) using DxWorks software (Vievorks Co., Ltd., 41–3, Burim–ro, 170beon–gil, Dongan–gu, Anyang–si, Gyeonggi–do, 14055 Korea) and saved as .jpg files (Figure 1B).

The study was approved by the II Local Ethical Committee on Animal Testing in Warsaw on behalf of the National Ethical Committees on Animal Testing (No WAW2/091/2020 approved on 29 July 2020). The owners agreed to use the horses' data in the current study.

2.2. Radiographs Classification

Based on the clinical and radiological signs achieved from the standard veterinary diagnostic procedure, four grade–related EOTRH groups (0–3) were annotated. The radiological classification system introduced by Hüls et al. [36] and modified by Rehl et al. [5] was used. This classification system includes the evaluation of shape, surface structure, contour, and consistency of incisor teeth as well as contour, radiodensity, and delineation of the periodontal space of incisor teeth. As the preliminary application of two–dimensional entropy measures in the radiographic–based detection of the signs of EOTRH syndrome was tested, the central maxillary incisor teeth showing the best presentation in the radiographs obtained in the dorsoventral projection and the lowest superimposition of rounding tissues, were selected for testing. Following the modified Triadan system for equine dental nomenclature [37], the test incisor teeth were numbered as 101 (the first upper right incisor tooth) and 201 (the first upper left incisor tooth). On each selected incisor tooth, the representative rectangular region of interest (ROI) was manually annotated. Each ROI covers the largest possible area of the tooth crown and the largest possible area of the tooth root. Each ROI was individually fitted to the consecutive, separate teeth as shown on Figure 1C. Each ROI was edged by four high–radiodensity lines representing: (i) the occlusal side of the incisor tooth, (ii) the medial side of the incisor tooth, (iii) the apical side of the incisor tooth, and (iv) the lateral side of the incisor tooth, respectively. The ROIs were annotated using the ImageJ software version 1.46r (Wayne Rasband, National Institutes of Mental Health, Bethesda, MD, USA) and saved as .png files.

Based on above criteria, 101 and 201 maxillary incisor teeth were classified to grade 0 (normal teeth; $n = 37$), grade 1 (mildly EOTRH affected teeth; $n = 94$), grade 2 (moderately EOTRH affected teeth; $n = 20$), and grade 3 (severely EOTRH affected teeth; $n = 8$). The total number of incisors for all groups was 159; as 1 incisor was excluded due to tooth fractures.

2.3. Digital Radiograph Processing

Radiographs were digitally processed in two steps including input image filtering (Figure 1D) and output image texture analysis (Figure 1E). For the image filtering, three filtering algorithms were chosen: Normalize, Median, and Laplacian Sharpening based on the previously described findings of equine incisor teeth radiographs evaluation [17]. For the image texture analysis, five entropy–based texture measures were considered: two–dimensional sample entropy (SampEn2D), two–dimensional fuzzy entropy (FuzzEn2D), two–dimensional permutation entropy (PermEn2D), two–dimensional dispersion entropy (DispEn2D), and two–dimensional distribution entropy (DistEn2D), based on the previously described applicability in the equine image evaluation [27,28]. Both processing steps were conducted one after the other for the annotated ROIs, so that for each ROI, fifteen filtering–entropy combinations were returned. Each ROI was considered separately. Additionally, the currently presented entropy–based texture measures were compared with the selected, previously reported Gray–Level Co–occurrence Matrix data [17].

One may observe in Górski et al. [17] that the data from the combination of nine filtering algorithms (Mean, Median, Normalize, Bilateral, Binomial, Curvature Flow, Laplacian Sharpening, Discrete Gaussian, and Smoothing Recursive Gaussian) and six texture analysis approaches (First Order Statistics (FOS), Gray–Level Co–occurrence Matrix (GLCM), Neighbouring Gray Tone Difference Matrix (NGTDM), Gray–Level Dependence Matrix (GLDM), Gray–Level Run Length Matrix (GLRLM), and Gray–Level Size Zone Matrix (GLSZM)) were returned using PyRadiomics—an open–source python package for the extraction of features from radiographic images [38]—and presented in relation to the radiological signs of EOTRH syndrome grades. The raw data of six selected GLCM features selected in a previous study [17] (Cluster Prominence, Contrast, Difference Average, Difference Entropy, Difference Variance, Inverse Variance) were used in the current study to find similarities with the current raw data of entropy–based texture measures. For the details of the protocol of GLCM features extraction, see Górski et al. [17].

2.3.1. Filtering

Three filtering algorithms were implemented to reduce the noise in the radiographs using SimpleITK toolkit in Python language [39,40]. The used filtering algorithms differ depending on the linearity of the filter, type of output image, and result of filtering, as shown in Table 1.

Table 1. The comparison of details (linearity of the filter, type of output image, and result of filtering) of three filtering algorithms (Normalize filter, Median filter, and Laplacian Sharpening filter) used in the study.

Filter	Linearity	Output Image	Result
Normalize filter [41]	Linear filter	A rescaled image in which the pixels have zero mean and unit variance	An increase in the contrast of the image
Median filter [41]	Non–linear filter	A recalculated image in which the pixels are represented by the medians of the pixels in the neighbourhood of the input pixel	A reduction in the noise
Laplacian Sharpening filter [42]	Non–linear filter	A produced image in which the pixels are convoluted with a Laplacian operator	A change of the regions of rapid intensity and highlights the edges

2.3.2. Extraction of the Entropy–Based Measures

The five entropy–based texture analyses were conducted separately, returning five entropy measures, using Python, version 3.8.5 64–bit using package EntopyHub [43]. The extracted entropy measures differed depending, i.e., on the definition, relations between the values and the irregularity/complexity of the image, and application of measures, as shown in Table 2. For more details and equations of the entropy measures extraction, see Domino et al. [28].

2.4. Statistical Analysis

Five entropy measures (SampEn2D, FuzzEn2D, PermEn2D, DispEn2D, DistEn2D) and six selected GLCM features (Cluster Prominence, Contrast, Difference Average, Difference Entropy, Difference Variance, Inverse Variance) were presented as a data series, where each tooth of each horse represented one realization. The entire data set was divided into four EOTRH grade–related groups, thus, four EOTRH grade–labelled data series were extracted. The extracted data series were tested independently for univariate distributions using a Shapiro–Wilk normality test.

EOTRH grade–labelled data series were then compared between EOTRH grades using the ordinary one–way ANOVA followed by Tukey's multiple comparisons test for Gaussian data and the Kruskal–Wallis test, followed by the Dunn's multiple comparisons test for non–Gaussian data, and for each entropy measure and GLCM feature independently. The alpha value was established as $\alpha = 0.05$. On the respective plot, when a measure value was found to significantly increase with the EOTRH grades, the red line was additionally marked. The entropy measures and GLCM features were presented on scatter plots with bars using mean $\pm$ SD and dots representing each realization, where lower case letters indicate differences between EOTRH grades.

EOTRH grade–labelled data series were then compared between used filtering algorithms using the ordinary one–way ANOVA followed, by Tukey's multiple comparisons test for Gaussian data and the Kruskal–Wallis test, followed by the Dunn's multiple comparisons test for non–Gaussian data, and for each entropy measure and GLCM feature independently. The alpha value was established as $\alpha = 0.05$. The entropy measures and GLCM features were presented on scatter plots with bars using mean $\pm$ SD and dots representing each realization, where lower case letters indicate differences between filtering algorithms.

Table 2. The comparison of details (definition, relations between the values and the irregularity/complexity of the image, and application of measures) of five entropy measures (SampEn2D, FuzzEn2D, PermEn2D, DispEn2D, DistEn2D) used in the study.

Entropy Measures	Definition	Values	Application
SampEn2D [29,44]	The negative natural logarithm of the probability of similarity of patterns of length m with patterns of length $m+1$ $$\text{SampEn2D} = -\ln \frac{\Phi^{m+1}}{\Phi^m}$$	Low: regular patterns or periodic structures, as they have the same number of patterns for both m and $m+1$ High: irregular patterns	A measure of the irregularity in the pixel patterns
FuzzEn2D [30,45]	The negative natural logarithm of the conditional probability $$\text{FuzzEn2D} = -\ln \frac{\Phi^{m+1}(r)}{\Phi^m(r)}$$	Low: regular patterns or periodic structures High: irregular patterns or non-periodic structures	A measure of the irregularity in pixel patterns but using a continuous exponential function to determine the degree of similarity
PermEn2D [31,46]	The concept of counting permutation patterns π, where the permutation patterns are obtained after ordering the positions of the initial image patterns $$\text{PermEn2D} = -\frac{1}{(n-d_n+1)(m-d_m+1)} \sum_{\pi=1}^{d_n! \times d_m!} p(\pi) \ln p(\pi)$$	Low: regular patterns with the pixels always appearing in the same order High: irregular patterns with the highly disordered image pixels	An identification of irregular structure of the image
DispEn2D [32,45]	The conception of using the sigmoid function relies on mapped to c classes and the values of image pixels form $z_{i,j}^c = round(c \times v(i,j) + 0.5)$, where $v(i,j)$ $$\text{DispEn2D} = -\frac{1}{(n-d_n+1)(m-d_m+1)} \sum_{\pi=1}^{d_n! \times d_m!} p(\pi_v) \ln p(\pi_v)$$	Low: regular patterns with the low probability of dispersion patterns High: irregular image with the high probability of dispersion patterns	An assessment of the regularity of images with no indeterminacy of small-sized images
DistEn2D [33,47]	The amount of similarity between two windows by measuring the distance between the corresponding windows based on the distance matrix used to estimate the empirical probability density function (ePDF) $$\text{DistEn2D} = -\sum_{t=1}^{M} p_t \log_2(p_t)$$	Low: regular patterns of the small size images High: irregular patterns of the small size images	A quantitative description of the irregularities of the images, taking into account the small size of the image

SampEn2D—two-dimensional sample entropy; FuzzEn2D—two-dimensional fuzzy entropy; PermEn2D—two-dimensional permutation entropy; DispEn2D—two-dimensional dispersion entropy; DistEn2D—two-dimensional distribution entropy.

Based on the received differences, only for the most EOTRH–related entropy measures and GLCM features were linear regressions calculated. On regression plots, two regression equations were displayed, including one selected entropy measure and one for Cluster Prominence, Contrast, Difference Average, Difference Entropy, Difference Variance, or Inverse Variance. Equations were supported with the measure of the difference of linearity. All the slopes were significantly non–zero ($p < 0.0001$). For non–significant differences between the slopes ($p > 0.05$), one slope was calculated and the intercepts were compared. For non–significant differences between the intercepts ($p > 0.05$), one intercept was calculated. When the slope value of the entropy measure was higher than the slope value of the GLCM features, the plot was additionally marked by dashed frames. GraphPad Prism6 software (GraphPad Software Inc., San Diego, CA, USA) was used for all statistical analyses.

Based on the received differences, for the most EOTRH–related entropy measures and GLCM features only, the detection accuracy of EOTRH 0 and EOTRH 3 was calculated using three thresholds for gradually increasing measures (mean, mean + SD, mean + 2SD). The radiograph was annotated as EOTRH 0 when the individually measured value was above the threshold and annotated as EOTRH 3 when below it. The same annotation was carried out for the both EOTRH grade–related groups. The sensitivity (Se), specificity (Sp), positive predictive value (PPV), and negative predictive value (NPV) were estimated. The values of Se, Sp, PPV, and NPV were calculated across the range from 0.1 to 1.0 using standard formulae [48].

3. Results

Among the 15 returned combinations of entropy measures ($n = 5$) and filtering algorithms ($n = 3$), three entropy measures for Normalize filtering output radiographs, four entropy measures for Median filtering output radiographs, and two entropy measures for Laplacian Sharpening filtering output radiographs differed significantly between the EOTRH grades (Figure 2). Although some EOTRH grade–related differences were noted for SampEn2D (Normalize filtering, $p = 0.0009$, Figure 2A and Median filtering, $p < 0.0001$, Figure 2F), FuzzEn2D (Normalize filtering, $p = 0.002$, Figure 2B; Median filtering, $p < 0.0001$, Figure 2G; and Laplacian Sharpening filtering, $p = 0.0014$, Figure 2L), and PermEn2D (Median filtering, $p = 0.005$, Figure 2H), only DistEn2D significantly increased with the EOTRH grades. DistEn2D extracted from the Normalize filtering output radiographs was the lowest in the EOTRH 0 group, higher in the EOTRH 1 and 2 groups, and the highest in the EOTRH 3 group, with no differences between the EOTRH 1 and 2 groups ($p < 0.0001$, Figure 2E). DistEn2D extracted from the Median filtering output radiographs was lower in the EOTRH 0 group compared to the EOTRH 3 group, with no differences between the EOTRH 0–2 groups and EOTRH 2–3 groups ($p < 0.0001$, Figure 2J). DistEn2D extracted from Laplacian Sharpening filtering output radiographs was lower in the EOTRH 0 group compared to EOTRH 1–3 groups with no differences between EOTRH 1–3 groups ($p < 0.0001$, Figure 2O). The significance of this step was to extract entropy–based measurements from the radiographs of equine incisor teeth, and select those combinations of measures and filters that changed with the EOTRH grades.

When comparing entropy measures between the filtering algorithms, the same differences in consecutive EOTRH groups were noted for SampEn2D ($p < 0.0001$, Figure 3A,F,K,P), FuzzEn2D ($p < 0.0001$, Figure 3B,G,L,Q), PermEn2D ($p < 0.0001$, Figure 3C,H,M,R), and DistEn2D ($p < 0.0001$, Figure 3E,J,O,T), respectively, but not for DispEn2D ($p > 0.05$, Figure 3D,I,N,S). In each EOTRH group, SampEn2D and FuzzEn2D were always the lowest after Median filtering, higher after Normalize filtering, and the highest after Laplacian Sharpening filtering. Similarly, in each EOTRH group, PermEn2D was higher after Median filtering than after Normalize and Laplacian Sharpening filtering, whereas DistEn2D was higher after Laplacian Sharpening filtering than after Normalize and Median filtering. This step demonstrates how the use of filtering algorithms affects the values of the entropy–based measurements received from the consecutive EOTRH groups.

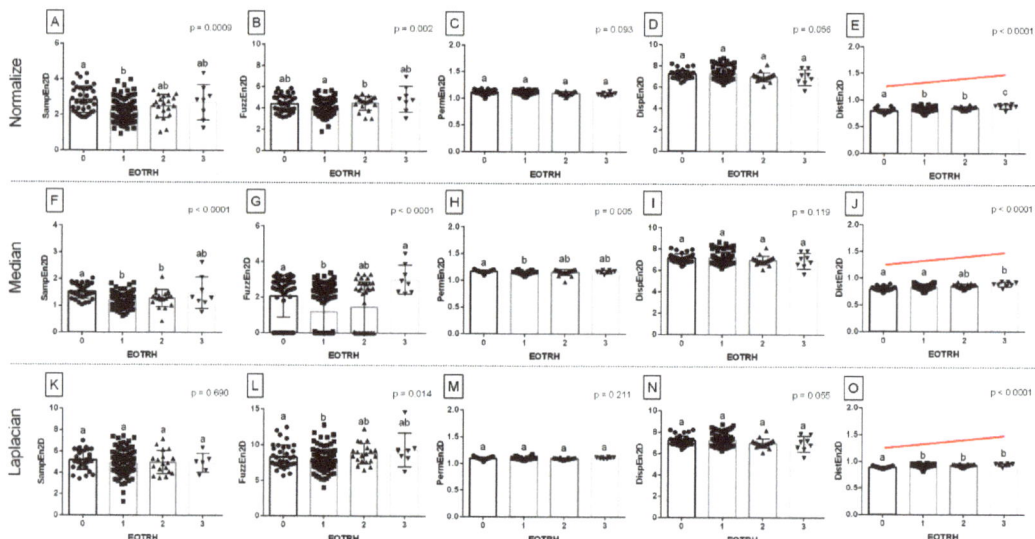

Figure 2. The comparison of the entropy measures between the EOTRH grades (0–3). The following entropy measures are considered: SampEn2D—two–dimensional sample entropy (**A,F,K**), FuzzEn2D—two–dimensional fuzzy entropy (**B,G,L**), PermEn2D—two–dimensional permutation entropy (**C,H,M**), DispEn2D—two–dimensional dispersion entropy (**D,I,N**), DistEn2D—two–dimensional distribution entropy (**E,J,O**). The output radiographs filtered by Normalize (**A–E**), Median (**F–J**), and Laplacian Sharpening (**K–O**) filtering algorithms are separated by dashed horizontal lines. Lower case letters (a–c) indicate differences between groups for $p < 0.05$ independently for each measure. The significant increase with the EOTRH grades is marked with a red line. Single realizations are marked with dots.

Among the 18 returned combinations of selected GLCM features ($n = 6$) and filtering algorithms ($n = 3$), all combinations differed significantly between the EOTRH grades and significantly increased with the EOTRH grades (Figure 4). Although some EOTRH grade–related increases were found between EOTRH 0 and 1 groups (Difference Variance after Median filtering, $p < 0.0001$, Figure 4K), between EOTRH 2 and 3 groups (Cluster Prominence after Median filtering, $p < 0.0001$, Figure 4G and Laplacian Sharpening filtering, $p < 0.0001$, Figure 4M; Contrast after Laplacian Sharpening filtering, $p = 0.010$, Figure 4N; Difference Average after Median filtering, $p = 0.004$, Figure 4I and Laplacian Sharpening filtering, $p = 0.029$, Figure 4O; Difference Entropy after Laplacian Sharpening filtering, $p = 0.006$, Figure 4P; Difference Variance after Laplacian Sharpening filtering, $p = 0.0009$, Figure 4Q; Inverse Variance after Median filtering, $p = 0.018$, Figure 4L and Laplacian Sharpening filtering, $p = 0.002$, Figure 4R), and EOTRH 1 and 3 groups (Contrast after Median filtering, $p = 0.0009$, Figure 4H; Difference Entropy after Median filtering, $p = 0.0002$, Figure 4J), all GLCM features significantly increased with the EOTRH grades from EOTRH 0 to 3 after Normalize filtering ($p < 0.0001$, Figure 4A–F). All examined GLCM features extracted from Normalize filtering output radiographs were the lowest in the EOTRH 0 group, higher in the EOTRH 1 and 2 groups, and the highest in the EOTRH 3 group, with no differences between the EOTRH 1 and 2 groups ($p < 0.0001$, Figure 4A–F). This step extracted the GLCM features from the radiographs of equine incisor teeth, and selected those combinations of features and filters that changed with each EOTRH grade.

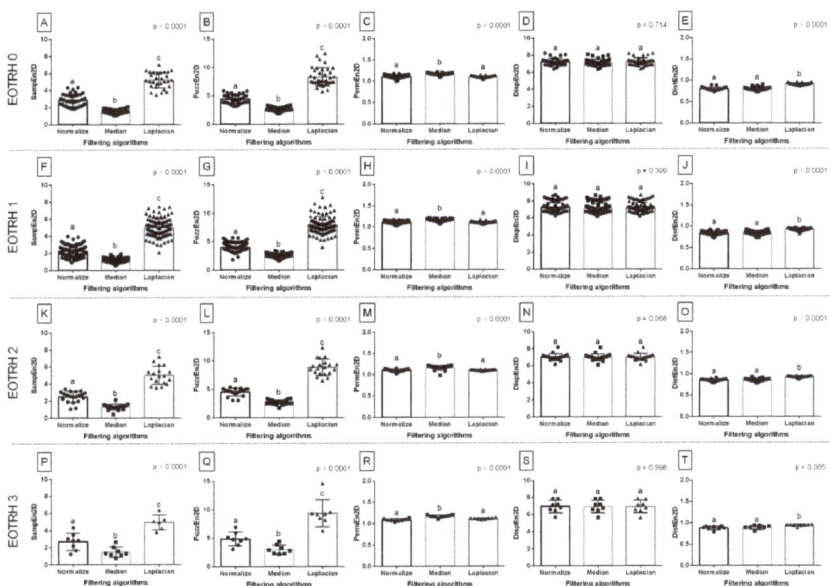

Figure 3. The comparison of the entropy measures between the filtering algorithms. The following entropy measures are considered: SampEn2D—two–dimensional sample entropy (**A,F,K,P**), FuzzEn2D—two–dimensional fuzzy entropy (**B,G,L,Q**), PermEn2D—two–dimensional permutation entropy (**C,H,M,R**), DispEn2D—two–dimensional dispersion entropy (**D,I,N,S**), DistEn2D—two–dimensional distribution entropy (**E,J,O,T**). The radiographs classified to EOTRH 0 grade (**A–E**), EOTRH 1 grade (**F–J**), EOTRH 2 grade (**K–O**), and EOTRH 3 grade (**P–T**) are separated by dashed horizontal lines. Lower case letters (a–c) indicate differences between groups for $p < 0.05$ independently for each measure. Single realizations are marked with dots.

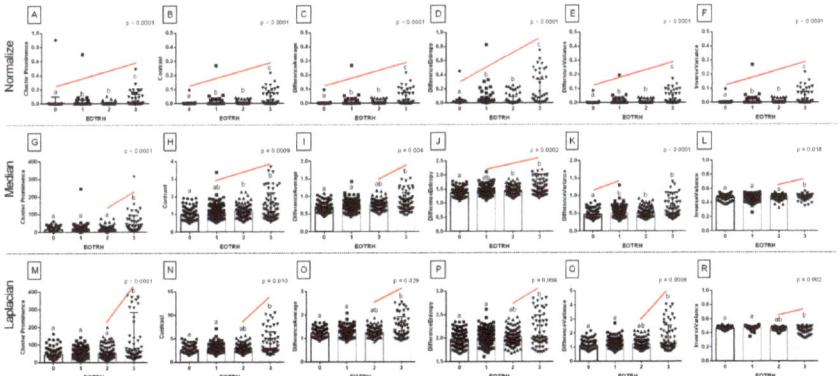

Figure 4. The comparison of the selected Gray–Level Co–occurrence Matrix (GLCM) features between the EOTRH grades (0–3). The following GLCM features are considered: Cluster Prominence (**A,G,M**), Contrast (**B,H,N**), Difference Average (**C,I,O**), Difference Entropy (**D,J,P**), Difference Variance (**E,K,Q**), Inverse Variance (**F,L,R**). The output radiographs filtered by Normalize (**A–F**), Median (**G–L**), and Laplacian Sharpening (**M–R**) filtering algorithms are separated by dashed horizontal lines. Lower case letters (a–c) indicate differences between groups for $p < 0.05$ independently for each feature. The significant increase with the EOTRH grades is marked with a red line. Single realizations are marked with dots.

When comparing selected GLCM features between the filtering algorithms, the same differences in consecutive EOTRH groups were noted for Cluster Prominence ($p < 0.0001$, Figure 5A,G,M,S), Contrast ($p < 0.0001$, Figure 5B,H,N,T), Difference Average ($p < 0.0001$, Figure 5C,I,O,U), Difference Entropy ($p < 0.0001$, Figure 5D,J,P,V), Difference Variance ($p < 0.0001$, Figure 5E,K,Q,W), and Inverse Variance ($p < 0.0001$, Figure 5F,L,R,X), respectively. In each EOTRH group, Cluster Prominence, Contrast, Difference Average, Difference Entropy, and Difference Variance were always the lowest after Normalize filtering, higher after Median filtering, and highest after Laplacian Sharpening filtering. Similarly, in each EOTRH group, Inverse Variance was higher after Median and Laplacian Sharpening filtering than after Normalize filtering. This demonstrated the effects that the filtering algorithms had on the select GLCM features received from the consecutive EOTRH groups.

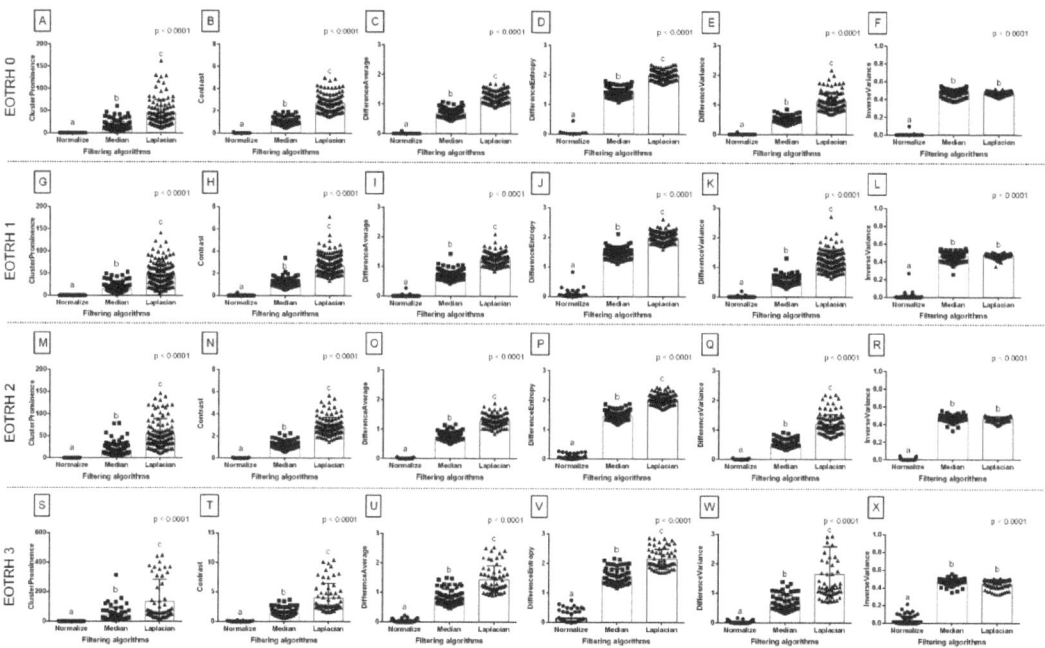

Figure 5. The comparison of the selected Gray–Level Co–occurrence Matrix (GLCM) features between the filtering algorithms. The following GLCM features are considered: Cluster Prominence (**A,G,M,S**), Contrast (**B,H,N,T**), Difference Average (**C,I,O,U**), Difference Entropy (**D,J,P,V**), Difference Variance (**E,K,Q,W**), Inverse Variance (**F,L,R,X**). The radiographs classified to EOTRH 0 grade (**A–F**), EOTRH 1 grade (**G–L**), EOTRH 2 grade (**M–R**), and EOTRH 3 grade (**S–X**) are separated by dashed horizontal lines. Lower case letters (a–c) indicate differences between groups for $p < 0.05$ independently for each measure. Single realizations are marked with dots.

Based on the received differences, the similarities were tested for DistEn2D and all six GLCM features, of which were only extracted from Normalize filtering output radiographs. The slope of the linear regression equations for DistEn2D compared to the slopes of GLCM features were not significantly different, and one slope measurement was calculated only for Difference Entropy ($p = 0.578$; one slope = 0.033; Figure 6D). The intercept within this data pair was compared and considered significant ($p < 0.0001$), thus, one intercept was not calculated. For all the other compared data pairs, the slopes were significantly different ($p < 0.05$; Figure 6A–C,E,F). The slope value of DistEn2D (slope = 0.028) was higher than the slope value of GLCM features for Cluster Prominence (slope = 0.009; Figure 6A), Contrast (slope = 0.007; Figure 6B), Difference Average (slope = 0.007; Figure 6C), Difference Entropy (slope = 0.006; Figure 6E), and Inverse Variance (slope = 0.007; Figure 6F); but not for Difference Entropy (slope = 0.034; Figure 6D). Here, similarities between the selected entropy measures and GLCM features after subsequent selected types of filtering can be observed.

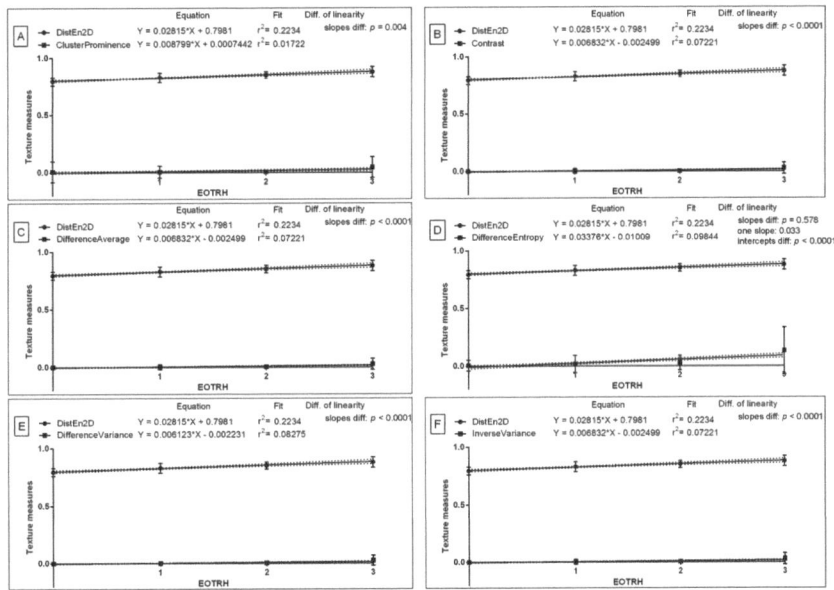

Figure 6. Comparison of selected entropy measure (DistEn2D–two–dimensional distribution entropy) and selected Gray–Level Co–occurrence Matrix (GLCM) features (Cluster Prominence (**A**), Contrast (**B**), Difference Average (**C**), Difference Entropy (**D**), Difference Variance (**E**), Inverse Variance (**F**)) throughout the EOTRH grades. Measure and features were extracted from the output radiographs after Normalize filtering. Similarity was tested using linear regressions. A $p < 0.05$ was considered significant. If the difference between slopes was not significant, a single slope measurement was calculated. Plot where the slope value of the entropy measure was higher than the slope value of the GLCM features was marked by dashed frames.

Based on the received differences, the detection accuracy of EOTRH 0 and EOTRH 3 was tested for DistEn2D and all six GLCM features extracted from Normalize filtering output radiographs (Table 3). For DistEn2D and all six GLCM features, a salient observation was made, identifying that the Se and NPV decreased with higher threshold values (mean > mean + SD > mean + 2SD) and the Sp and PPV increased with higher threshold values (mean > mean + SD > mean + 2SD). For the first threshold (mean), Se ranged from 0.50 for DistEn2D; 0.27 for Difference Entropy; to 0.25 for the remaining five GLCM features. Additionally, Sp ranged from 0.95 for DistEn2D to 0.99 for all GLCM features. For the second threshold (mean + SD), Se ranged from 0.13 for DistEn2D; to 0.22 for Difference Entropy; through 0.17 for the remaining five GLCM features. Moreover, Sp ranged from 1.00 for DistEn2D; to 0.98 for Difference Entropy; through to 0.99 for the remaining five GLCM features. For the third threshold (mean + SD), Se ranged from 0.00 for DistEn2D; 0.03 for Cluster Prominence; to 0.07 for the remaining five GLCM features. Furthermore, Sp ranged from 0.99 for Cluster Prominence to 1.00 DistEn2D and the remaining five GLCM features. This step allowed for the summarization of the detection accuracy of the radiographic signs of EOTRH syndrome based on the selected entropy measures and GLCM features.

Table 3. The accuracy (Se—sensitivity; Sp—specificity; PPV—positive predictive value; NPV—negative predictive value) of the detection of EOTRH 0 and EOTRH 3 based on the selected entropy measure (DistEn2D—two-dimensional distribution entropy) and the selected Gray–Level Co–occurrence Matrix (GLCM) features (ClusterProminence; Contrast; DifferenceAverage; DifferenceEntropy; DifferenceVariance; Inverse Variance) extracted from the output images filtered by Normalize filter. Three thresholds (mean; mean + SD; mean + 2SD) were used.

Measures	DistEn2D	Cluster Prominence	Contrast	Difference Average	Difference Entropy	Difference Variance	Inverse Variance
Threshold				mean			
Se	0.50	0.25	0.25	0.25	0.27	0.25	0.25
Sp	0.95	0.99	0.99	0.99	0.99	0.99	0.99
PPV	0.67	0.94	0.94	0.94	0.94	0.94	0.94
NPV	0.90	0.70	0.70	0.70	0.70	0.70	0.70
Threshold				mean + SD			
Se	0.13	0.17	0.17	0.17	0.22	0.17	0.17
Sp	1.00	0.99	0.99	0.99	0.98	0.99	0.99
PPV	1.00	0.91	0.91	0.91	0.93	0.91	0.91
NPV	0.84	0.68	0.68	0.68	0.58	0.68	0.68
Threshold				mean + 2SD			
Se	0.00	0.03	0.07	0.07	0.07	0.07	0.07
Sp	1.00	0.99	1.00	1.00	1.00	1.00	1.00
PPV	-	0.67	1.00	1.00	1.00	1.00	1.00
NPV	0.82	0.65	0.66	0.66	0.66	0.66	0.66

4. Discussion

The benefit of using imaging processing in the radiological assessment of EOTRH will come from the enhanced automated detection of early signs of the disease that might be missed by a mere personal evaluation. As the formation of the computed–aided detector is a multi-stage process requiring extensive basic research, the current study presents the second step towards achieving this main goal. In this paper, the novel quantitative description of incisor tooth radiographs was used to enhance the quality of the radiograph to make identifying the radiographic signs of EOTRH syndrome easier, and if possible, to enhance the specific detection of the radiological signs of grade 1, grade 2, and grade 3 EOTRH syndrome.

Recently, filtering algorithms and texture analysis based on the first– and second–order statistics have been successfully used in the digital processing of the equine maxillary incisor teeth radiographs [17]. As the recent report was focused only on maxillary, not maxillary and mandibulary incisor teeth, the current study was focused similarly to provide the appropriate data sets required for the evaluation of similarities. In the previous study, the GLCM application—supported by filtering by the Normalize filter—improved edge delimitation, and was concluded to be the most advisable for the quantification of radiographic signs of EOTRH syndrome [17]. In the current study, the EOTRH grade–related increase level and accuracy of the EOTRH grade differentiation were compared between the previous digital processing approach and the new one, showing a higher slope of the linear regression equations and a higher sensitivity of radiographic sign detection for entropy–based measures than gray–level matrix–based features. As the same radiographs were used in both approaches, one may uphold the current hypothesis, that digital radiograph processing, including filtering and entropy measures extraction, may be considered as the enhancement of the quantitative description of incisor teeth radiographs and the advancement of field dental radiography. The research undertaken meets Zarychta's [26] statement that the applicability of entropy measures should be evaluated for various specimens and should highlight advances in the development, testing, and application of radiograph–processing algorithms to standard veterinary dental radiography.

In the case of EOTRH syndrome, two opposing pathological processes, resorption and hypercementosis, affect the incisor teeth [5,11]. In both processes, a variable grade of tooth resorption and mild-to-severe hypercementosis were radiographically recognized in most publications devoted to the radiological diagnosis of EOTRH syndrome [5,6,15,49,50]—resorption shows low radiopaque signs, whereas hypercementosis shows high radiopaque signs on the background of the high radiodensity tooth structure [16,17]. Both processes may involve the whole tooth structure, although resorption signs mainly appear in the enamel, cementum, dentine, and pulp cavity [11], whereas hypercementosis is most commonly found in the apex of the tooth, with bulbous enlargements of cement accumulation [51]. The alternating occurrence of radiological signs of resorption and hypercementosis gives a mosaic pattern of the tooth structure that is separable visually [5,6,15] and quantifiable with second-order descriptive statistics [17]. This quantification, based on the Gray-Level Co-occurrence Matrix evaluation, counts the randomness in the radiograph using the differences in the intensity value of the respective pixels or their surroundings [17]. Precisely, the irregularity of pixels in a given window and the likelihood of similarity of these pixels and the pixels of the next window are the basis of the creation of a matrix where the occurrence of a given pixel is counted [52,53]. Contrarily, all currently used entropy measures are calculated directly on the image [24], returning the repeatability of pixel patterns of the image, which in this application, is related to the texture properties of the radiograph [25]. In a currently considered type of application, the values returned from the radiographs are directly related to the predictability or uncertainty of the radiograph's spatial patterns and are directly related to the radiograph's irregularity or complexity [29–32]. Therefore, one may observe that the approaches based on calculating features from the matrix obtained from the processing step applied to the image, such as GLCM, represent the disorder of the intermediate matrix rather than the irregularity of the image [54], whereas, in the case of the EOTRH radiological signs, measures of irregularity and complexity [29–32] rather than features of disorder [52] of radiograph texture may be extracted as more relevant and insightful. This hypothesis is supported by the current results, which indicate that measures of irregularity and complexity, such as DispEn2D, are more accurate in the differentiation of the EOTRH radiological signs than the features of the disorder, such as Cluster Prominence, Contrast, Difference Average, Difference Entropy, Difference Variance, and Inverse Variance. It should be highlighted that DispEn2D, rather than GLCM features, may be considered in further automated detection developments, which ultimately aim to improve EOTRH detection.

In the current study, the ROIs annotated on the incisor teeth pass the criterion of being a small size image, thus, one may suspect DispEn2D and DistEn2D rather than SampEn2D, FuzzEn2D, and PermEn2D to be effective in this type of application, especially considering that both DispEn2D and DistEn2D have been shown to be the most suitable for the entropy-based texture analysis of small ROIs which were extracted from thermographs in the equine applications of pregnancy [27] and back load [28] detection. Interestingly, in the current study, only DistEn2D, not DispEn2D, demonstrated the most favourable EOTRH grade-related differences. DistEn2D extracted from Normalize filtering output radiographs was the lowest in the EOTRH 0 group, higher in the EOTRH 1 and 2 groups, and the highest in the EOTRH 3 group. One may observe that the concept of counting the amount of similarity between two windows by measuring the distance between the corresponding windows, used in DistEn2D [33,47], is more suitable for the texture analysis of small regions of the radiographs of equine incisor teeth than the concept of using the sigmoid function, as used in DispEn2D [32,45]. The DistEn2D algorithm is invariant to rotation [33,44], whereas the DispEn2D algorithm is the least sensitive to rotation, translation, and image size, out of the five currently studied measures of entropy [45]. Thus, it appears that the concept of a measure, and not the rotation, is essential to the usefulness of the DistEn2D algorithm in this application. These findings justified the choice to use the DispEn2D for further automated detection development.

One may note that the DistEn2D value was lower after Normalize and Median filtering than after Laplacian Sharpening filtering, and the DispEn2D algorithm was the least sensitive to filtering out of the five currently studied measures of entropy [29–32]. This can be considered a benefit over the GLCM approach. All GLCM features considered in the current study differed between EOTRH grades 0–3 after filtering by the Normalize filter but not after Median and Laplacian Sharpening filtration. The Laplacian Sharpening filter returns the output radiographs with a sharper quality than the input radiograph [55], and has been considered more suitable for the first–order than the second–order statistic extracted from equine radiographs [17]. The Normalize filter increases the contrast of the radiographs [56], which seems to be more favourable for the GLCM approaches than other filtering algorithms [17]. As the GLCM approach returns the spatial distribution of the pixel disorder [57], the output radiograph, after filtering by the contrast–improved algorithm, demonstrates a greater grade of differentiation [58,59]. Contrarily, as the DispEn2D measure returns a quantitative description of the irregularities of the images [33], both the contrast improvement by Normalize filter and the noise reduction by Median [48] may provide a good grade of differentiation for EOTRH radiological signs. One may also observe that for the Normalize filtering output radiograph, the slope value of DistEn2D was higher than the slope value of five from six compared GLCM features. These differences in the slopes of the regression curves indicate a greater increase in the value of the entropy measure than GLCM features with regard to the severity of the radiological signs of EOTRH, and suggest a greater usefulness of DistEn2D than GLCM, which was confirmed by the detection accuracy of EOTRH 0 and EOTRH 3. These findings justified the choice of the Normalize and Median filtering for the further automated detection development.

Finally, one may discern that the proposed method of digital processing of radiographs allows to detect the radiological signs of all grades of EOTRH syndrome, although it does not adequately support the differentiation between EOTRH 0 and 1, EOTRH 1 and 2, as well as EOTRH 2 and 3. Although the DistEn2D–based differentiation between EOTRH 0 and 3 was more accurate than GLCM–based differentiation, further studies on a bigger data set are required to verify the applicability of the proposed algorithms. Within the benefit of using imaging processing in the radiological assessment of EOTRH in horses, the enhancement of the quality of the radiograph to facilitate the identification of identifying the radiographic signs of EOTRH syndrome should be highlighted.

5. Conclusions

From the entropy measures recently applied in the equine image analysis, only DistEn2D showed the EOTRH grade–related differences which could be introduced to the advanced veterinary diagnostic procedure for incisor teeth disorders. These observed differences were the least susceptible to the use of radiograph filtering algorithms, returning the same values after Normalize and Median filtering. As the EOTRH grade–related differences were the most favourable for DistEn2D extraction from the Normalize filtering output radiographs, this combination of digital radiograph processing may be carefully advised in equine incisor teeth radiography. Interestingly, the considered GLCM features demonstrated a higher susceptibility for filtering than the entropy measures, showing, similar to DistEn2D, the most favourable differences after Normalize filtering. Moreover, both the evidence of similarity and the highest EOTRH grade–related increase level were noted for DistEn2D and Difference Entropy after Normalize filtering. As these two measures also demonstrated the highest accuracy of the EOTRH grade differentiation, one may suggest that they could be introduced as advancements into the field equine dentistry.

Author Contributions: Conceptualization, K.G. and M.D.; methodology, K.G., M.B. and M.D.; software, M.B.; validation, E.S. and I.P.; formal analysis, K.G., M.B. and M.D.; investigation, K.G., M.B., E.S., I.P., B.T., A.B. and M.D.; resources, K.G. and M.B.; data curation, K.G. and M.D.; writing—original draft preparation, K.G., M.B., E.S. and M.D.; writing—review and editing, I.P., B.T. and A.B.; visualization, K.G. and M.D.; supervision, I.P.; project administration, K.G. and M.D.; funding acquisition, K.G. All authors have read and agreed to the published version of the manuscript.

Funding: The study was supported by the National Science Centre, Poland, "Miniatura 6" Project, No. 2022/06/X/ST6/00431.

Institutional Review Board Statement: The animal protocols used in this work were evaluated and approved by the II Local Ethical Committee on Animal Testing in Warsaw on behalf of the National Ethical Committees on Animal Testing (protocol code WAW2/091/2020 approved on 29 July 2020). They are in accordance with FELASA guidelines and the National law for Laboratory Animal Experimentation (Dz. U. 2015 poz. 266 and 2010–63–EU directive).

Informed Consent Statement: Not applicable.

Data Availability Statement: The data presented in this study are available on request from the corresponding author.

Conflicts of Interest: The authors declare no conflict of interest. The funders had no role in the design of the study; in the collection, analyses, or interpretation of data; in the writing of the manuscript, or in the decision to publish the results.

References

1. Dixon, P.M.; Dacre, I. A review of equine dental disorders. *Vet. J.* **2005**, *169*, 165–187. [CrossRef] [PubMed]
2. Dixon, P.M. The Gross, Histological, and Ultrastructural Anatomy of Equine Teeth and Their Relationship to Disease. In Proceedings of the 49th Annual Convention of the American Association of Equine Practitioners, New Orleans, LA, USA, 21–25 November 2003; Volume 48, pp. 421–437.
3. Brigham, E.J.; Duncanson, G.R. An equine postmortem dental study: 50 cases. *Equine Vet. Educ.* **2000**, *12*, 59–62. [CrossRef]
4. Limone, L. General clinical, oral and dental examination. In *Equine Dentistry and Maxillofacial Surgery*; Cambridge Scholars Publishing: Newcastle upon Tyne, UK, 2022; p. 302.
5. Rehrl, S.; Schröder, W.; Müller, C.; Staszyk, C.; Lischer, C. Radiological prevalence of equine odontoclastic tooth resorption and hypercementosis. *Equine Vet. J.* **2018**, *50*, 481–487. [CrossRef] [PubMed]
6. Henry, T.J.; Puchalski, S.M.; Arzi, B.; Kass, P.H.; Verstraete, F.J.M. Radiographic evaluation in clinical practice of the types and stage of incisor tooth resorption and hypercementosis in horses. *Equine Vet. J.* **2016**, *49*, 486–492. [CrossRef] [PubMed]
7. Easley, J. A new look at dental radiography. In Proceedings of the 48th Annual Convention of the American Association of Equine Practitioners, Orlando, FL, USA, 4–8 December 2002; Volume 48, pp. 412–420.
8. Barakzai, S.Z.; Dixon, P.M. A study of open-mouthed oblique radiographic projections for evaluating lesions of the erupted (clinical) crown. *Equine Vet. Edu.* **2003**, *15*, 143–148. [CrossRef]
9. Greet, T.R.C. Oral and dental trauma. In *Equine Dentistry*, 1st ed.; Baker, G.J., Easley, J., Eds.; W.B. Saunders: London, UK, 1999; pp. 60–69.
10. Dixon, P.M.; Tremaine, W.H.; Pickles, K.; Kuhns, L.; Hawe, C.; McCann, J.; McGorum, B.; Railton, D.I.; Brammer, S. Equine dental disease Part 1: A longterm study of 400 cases: Disorders of incisor, canine and first premolar teeth. *Equine Vet. J.* **1999**, *31*, 369–377. [CrossRef]
11. Staszyk, C.; Bienert, A.; Kreutzer, R.; Wohlsein, P.; Simhofer, H. Equine odontoclastic tooth resorption and hypercementosis. *Vet. J.* **2008**, *178*, 372–379. [CrossRef] [PubMed]
12. Pearce, C.J. Recent developments in equine dentistry. *N. Z. Vet. J.* **2020**, *68*, 178–186. [CrossRef]
13. Barrett, M.F.; Easley, J.T. Acquisition and interpretation of radiographs of the equine skull. *Equine Vet. Educ.* **2013**, *25*, 643–652. [CrossRef]
14. Moore, N.T.; Schroeder, W.; Staszyk, C. Equine odontoclastic tooth resorption and hypercementosis affecting all cheek teeth in two horses: Clinical and histopathological findings. *Equine Vet. Educ.* **2016**, *28*, 123–130. [CrossRef]
15. Górski, K.; Tremaine, H.; Obrochta, B.; Buczkowska, R.; Turek, B.; Bereznowski, A.; Rakowska, A.; Polkowska, I. EOTRH syndrome in polish half-bred horses-two clinical cases. *J. Equine Vet. Sci.* **2021**, *101*, 103428. [CrossRef] [PubMed]
16. Saccomanno, S.; Passarelli, P.C.B.; Oliva, B.; Grippaudo, C. Comparison between two radiological methods for assessment of tooth root resorption: An in vitro study. *BioMed Res. Int.* **2018**, *2018*, 5152172. [CrossRef]
17. Górski, K.; Borowska, M.; Stefanik, E.; Polkowska, I.; Turek, B.; Bereznowski, A.; Domino, M. Selection of Filtering and Image Texture Analysis in the Radiographic Images Processing of Horses' Incisor Teeth Affected by the EOTRH Syndrome. *Sensors* **2022**, *22*, 2920. [CrossRef]
18. Manso-Díaz, G.; García-López, J.M.; Maranda, L.; Taeymans, O. The role of head computed tomography in equine practice. *Equine Vet. Educ.* **2015**, *27*, 136–145. [CrossRef]
19. Baratt, R.M. Dental Radiography and Radiographic Signs of Equine Dental Disease. *Vet. Clin. N. Am. Equine Pract.* **2020**, *36*, 445–476. [CrossRef] [PubMed]
20. Dakin, S.G.; Lam, R.; Rees, E.; Mumby, C.; West, C.; Weller, R. Technical Set-up and Radiation Exposure for Standing Computed Tomography of the Equine Head: Standing CT of the Equine Head. *Equine Vet. Educ.* **2014**, *26*, 208–215. [CrossRef]
21. van der Stelt, P.F. Filmless imaging: The uses of digital radiography in dental practice. *J. Am. Dent. Assoc.* **2005**, *136*, 1379–1387. [CrossRef]
22. Tan, T.; Platel, B.; Mus, R.; Tabar, L.; Mann, R.M.; Karssemeijer, N. Computer-aided detection of cancer in automated 3-D breast ultrasound. *IEEE TMI* **2013**, *32*, 1698–1706. [CrossRef] [PubMed]

23. Vidal, P.L.; de Moura, J.; Novo, J.; Ortega, M. Multi-stage transfer learning for lung segmentation using portable X-ray devices for patients with COVID-19. *Expert Syst. Appl.* **2021**, *173*, 114677. [CrossRef]
24. Humeau-Heurtier, A. Texture feature extraction methods: A survey. *IEEE Access* **2019**, *7*, 8975–9000. [CrossRef]
25. Silva, L.E.; Duque, J.J.; Felipe, J.C.; Murta, L.O., Jr.; Humeau-Heurtier, A. Two-dimensional multiscale entropy analysis: Applications to image texture evaluation. *Signal Process.* **2018**, *147*, 224–232. [CrossRef]
26. Zarychta, P. Application of fuzzy image concept to medical images matching. In *Information Technology in Biomedicine. ITIB 2018. Advances in Intelligent Systems and Computing*, 1st ed.; Pietka, E., Badura, P., Kawa, J., Wieclawek, W., Eds.; Springer: Cham, Switzerland, 2019; Volume 762, pp. 27–38.
27. Borowska, M.; Maśko, M.; Jasiński, T.; Domino, M. The Role of Two-Dimensional Entropies in IRT-Based Pregnancy Determination Evaluated on the Equine Model. In *Information Technology in Biomedicine. ITIB 2022. Advances in Intelligent Systems and Computing*, 1st ed.; Pietka, E., Badura, P., Kawa, J., Wieclawek, W., Eds.; Springer: Cham, Switzerland, 2022; Volume 1429, pp. 54–65.
28. Domino, M.; Borowska, M.; Zdrojkowski, Ł.; Jasiński, T.; Sikorska, U.; Skibniewski, M.; Maśko, M. Application of the Two-Dimensional Entropy Measures in the Infrared Thermography-Based Detection of Rider: Horse Bodyweight Ratio in Horseback Riding. *Sensors* **2022**, *22*, 6052. [CrossRef]
29. Da Silva, L.E.; Senra Filho, A.C.; Fazan, V.P.; Felipe, J.C.; Murta, L.O., Jr. Two-dimensional sample entropy analysis of rat sural nerve aging. In Proceedings of the 2014 36th Annual International Conference of the IEEE Engineering in Medicine and Biology Society, Chicago, IL, USA, 26–30 August 2014; pp. 3345–3348.
30. Hilal, M.; Berthin, C.; Martin, L.; Azami, H.; Humeau-Heurtier, A. Bidimensional multiscale fuzzy entropy and its application to pseudoxanthoma elasticum. *IEEE Trans. Biomed. Eng.* **2019**, *67*, 2015–2022. [CrossRef] [PubMed]
31. Ribeiro, H.V.; Zunino, L.; Lenzi, E.K.; Santoro, P.A.; Mendes, R.S. Complexity-entropy causality plane as a complexity measure for two-dimensional patterns. *PLoS ONE* **2012**, *7*, e40689. [CrossRef]
32. Azami, H.; da Silva, L.E.V.; Omoto, A.C.M.; Humeau-Heurtier, A. Two-dimensional dispersion entropy: An information-theoretic method for irregularity analysis of images. *Signal. Process. Image Commun.* **2019**, *75*, 178–187. [CrossRef]
33. Azami, H.; Escudero, J.; Humeau-Heurtier, A. Bidimensional Distribution Entropy to Analyze the Irregularity of Small-Sized Textures. *IEEE Signal. Proc. Lett.* **2017**, *24*, 1338–1342. [CrossRef]
34. Radostits, O.M.; Gay, C.; Hinchcliff, K.W.; Constable, P.D. (Eds.) *Veterinary Medicine E-Book: A Textbook of the Diseases of Cattle, Horses, Sheep, Pigs and Goats*; Elsevier: Amsterdam, The Netherlands, 2006.
35. Salem, S.E.; Townsend, N.B.; Refaai, W.; Gomaa, M.; Archer, D.C. Prevalence of oro-dental pathology in a working horse population in Egypt and its relation to equine health. *Equine Vet. J.* **2017**, *49*, 26–33. [CrossRef]
36. Hüls, I.; Bienert, A.; Staszyk, C. Equine odontoclastic tooth resorption and hyper-cementosis (EOTRH): Röntgenologische und makroskopisch-anatomische Befunde. In Proceedings of the 10 Jahrestagung der Internationalen Gesellschaft zur Funktionsverbesserung der Pferdezähne, Wiesbaden, Germany, 3–4 March 2012.
37. Floyd, M.R. The modified Triadan system: Nomenclature for veterinary dentistry. *J. Vet. Dent.* **1991**, *8*, 18–19. [CrossRef] [PubMed]
38. van Griethuysen, J.J.M.; Fedorov, A.; Parmar, C.; Hosny, A.; Aucoin, N.; Narayan, V.; Beets-Tan, R.G.H.; Fillon-Robin, J.C.; Pieper, S.; Aerts, H.J.W.L. Computational radiomics system to decode the radiographic phenotype. *Cancer Res.* **2017**, *77*, e104–e107. [CrossRef]
39. Lowekamp, B.C.; Chen, D.T.; Ibáñez, L.; Blezek, D. The design of SimpleITK. *Front. Neuroinform.* **2013**, *7*, 45. [CrossRef]
40. Yaniv, Z.; Lowekamp, B.C.; Johnson, H.J.; Beare, R. SimpleITK image-analysis notebooks: A collaborative environment for education and reproducible research. *J. Digit. Imaging* **2018**, *31*, 290–303. [CrossRef]
41. Lim, J.S. *Two-Dimensional Signal and Image Processing*, 1st ed.; Prentice Hall: Englewood Cliffs, NJ, USA, 1990.
42. Gonzalez, R.C.; Eddins, S.L.; Woods, R.E. *Digital Image Publishing Using MATLAB*, 1st ed.; Prentice Hall: Upper Saddle River, NJ, USA, 2004.
43. Flood, M.W.; Grimm, B. EntropyHub: An open-source toolkit for entropic time series analysis. *PLoS ONE* **2021**, *16*, e0259448.
44. Silva, L.E.V.; Senra Filho, A.C.S.; Fazan, V.P.S.; Felipe, J.C.; Murta Junior, L.O. Two-dimensional sample entropy: Assessing image texture through irregularity. *Biomed. Phys. Eng. Express* **2016**, *2*, 045002. [CrossRef]
45. Furlong, R.; Hilal, M.; O'brien, V.; Humeau-Heurtier, A. Parameter Analysis of Multiscale Two-Dimensional Fuzzy and Dispersion Entropy Measures Using Machine Learning Classification. *Entropy* **2021**, *23*, 1303. [CrossRef] [PubMed]
46. Morel, C.; Humeau-Heurtier, A. Multiscale permutation entropy for two-dimensional patterns. *Pattern Recognit. Lett.* **2021**, *150*, 139–146. [CrossRef]
47. He, J.; Shang, P.; Zhang, Y. PID: A PDF-induced distance based on permutation cross-distribution entropy. *Nonlinear Dyn.* **2019**, *97*, 1329–1342. [CrossRef]
48. Dohoo, I.; Martin, W.; Stryhn, H. *Veterinary Epidemiologic Research*, 2nd ed.; VER Inc.: Charlottetown, PE, Canada, 2009.
49. Sykora, S.; Pieber, K.; Simhofer, H.; Hackl, V.; Brodesser, D.; Brandt, S. Isolation of Treponema and Tannerella spp. from equine odontoclastic tooth resorption and hypercementosis related periodontal disease. *Equine Vet. J.* **2014**, *46*, 358–363. [CrossRef]
50. Zhang, H.; Hung, C.L.; Min, G.; Guo, J.P.; Liu, M.; Hu, X. GPU-accelerated GLRLM algorithm for feature extraction of MRI. *Sci. Rep.* **2019**, *9*, 10883. [CrossRef]
51. Smedley, R.C.; Earley, E.T.; Galloway, S.S.; Baratt, R.M.; Rawlinson, J.E. Equine odon-toclastic tooth resorption and hypercementosis: Histopathologic features. *Vet. Pathol.* **2015**, *52*, 903–909. [CrossRef]

52. Szczypiński, P.; Klepaczko, A.; Pazurek, M.; Daniel, P. Texture and color based image segmentation and pathology detection in capsule endoscopy videos. *Comput. Methods Programs Biomed.* **2014**, *113*, 396–411. [CrossRef]
53. Szczypinski, P.M.; Klepaczko, A.; Kociołek, M. QMaZda—Software tools for image analysis and pattern recognition. In Proceedings of the 2017 Signal Processing: Algorithms, Architectures, Arrangements, and Applications (SPA), Poznan, Poland, 20–22 October 2017; pp. 217–221.
54. Depeursinge, A.; Al-Kadi, O.S.; Mitchell, J.R. *Biomedical Texture Analysis: Fundamentals, Tools and Challenges*; Academic Press: Cambridge, MA, USA, 2017.
55. Al-Ameen, Z.; Sulong, G.; Gapar, M.D.; Johar, M.D. Reducing the Gaussian blur artifact from CT medical images by employing a combination of sharpening filters and iterative deblurring algorithms. *J. Theor. Appl. Inf. Technol.* **2012**, *46*, 31–36.
56. Heidari, M.; Mirniaharikandehei, S.; Khuzani, A.Z.; Danala, G.; Qiu, Y.; Zheng, B. Improving the performance of CNN to predict the likelihood of COVID-19 using chest X-ray images with preprocessing algorithms. *Int. J. Med. Inform.* **2020**, *144*, 104284. [CrossRef] [PubMed]
57. Jusman, Y.; Tamarena, R.I.; Puspita, S.; Saleh, E.; Kanafiah, S.N.A.M. Analysis of features extraction performance to differentiate of dental caries types using gray level co-occurrence matrix algorithm. In Proceedings of the 2020 10th IEEE International Conference on Control System, Computing and Engineering (ICCSCE), Penang, Malaysia, 21–22 August 2020; pp. 148–152.
58. Nagarajan, M.B.; Coan, P.; Huber, M.B.; Diemoz, P.C.; Glaser, C.; Wismüller, A. Computer-aided diagnosis for phase-contrast X-ray computed tomography: Quantitative characterization of human patellar cartilage with high-dimensional geometric features. *J. Digit. Imaging* **2014**, *27*, 98–107. [CrossRef] [PubMed]
59. Kociołek, M.; Strzelecki, M.; Obuchowicz, R. Does image normalization and intensity resolution impact texture classification? *Comput. Med. Imaging Graph.* **2020**, *81*, 101716. [CrossRef] [PubMed]

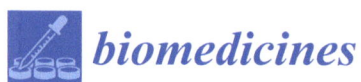 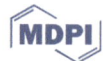

Case Report

Method Presentation of a New Integrated Orthodontic-Conservative Approach for Minimally Invasive Full Mouth Rehabilitation: Speed Up Therapy

Davide Foschi [1,†], Andrea Abate [2,3,*,†], Cinzia Maspero [2,3,*], Luca Solimei [4], Claudio Lanteri [5] and Valentina Lanteri [2,3]

1. Private Practice, 40100 Bologna, Italy
2. Department of Biomedical Surgical and Dental Sciences, University of Milan, 20142 Milan, Italy
3. Fondazione IRCCS Cà Granda, Ospedale Maggiore Policlinico, 20142 Milan, Italy
4. Department of Surgical Science and Integrated Diagnostics (DISC), University of Genova, 16126 Genova, Italy
5. Private Practice, Casale Monferrato, 15033 Alessandria, Italy
* Correspondence: andreabate93@gmail.com (A.A.); cinzia.maspero@unimi.it (C.M.); Tel.: +39-(33)-17712541 (A.A.)
† These authors contributed equally to this work.

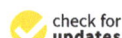

Citation: Foschi, D.; Abate, A.; Maspero, C.; Solimei, L.; Lanteri, C.; Lanteri, V. Method Presentation of a New Integrated Orthodontic-Conservative Approach for Minimally Invasive Full Mouth Rehabilitation: Speed Up Therapy. *Biomedicines* **2022**, *10*, 2536. https://doi.org/10.3390/biomedicines10102536

Academic Editor: Giuseppe Minervini

Received: 22 September 2022
Accepted: 5 October 2022
Published: 11 October 2022

Publisher's Note: MDPI stays neutral with regard to jurisdictional claims in published maps and institutional affiliations.

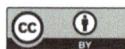

Copyright: © 2022 by the authors. Licensee MDPI, Basel, Switzerland. This article is an open access article distributed under the terms and conditions of the Creative Commons Attribution (CC BY) license (https://creativecommons.org/licenses/by/4.0/).

Abstract: The materials available today allow for extensive oral rehabilitations in a non-invasive way, and often an orthodontic preparation is useful and, thanks to the use of clear aligners, is predictable and comfortable. A preliminary study of the wax-up, mock-up, and set-up allow the clinician to plan every aspect of the treatment in detail. Furthermore, the procedure offers the patient an intuitive and understandable view of the expected final result. The new proposed method, called "speed up therapy", allows for the integration of the orthodontic set-up with the mock-up technique, simulating the occlusal and aesthetic components of the planned restoration, in all details. The clinical case presented, demonstrates step by step the predictability and clinical reliability of the proposed procedure. The final clinical result coincides exactly with the initial mock-up and demonstrates that the proposed method is predictable and reliable. The correct execution of the technique is rigorously customized, and its success is operator dependent, both for the clinical aspects and for the dental laboratory. Thus, the visualization of the objectives of the treatment constitutes a decisive support for the clinician and provides the patient with the possibility of benefiting from an immediate improvement by making it easier for them to accept a treatment plan. The visualization also includes an orthodontic phase that potentially lengthens the treatment but makes the realization more conservative and predictable.

Keywords: speed-up therapy; set-up; mock-up; clear aligners; smile aesthetics; orthodontics; full mouth rehabilitation

1. Introduction

Dentists are often called upon to care for adult patients who, not conscious of the complexity of their problems, wish to improve their appearance. The causes of smile imperfections are manifold and are associated with each other [1]. Some of these causes are, for example, the evolution of untreated malocclusions at a suitable age, tooth loss not replaced by prostheses, tooth movement secondary to loss of periodontal support, occlusal changes due to inadequate conservative or prosthetic therapies, and tooth wear due to erosion and parafunctions. Dental erosion is a constantly increasing phenomenon, related to both environmental factors (mainly dietary and/or volitional) and organic factors of intrinsic origin (gastro-esophageal reflux) [2–5]. Due to the overlapping of hard tissue lesions of different etiology and the lack of homogeneous and universally accepted classification criteria, it is often difficult to diagnose [6,7]. Instead, its destructive potential is evident, in the most severe cases it can cause vertical dimension collapse, resulting in the occurrence of aesthetic impairment and functional alterations that require multidisciplinary interventions [8]. The traditional therapeutic approach involves the preparation of damaged dental elements and their prosthetic recovery, sacrificing parts of intact dental tissue and resorting not infrequently to endodontic therapy.

Thanks to adhesive techniques, vertical dimension and the correct occlusal morphology can be restored by minimally invasive techniques (direct or indirect additive approaches) that allow for a significant savings in biological tissue [8]. In many cases, preliminary orthodontic treatment can help to resolve various types of dental incongruities and correct irregularities in arch shape and occlusal plane or loss of vertical dimension, reducing the need for compromise solutions that could have negative repercussions on prosthetic work prognosis and customer satisfaction [9,10].

In orthodontics, it can be considered "adult" when the patient has completed the permutation of teeth and, above all, their skeletal growth potential, in relation to both sex and individual variables. Tissue modifications that occur at the end of growth and slow the biological response to orthodontic forces are characterized by the numerical reduction of connective cells in the ligament and alveolar bone, which acquires a more compact appearance due to the reduction of medullary spaces and vascular network [11,12]. The end of growth coincides with the inactivation and progressive synostosis of the sutures [13,14]; thus, the orthodontic approach of the adult can only contemplate dento-alveolar problems, without being able to address skeletal discrepancies; in cases of severity, these must be corrected surgically [15].

The choice of therapeutic devices is largely conditioned by the treatment goals and the requirements of performing complex root movements. The ideal ones should accomplish the required movements in a short time and with the best possible aesthetics. They should also have a simple structure to ensure the best comfort and predict the absence of pain to allow for easy management of orthodontic forces as well as accurate hygiene [16]. To perform orthodontic treatment, the cooperation of the adult patient is important: First, they must accept the equipment used, which can lead to aesthetic and social problems. In addition, they must have acquired complete control of the bacterial plaque and gingival inflammation before starting the treatment by carefully observing hygiene rules [17].

In response to these multiple needs, the usual choice is clear aligners that, thanks to today's customized technologies, allow for a high three-dimensional control of the teeth that is adequate for the treatment of most cases [18–20]. In the presence of an important cross-sectional deficit of the palate, dental alignment will normally be preceded by a dental-alveolar expansion, by devices producing light and constant force [21,22].

From the point of view of the prosthetic treatment plan, the preliminary orthodontic preparation can reduce the spacing present in the arch and/or convey them in a single district (preferably in the posterior areas of the arch) in order to reduce the size of the restorations, optimize the shape of the coronal reconstruction, and allow a more conservative approach, with reduction of the subtractive preparation and therefore saving the biological heritage of the patient. In other words, the correct positioning of the teeth can facilitate the morphology of the conservative-prosthetic restoration and reduce the invasiveness of the preparation, while respecting the biological heritage of the patient [23–25].

The aim of this report was to present a new orthodontic-conservative integrated method for the minimally invasive rehabilitation of the full mouth, considering the most recent method reported in the scientific literature, and in terms of etiology, diagnosis, and treatment of lesions of erosive origin.

2. Case Report

A 54-year-old man came to the dental clinic reporting functional and aesthetic complications in relation to the numerous erosive lesions present in the upper and lower arch (Figure 1). At the clinical examination, the patient's dentition showed extensive erosions at the palatal surfaces of the frontal elements and wear on the occlusal surface of the posterior sectors, resulting in loss of vertical dimension and tilting of the occlusal plane to the right.

In addition, posterior cross bite and misalignment of the anterior sector were present in the upper arch, while in the lower arch, there was anterior crowding. Moreover, incongruous conservative and prosthetic treatments were visible at the occlusal surface of the posterior sectors (Figure 2). It was also observed that occlusal changes that occurred because of the extensive tooth erosions compromised the physiological occlusal dynamics in protrusion and lateral movements (Figure 3).

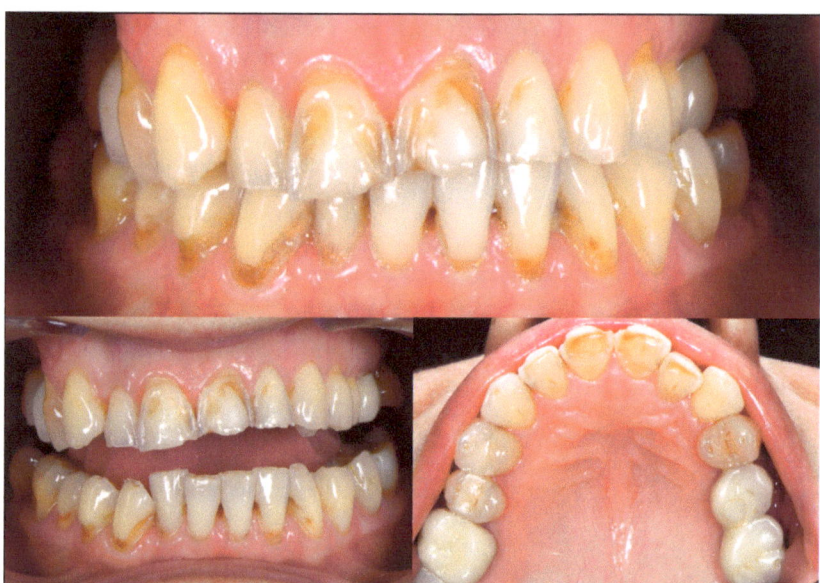

Figure 1. Intra-oral photos showing the extensive erosion of the frontal teeth.

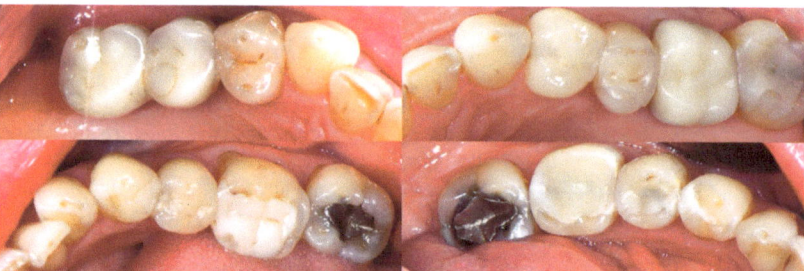

Figure 2. Incongruous conservative and prosthetic treatments visible at the occlusal surface of the posterior sectors.

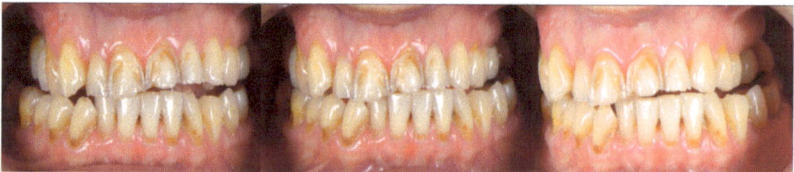

Figure 3. Occlusal changes that occurred as a result of the extensive tooth erosions compromised the physiological occlusal dynamics in protrusion and lateral movements.

Clinical and radiographic examinations revealed a good status of the periodontal tissue (Figures 4 and 5).

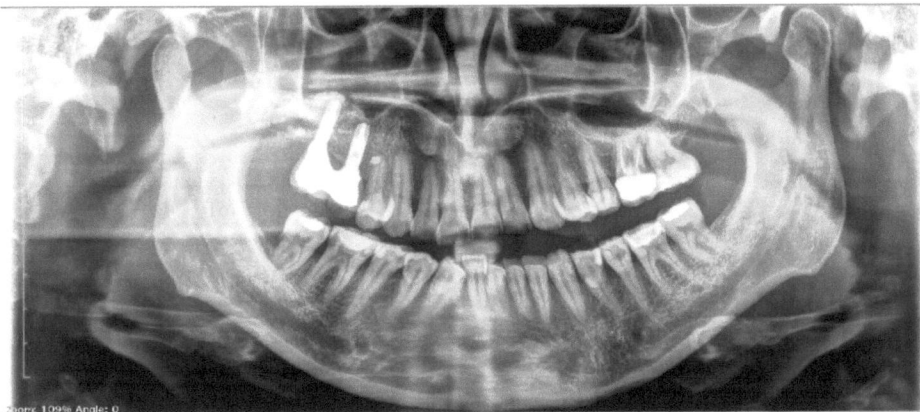

Figure 4. Pretreatment panoramic radiograph.

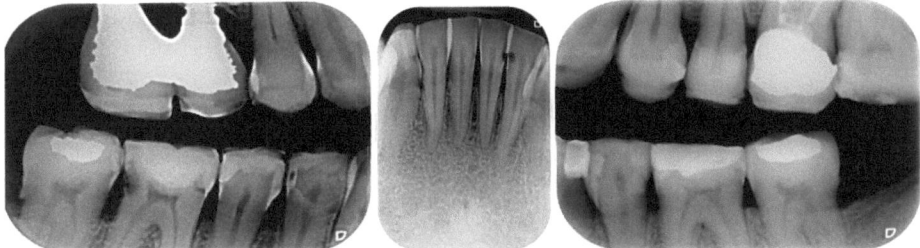

Figure 5. Pre-treatment evaluations by endoral radiographs.

2.1. Therapeutic Plan

In complex cases requiring an initial phase of pre-prosthetic orthodontics, it is useful to perform a set-up that, by simulating the outcome of orthodontic therapy, allows the dentist and orthodontist to plan together the final position of individual teeth and the distribution of spaces in the arches. Three-dimensional visualization of the result makes the treatment goals immediately understandable even to the patient, who can thus clearly understand the expected result and thus become more aware and cooperative. The shortcoming of the conventional orthodontic set-up is that it only visualizes the final position of the teeth without reference to other aspects that are fundamental to esthetic recovery, especially shape and color.

Our contribution to solving this problem is drawn from the already well-known "three-step technique" of Vailati et al. [26–28], but differs from it in materials and operative protocols. The most significant feature consists in integrating the diagnostic wax-up (wax-up) and mock-up with the orthodontic set-up, thus offering an anticipation of the result, complete with all details, through the close coordination of the dental team with the dental laboratory.

Step I: the diagnostic wax-up or wax-up: The first step is diagnostic wax-up, performed on the patient's models for preliminary visualization of the final result regarding tooth position, crown morphology, and occlusion characteristics. Treatment simulation facilitates interdisciplinary communication and planning the timing of the different treatments required [27].

Step II: the mock-up: In the second step, on the basis of the wax-up, the composite mock-up is created directly in the mouth, which also allows for the aesthetic and functional components of the planned restoration to be accurately simulated, on the basis of individual anatomical and functional parameters [29,30]. According to the literature, if the vertical dimension loss is less than 0.5 mm, it is possible to intervene with direct restorations to protect the exposed dentin; if the loss is less than 2 mm, the choice will fall on direct composite restoration of both the occlusal surface of posterior elements and the palatal and vestibular surface of anterior elements; for defects greater than 2 mm, the prevailing indication suggests indirect restorations; finally, if the loss is more than 4 mm, the classical choice fell on conventional fixed prosthesis, but today it can also be achieved through the use of partial restorations [31].

The practitioner's sensitivity will guide them in transferring the patient's expectations into solutions of immediate understanding. The expectations of the dentist must also find a place in this phase, and the dentist will be able to make the patient aware of the details of the morphological customization. This phase ends when the functional and aesthetic feedback of the provisional solution reaches the full satisfaction of both parties.

Step III: the set-up: In the third step, the orthodontic set-up is performed. It aims to realize the mock-up that has already been evaluated and approved, changing the position of the teeth from a pre-prosthetic and not abstractly orthodontic perspective. In other words, in speed up therapy, the purpose of the set-up is to bring the natural teeth into the most favorable positions to minimize the final prosthetic preparation required by the realization of the mock-up. For example, in II/II malocclusion with proclined lateral incisors and retroinclined central incisors, an alignment with veneers would require very aggressive preparations that can be significantly reduced by preliminary orthodontic treatment of the mispositioned and abraded teeth. The mock-up represents the goal of the treatment, while the orthodontic set-up aims to bring the teeth (underlying the mock-up) into the optimal position for the purposes of ensuring the best biological sparing of the tissues that are to be reconstructed by prosthetic intervention and will therefore have to take on peculiar characteristics by design and clinical implementation. In essence, the orthodontic laboratory performs a series of aligners, of which one will impart a small movement to the affected teeth, programmed in consultation with the orthodontist. Individual teeth's movements are broken down into fractions of 0.20 mm, and then aligners will be produced in the number necessary to achieve the programmed result [18]. The design of each aligner will be developed as if working on natural dentition, but the clinician will have to provide for the retouches of the mock-up-coated surfaces that will be necessary progressively, because of the change in position/relation of the teeth caused by the programmed orthodontic movements. During the creation of set-up, therefore, the vestibular aspect of the mock-up is considered as the final reference point for orthodontic correction.

Step IV: the orthodontic treatment: The special feature is that, during orthodontic movement, the initial provisional alignment obtained by mock-up will tend to become incongruous. It follows that any change of aligner will have to be accompanied by a modification of the mock-up equal to the planned movement. Perfecting the position of the natural tooth will ensure that the need for reconstruction/preparation is finally minimized and made perfectly predictable. A special aspect of the orthodontic phase, which is highly appreciated by patients, is that the teeth are moved without removing the mock-up, thus maintaining the esthetic benefit gained already at the beginning of treatment.

Step V: prosthetic finalization: At the end of orthodontic treatment, the alignment of the teeth will be optimal while the morphology of the mock-up will be significantly reworked, because of the retouching required to accommodate tooth movement. With the introduction of new materials available for modern conservative dentistry, it is possible to rehabilitate with direct or indirect technique elements affected by blemishes, discoloration, and wear with a satisfactory functional and esthetic result [8,9,26]. At this point, the clinician proceeds with the removal of the residual mock-up and performs the definitive reconstruction, choosing the technique that they prefer and taking care to reproduce the clinical, functional, and esthetic outcome, which is liked by the patient, even before the start of therapy.

Thus, the steps involved in our proposed technique follow the following order: diagnostic wax-up, mock-up, orthodontic set-up based on the mock-up, orthodontic treatment with clear aligners (without removing the mockup), and prosthetic finalization (possibly preceded by sectional temporaries).

2.2. Clinical Example

To describe the details of the proposed method, regarding the treatment of the frontal sectors of both arches, we report below a demonstration clinical case. The treatment plan proposed in this clinical case perfectly mirrors the procedure proposed in the previous paragraph (Steps I-II): treatment planning by wax-up, mock-up, and set-up: the performance of wax-up and mock-up allows for the visualization of the final result and three-dimensional assessment of the orthodontic movements required for the purpose of optimal use of the available dental structures, minimizing the invasiveness of the final restoration (Figures 6 and 7).

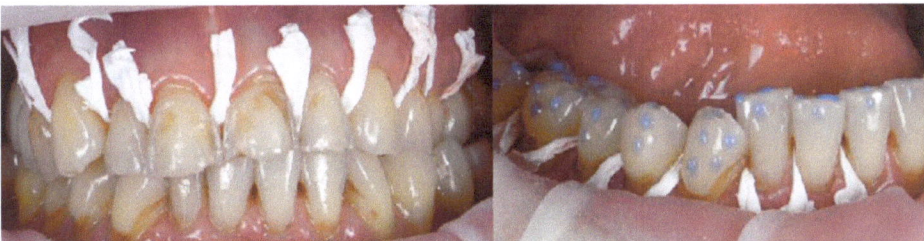

Figure 6. Selective etching of surfaces and application of adhesive system for better mock-up stability.

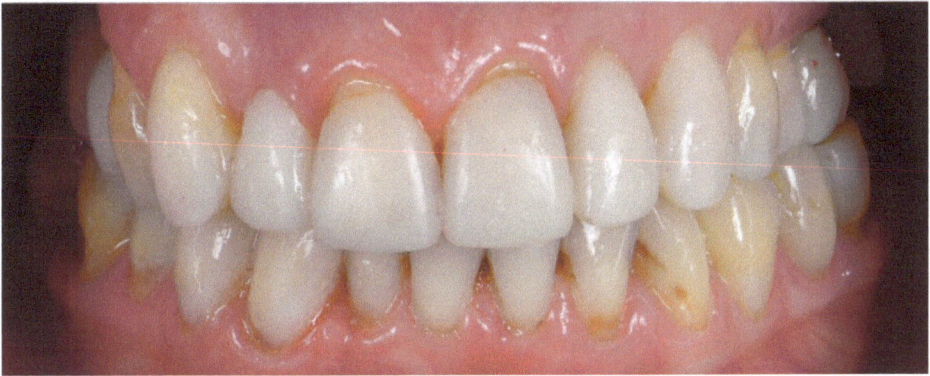

Figure 7. Initial mock-up made without tooth preparation (additive approach) through the use of a self-curing composite resin.

Set-up and orthodontics (Steps III-IV): The orthodontic step is the next step after mock-up creation and the creation of a clinical validity of vertical dimension elevation. Each new aligner will exert different pressure on individual teeth, programmed with the digital set-up. It will be the clinician's job to perform stripping and occlusal retouching of the mock-up to allow the teeth to move in the predetermined direction and amount (Figure 8). After 6 months of aligners, the goals of orthodontic treatment have been achieved, and the case is ready for finalization (Figure 9).

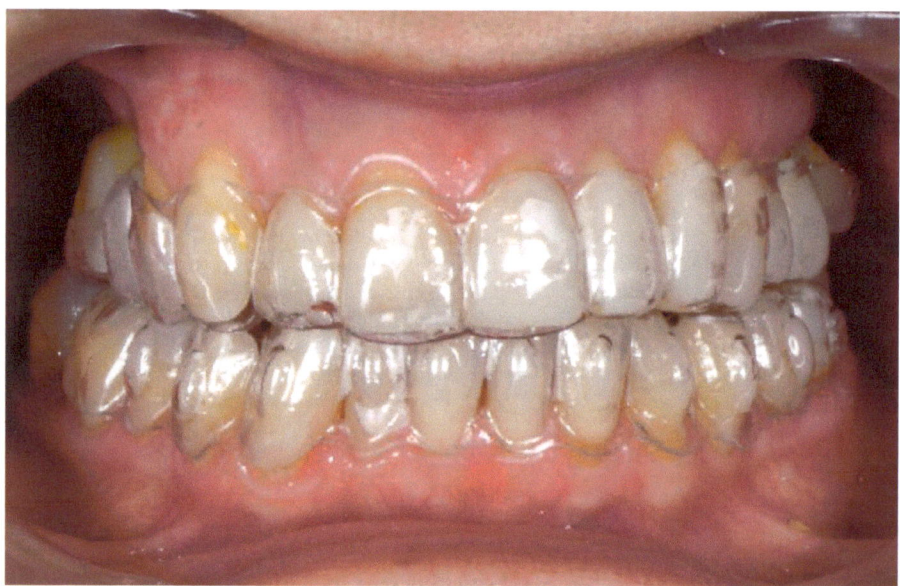

Figure 8. Orthodontic treatment with customized aligners based on the mock-up.

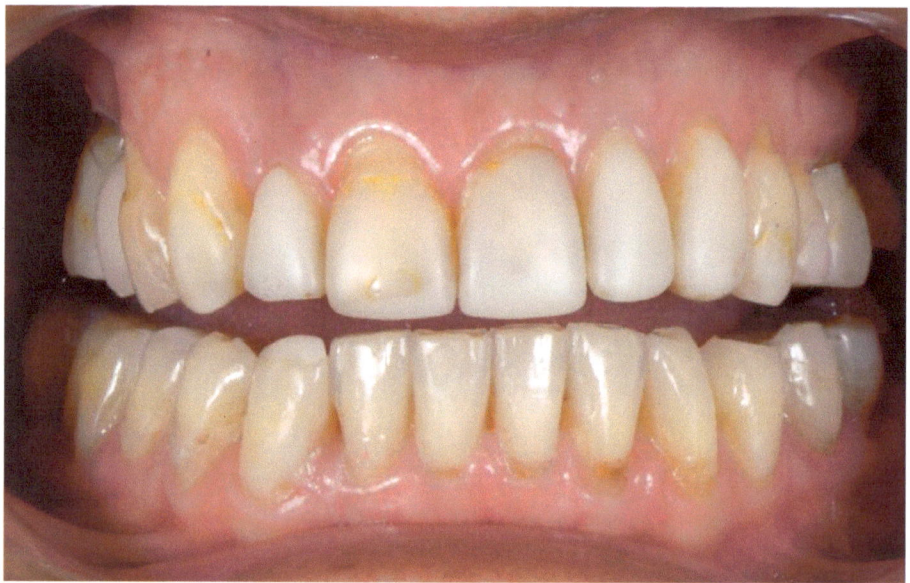

Figure 9. Result after 6 months of aligners.

Prosthetic finalization (Step V): This phase involves the aesthetic and functional reconstruction of the arches through the placement of definitive restorations by employing adhesive techniques. The choice of materials for reconstruction is a point of fundamental importance, in order to be evaluated according to the needs of the individual patient, favoring an attitude as conservative as possible. If the technique has been correctly performed in each step, the exact correspondence with the functionalized mock-up will be verified (Figure 10).

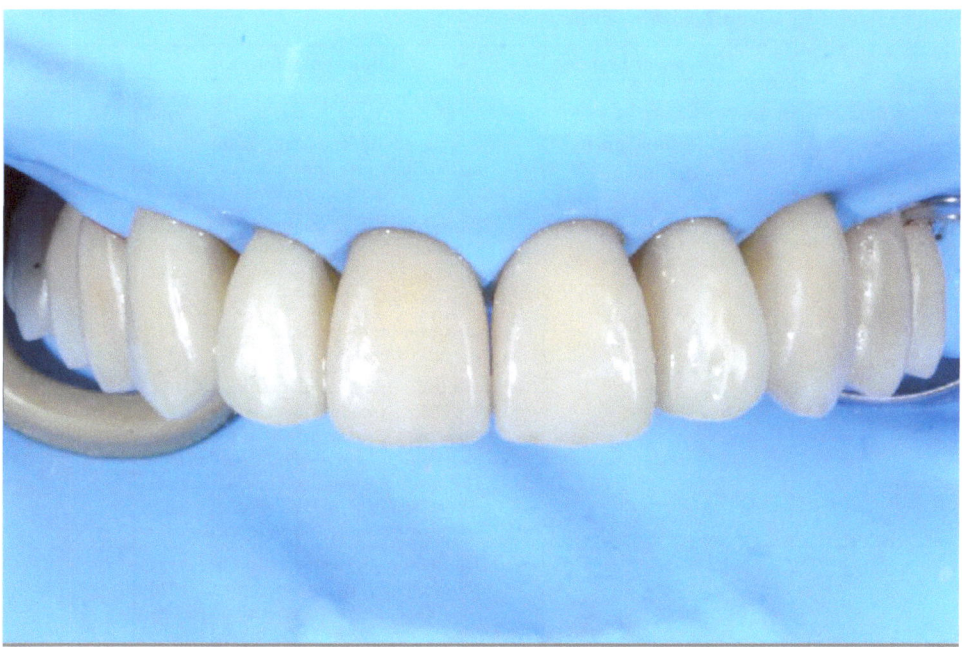

Figure 10. Adhesive cementation of prosthetic artifacts (overlays, onlays, and veneers) using an adhesive technique, dry field.

2.3. Outcome Achieved

With the aim of objectively evaluating the achieved results, we used as a reference a checklist that reports the anatomo-functional and aesthetic conditions that most frequently induce the adult patient to undergo more or less complex rehabilitative treatment (Tables 1 and 2). The correct execution of the orthodontic-conservative procedure allowed us to achieve, with excellent approximation, the planned result, both from the functional point of view and from the point of view of smile aesthetics (Figures 9–11).

Table 1. Summary objective examination of the patient before and after treatment.

	Before	After
Disharmonious smile	Yes	No
Dyschromia, dysmorphia, abrasions, and erosions of teeth	Yes	No
Anterior crowding in the upper arch	Yes	No
Anterior crowding in the lower arch	Yes	No
Upper transverse discrepancy	Yes	No
Presence of buccal corridors or black tunnels	Yes	No
Curve of Spee alteration	Yes	No
Curve of Wilson alteration	Yes	No
Functional movements with altered guides	Yes	No
Pain and/or noise ATM	Yes	No

Table 2. Smile aesthetic parameters.

Parameter Examined	Clinical Significance	Result Obtained
Smile symmetry	Smile symmetry refers to the mirror agreement between the two sides of the mouth but can also consider the bi-pupillary line, the incisal line, and the labial commissure.	YES
Horizontal symmetry	It originates from the presence of similar elements placed in a regular sequence, as verified in a dentition with teeth well aligned in the horizontal plane.	YES
Vertical symmetry	Recall the same principle as above, referring to the vertical direction.	YES
Repeated report	It indicates the division of space into portions that may not be identical in shape and size but arranged to generate a harmonious connection between them. This is what is verified between opposing hemiarches with well-arranged teeth, inspiring a sense of order and balance.	YES
Prospective effect	The contour of the buccal surface and the alignment of the inclined planes of the teeth is decisive in generating a correct perspective effect. The different length or strong color difference of even one element can impair the perspective effect and compromise the sense of harmony of the whole.	YES
Lip height	Useful distinction in static and dynamic harmony. The average height of the upper vermilion is 7.1 mm in the male and 7.7 mm in the female. The lower vermilion is normally more extensive, about 10 mm on average; these are statistical values, with wide individual variations.	YES
Lip line	The height of the upper lip, relative to the upper central incisors, can be classified as low, medium, or high, on the basis of the amount of crown exposure.	YES
Smile line	Smile line is a curved line passing through the incisal margin of the upper incisors, parallel to the inner margin of the lower lip.	YES
Curvature of the upper lip	With superior convexity, it extends from the center toward the lateral triangular spaces. When rectilinear or worse with inverted convexity, it gives the subject a sad and unattractive expression.	YES
Frontal axial alignment	The smooth slope of the long axis of the front elements helps generate a sense of regularity.	YES

Table 2. *Cont.*

Parameter Examined	Clinical Significance	Result Obtained
Tooth alignment in the arch	Recalls the anatomical harmony represented by the correct positioning of teeth in the center of the alveolar ridge.	YES
Contact point alignment	In the anterior sectors, the contact points are located near the incisal third and their sequence defines a curvilinear pattern.	YES
Color	Color is one of the cardinal elements of dental aesthetic recovery. It must always be evaluated in a much broader context, involving many other periodontal, labial, and skin parameters of the patient.	YES
Gingival scalloping	Gingival parabolas are decisive for the aesthetic effect of the frontal group. Orthodontic treatment can contribute to their harmonization.	YES
Negative space	A restrained smile enhances the characteristics of the teeth, while an excessive smile imparts an unattractive sense of emptiness.	YES
Arch geometry	There are several types of arch form related to individual craniofacial conformation that must be recreated or respected by orthodontic treatment.	YES
Buccal corridors o black tunnels	A restrained smile enhances the characteristics of the teeth, while an excessive smile imparts an unattractive sense of emptiness.	YES
Fibonacci golden proportion	It evaluates proportions by relating harmony to numerical values. In the dental field, it can find application in the evaluation of various dental and facial morphological parameters.	YES

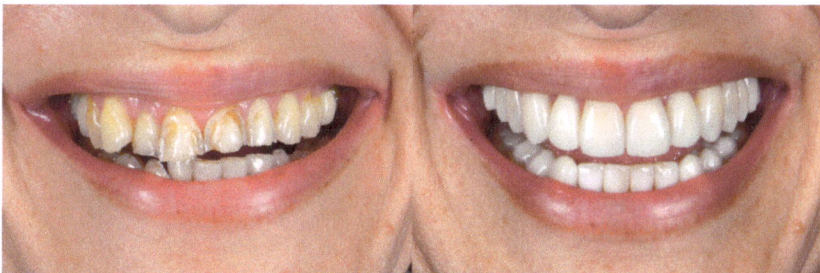

Figure 11. Comparison of the initial and final situation.

Orthodontic treatment and anatomical reconstruction of eroded teeth allowed us to create the reconstitution of physiological occlusal dynamics (Figures 12 and 13).

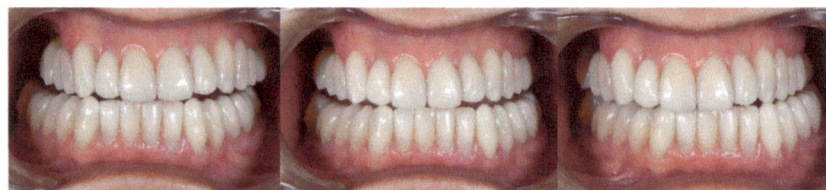

Figure 12. Physiological occlusal dynamics in protrusion and lateral movements.

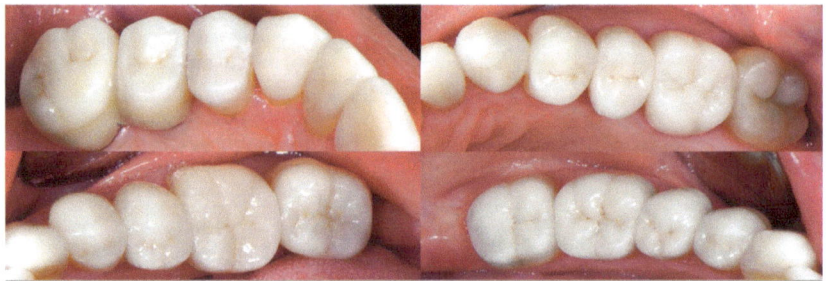

Figure 13. Details of posterior quadrant reconstruction with recovery of the vertical dimension, chewing efficiency, and aesthetics.

The correct execution of the orthodontic-conservative procedure allowed us to achieve, with excellent approximation, all the planned goals (Figure 14). Stability of outcome was confirmed by a clinical and radiographical follow-up at 2 years after the finish of therapy (Figures 15 and 16).

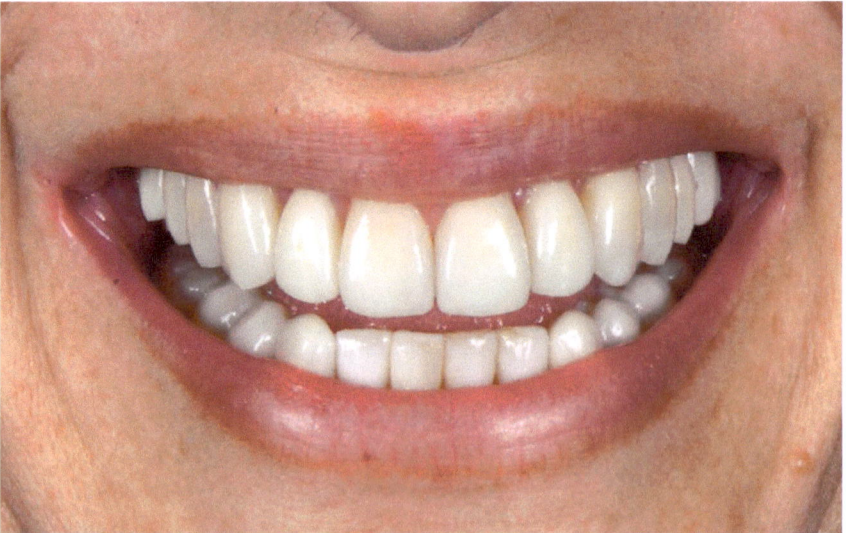

Figure 14. Details of posterior quadrant reconstruction with recovery of the vertical dimension, chewing efficiency, and aesthetics.

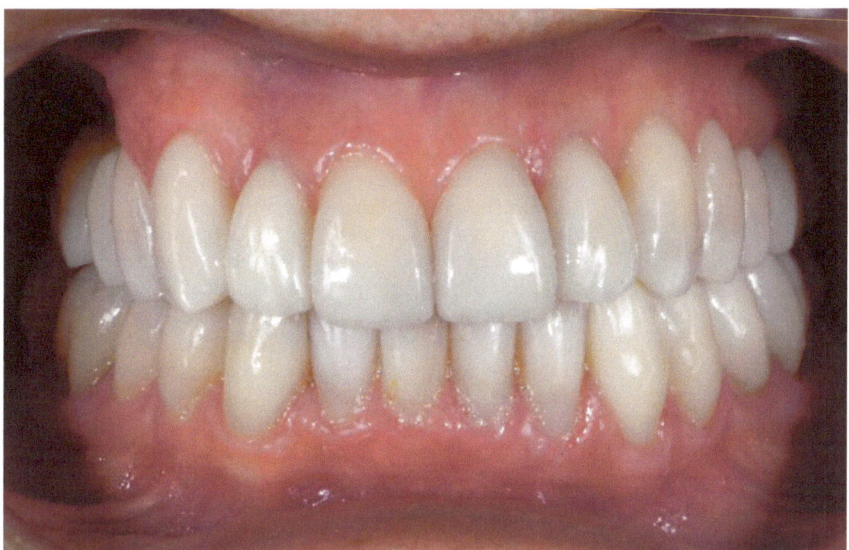

Figure 15. Clinical follow-up at 24 months.

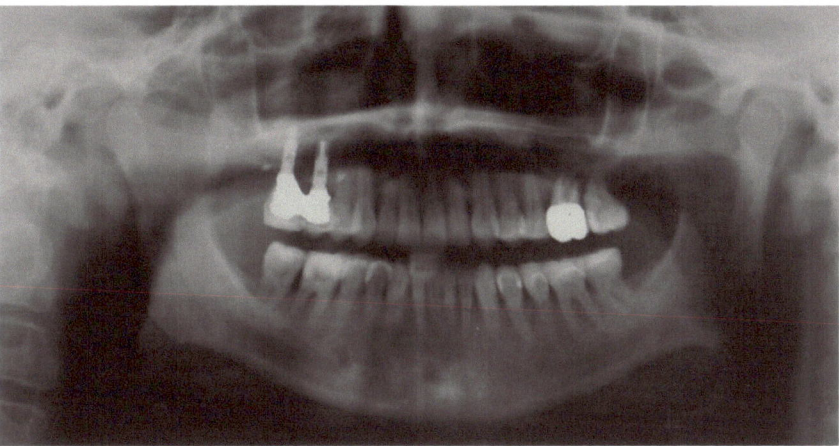

Figure 16. Orthopantomography at 24 months.

3. Discussion

Several authors have proposed different criteria to define the aesthetic canons of a harmonious smile [1,29]. The ideal smile is an individual datum, generated by the integration of numerous components capable of stimulating a wide range of emotional reactions. Our case provides us the opportunity to summarize the most well-known ones, in order to be able to identify whether the correct dento-labial ratios have been achieved. We therefore obtained some of the best-known esthetic parameters from the literature and then subjected our results to verification (see Table 2—Aesthetic parameters of the smile). The presented clinical case, considering the parameters listed in Table 1, demonstrated that the planned goals were achieved. In particular, the final clinical image coincides with the initial mock-up, demonstrating that the proposed method proved to be predictable and reliable [30,32].

One of the greatest advantages in such particular case is that the "eroded" teeth with exposed dentin do not suffer any more sensitivity and possible worse degenerations due to the application of the segmented full mock-up at the beginning of the treatment [4,33,34]. Every mock-up/set-up modification was tested and functionalized directly in the mouth using the same reversible approach: sandblast of the existence surfaces, bonding application, and self-curing/light curing resin application without the need to anesthetize the patient, which were very helpful in regulating the occlusal contacts differently from what occurs in a classical prosthodontics approach. From the patient's point of view, the most appreciated aspects were the aesthetics and the comfort during the provisional phase, so we could say that the immediate aesthetic improvement and the possibility to be additive and not subtractive were the real benefits given by this combination of treatments. The choice of the transparent aligners was the perfect integration of the orthodontic treatment, given the same concept: additive appliances, soft forces, preview of the final result, and more comfort for the patient. Moreover, the choice to use clear aligners stems from the fact that they do not significantly affect the periodontal and microbiological conditions of the oral cavity. The literature reported that the use of clear aligners should be considered as a valuable therapeutic option that has no significant impact on oral and microbiological parameters if compared with untreated patients [35–37].

The proper execution of the technique is rigorously customized, and its success is certainly operator dependent, both for the clinical aspects and for the dental laboratory. The present case report allows us to emphasize the importance of the treatment plan, which must be planned in detail for procedures and timing, being aimed at achieving therapeutic objectives in the shortest possible time. It is also very important that the orthodontic phase involves the use of simple appliances to minimize patient discomfort and difficulties in maintaining oral hygiene, which must always be kept impeccable. The particularity of this type of patient, characterized by great variability in individual clinical photos, makes it effectively impossible to have homogeneous samples on which to base statistically significant studies for the purposes of evidence-based medicine. Rather, the evidence of reference will be based on clinical observations and customer satisfaction.

Our patients are increasingly exigent about medical and dental care in general, with particular regard to treatments with significant esthetic implications. Preliminary visualization of treatment goals, detailed and immediately understandable, introduces an extraordinary new communication instrument that brings significant added value into our relationships with our patients. From a marketing point of view, such a concrete visualization of the planned result facilitates acceptance by patients, who show that they greatly appreciate the realistic and rapid response to their aesthetic requests. Moreover, of note is the full respect for individual biological characteristics and the preventive aspects towards possible iatrogenic damage inherent in the technique [38]. The additive approach is today the first option to be considered when treating serious problems of dental wear. The adhesive prosthesis characterized using partial restorations, such as onlays, overlays, and veneers, is now preferred and sought not only by professionals, but also by patients. Exploiting the variation of the vertical dimension of the occlusion allows for operations to occur whilst preserving the residual dental structures to the maximum and reducing the subtractive procedures to a minimum. Whatever gnathological philosophy the clinician may prefer, the idea "to test" the project in a totally reversible way, using complete mockups, represents a reliable, dynamic, cost-effective, and comfortable method for patients.

4. Conclusions

In conclusion, the correct execution of the present orthodontic-conservative approach allowed us to obtain, with excellent approximation, the planned results, both from the aesthetics and functional point of view. The collaboration between dental office and laboratory plays a key role in the planning and achievement of the rehabilitation process. The comparison between the needs of the clinician and those of the dental technician allows for a rationalization for situations where it is preferable to segment the realization of final restorations, rather than proceed with the simultaneous realization of complete arches.

The development of new hybrid materials and digital workflow procedures allows us today to make completely adhesive rehabilitations, pushing the limit of the additive approach beyond what seemed impossible only few years ago. The challenge for the coming years will be to obtain therapeutic results that can come as close as possible to the patient's expectations.

Author Contributions: Conceptualization, D.F., C.M. and C.L.; methodology, D.F.; software, A.A. and C.M.; validation, C.L., V.L. and D.F.; formal analysis, A.A. and L.S.; investigation, D.F.; resources, A.A.; data curation, A.A.; writing—original draft preparation, C.L.; writing—review and editing, A.A.; supervision, V.L.; project administration, D.F. and V.L. All authors have read and agreed to the published version of the manuscript.

Funding: This research received no external funding.

Institutional Review Board Statement: The patient provided written informed consent to carry out an anonymous analysis of his anamnesis for research purposes. The study protocol was approved by the Ethical Committee of the Fondazione IRCCS Ca'Granda, Ospedale Maggiore, Milan, Italy (protocol no. 573/15). This study was performed in compliance with the Declaration of Helsinki for human studies.

Informed Consent Statement: Written informed consent was obtained from the patient(s) to publish this paper.

Data Availability Statement: Not applicable.

Acknowledgments: The authors want to thank Giovanni Favara and Nicola Gondoni.

Conflicts of Interest: The authors declare no conflict of interest.

References

1. Redi, F.; Marchio, V.; Derchi, G.; Lardani, L.; Redi, L.; Lanteri, V. Aesthetic parameters of the human profile through the 20th century as an aid for orthodontic treatment. *Int. J. Clin. Dent.* **2021**, *14*, 253–261.
2. Schlueter, N.; Tveit, A.B. Prevalence of erosive tooth wear in risk groups. *Monogr. Oral Sci.* **2014**, *25*, 74–98. [CrossRef] [PubMed]
3. Bartlett, D. Intrinsic causes of erosion. *Monogr. Oral Sci.* **2006**, *20*, 119–139. [CrossRef]
4. Jaeggi, T.; Lussi, A. Prevalence, incidence and distribution of erosion. *Monogr. Oral Sci.* **2014**, *25*, 55–73. [CrossRef]
5. Abate, A.; Gaffuri, F.; Lanteri, V.; Fama, A.; Ugolini, A.; Mannina, L.; Maspero, C. A CBCT based analysis of the correlation between volumetric morphology of the frontal sinuses and the facial growth pattern in caucasian subjects. A cross-sectional study. *Head Face Med.* **2022**, *18*, 4. [CrossRef] [PubMed]
6. Larsen, I.B.; Westergaard, J.; Stoltze, K.; Larsen, A.I.; Gyntelberg, F.; Holmstrup, P. A clinical index for evaluating and monitoring dental erosion. *Community Dent. Oral Epidemiol.* **2000**, *28*, 211–217. [CrossRef] [PubMed]
7. Smith, B.G.; Knight, J.K. An index for measuring the wear of teeth. *Br. Dent. J.* **1984**, *156*, 435–438. [CrossRef]
8. Freitas, A.C.J.; Silva, A.M.; Lima Verde, M.A.R.; Jorge de Aguiar, J.R.P. Oral rehabilitation of severely worn dentition using an overlay for immediate re-establishment of occlusal vertical dimension. *Gerodontology* **2012**, *29*, 75–80. [CrossRef]
9. Derchi, G.; Marchio, V.; Borgia, V.; Özcan, M.; Giuca, M.R.; Barone, A. Twelve-year longitudinal clinical evaluation of bonded indirect composite resin inlays. *Quintessence Int.* **2019**, *50*, 448–454. [CrossRef]
10. Didier, H.; Assandri, F.; Gaffuri, F.; Cavagnetto, D.; Abate, A.; Villanova, M.; Maiorana, C. The Role of Dental Occlusion and Neuromuscular Behavior in Professional Ballet Dancers' Performance: A Pilot Study. *Healthcare* **2021**, *9*, 251. [CrossRef]
11. Sim, H.-Y.; Kim, H.-S.; Jung, D.-U.; Lee, H.; Lee, J.-W.; Han, K.; Yun, K.-I. Association between orthodontic treatment and periodontal diseases: Results from a national survey. *Angle Orthod.* **2017**, *87*, 651–657. [CrossRef] [PubMed]
12. Choi, J.-I.; Park, S.-B. A multidisciplinary approach for the management of pathologic tooth migration in a patient with moderately advanced periodontal disease. *Int. J. Periodontics Restor. Dent.* **2012**, *32*, 225–231.
13. Gupta, S.; Jain, S.; Gupta, P.; Deoskar, A. Determining skeletal maturation using insulin-like growth factor I (IGF-I) test. *Prog. Orthod.* **2012**, *13*, 288–295. [CrossRef] [PubMed]
14. Baccetti, T.; Franchi, L.; McNamara, J.A.J. An improved version of the cervical vertebral maturation (CVM) method for the assessment of mandibular growth. *Angle Orthod.* **2002**, *72*, 316–323. [CrossRef]
15. Downs, W.B. Variations in facial relationships: Their significance in treatment and prognosis. *Am. J. Orthod.* **1948**, *34*, 812–840. [CrossRef]

16. Cossellu, G.; Lanteri, V.; Lione, R.; Ugolini, A.; Gaffuri, F.; Cozza, P.; Farronato, M. Efficacy of ketoprofen lysine salt and paracetamol/acetaminophen to reduce pain during rapid maxillary expansion: A randomized controlled clinical trial. *Int. J. Paediatr. Dent.* **2019**, *29*, 58–65. [CrossRef] [PubMed]
17. Matarese, G.; Isola, G.; Ramaglia, L.; Dalessandri, D.; Lucchese, A.; Alibrandi, A.; Fabiano, F.; Cordasco, G. Periodontal biotype: Characteristic, prevalence and dimensions related to dental malocclusion. *Minerva Stomatol.* **2016**, *65*, 231–238.
18. Lanteri, V.; Farronato, G.; Lanteri, C.; Caravita, R.; Cossellu, G. The efficacy of orthodontic treatments for anterior crowding with Invisalign compared with fixed appliances using the Peer Assessment Rating Index. *Quintessence Int.* **2018**, *49*, 581–587. [CrossRef]
19. Lanteri, V.; Poggi, S.; Blasi, S.; De Angelis, D.; Gangale, S.; Farronato, M.; Maiorani, C.; Butera, A. Periodontal aspects of orthodontic treatment with invisalign® versus fixed appliances in the same patients—A pilot study. *Int. J. Clin. Dent.* **2020**, *13*, 419–447.
20. Rossini, G.; Parrini, S.; Castroflorio, T.; Deregibus, A.; Debernardi, C.L. Efficacy of clear aligners in controlling orthodontic tooth movement: A systematic review. *Angle Orthod.* **2015**, *85*, 881–889. [CrossRef]
21. Lanteri, V.; Cavagnetto, D.; Abate, A.; Mainardi, E.; Gaffuri, F.; Ugolini, A.; Maspero, C. Buccal Bone Changes Around First Permanent Molars and Second Primary Molars after Maxillary Expansion with a Low Compliance Ni-Ti Leaf Spring Expander. *Int. J. Environ. Res. Public Health* **2020**, *17*, 9104. [CrossRef] [PubMed]
22. Lanteri, V.; Abate, A.; Cavagnetto, D.; Ugolini, A.; Gaffuri, F.; Gianolio, A.; Maspero, C. Cephalometric Changes Following Maxillary Expansion with Ni-Ti Leaf Springs Palatal Expander and Rapid Maxillary Expander: A Retrospective Study. *Appl. Sci.* **2021**, *11*, 5748. [CrossRef]
23. Acharya, V.; Victor, D. Orthodontic management of patients undergoing prosthetic rehabilitation. *J. Calif. Dent. Assoc.* **2015**, *43*, 185–191. [PubMed]
24. Small, B.W. Pre-prosthetic orthodontics for esthetics and function in restorative dentistry. *Gen. Dent.* **2011**, *59*, 91–94. [PubMed]
25. Maspero, C.; Abate, A.; Inchingolo, F.; Dolci, C.; Cagetti, M.G.; Tartaglia, G.M. Incidental Finding in Pre-Orthodontic Treatment Radiographs of an Aural Foreign Body: A Case Report. *Children* **2022**, *9*, 421. [CrossRef] [PubMed]
26. Vailati, F.; Carciofo, S. Treatment planning of adhesive additive rehabilitations: The progressive wax-up of the three-step technique. *Int. J. Esthet. Dent.* **2016**, *11*, 356–377. [PubMed]
27. Vailati, F.; Belser, U.C. Full-mouth adhesive rehabilitation of a severely eroded dentition: The three-step technique. Part 1. *Eur. J. Esthet. Dent. Off. J. Eur. Acad. Esthet. Dent.* **2008**, *3*, 30–44.
28. Vailati, F.; Belser, U.C. Classification and treatment of the anterior maxillary dentition affected by dental erosion: The ACE classification. *Int. J. Periodontics Restorative Dent.* **2010**, *30*, 559–571. [PubMed]
29. Lo Giudice, A.; Ortensi, L.; Farronato, M.; Lucchese, A.; Lo Castro, E.; Isola, G. The step further smile virtual planning: Milled versus prototyped mock-ups for the evaluation of the designed smile characteristics. *BMC Oral Health* **2020**, *20*, 165. [CrossRef] [PubMed]
30. Vailati, F.; Belser, U.C. Full-mouth adhesive rehabilitation of a severely eroded dentition: The three-step technique. Part 3. *Eur. J. Esthet. Dent. Off. J. Eur. Acad. Esthet. Dent.* **2008**, *3*, 236–257.
31. Belser, U.C.; Magne, P.; Magne, M. Ceramic laminate veneers: Continuous evolution of indications. *J. Esthet. Dent.* **1997**, *9*, 197–207. [CrossRef]
32. Vailati, F.; Belser, U.C. Full-mouth adhesive rehabilitation of a severely eroded dentition: The three-step technique. Part 2. *Eur. J. Esthet. Dent. Off. J. Eur. Acad. Esthet. Dent.* **2008**, *3*, 128–146.
33. Grippo, J.O.; Simring, M.; Schreiner, S. Attrition, abrasion, corrosion and abfraction revisited: A new perspective on tooth surface lesions. *J. Am. Dent. Assoc.* **2004**, *135*, 1105–1109. [CrossRef] [PubMed]
34. Lussi, A.; Carvalho, T.S. Erosive tooth wear: A multifactorial condition of growing concern and increasing knowledge. *Monogr. Oral Sci.* **2014**, *25*, 1–15. [CrossRef] [PubMed]
35. Sfondrini, M.F.; Butera, A.; Di Michele, P.; Luccisano, C.; Ottini, B.; Sangalli, E.; Gallo, S.; Pascadopoli, M.; Gandini, P.; Scribante, A. Microbiological Changes during Orthodontic Aligner Therapy: A Prospective Clinical Trial. *Appl. Sci.* **2021**, *11*, 6758. [CrossRef]
36. Butera, A.; Maiorani, C.; Morandini, A.; Simonini, M.; Morittu, S.; Barbieri, S.; Bruni, A.; Sinesi, A.; Ricci, M.; Trombini, J.; et al. Assessment of Genetical, Pre, Peri and Post Natal Risk Factors of Deciduous Molar Hypomineralization (DMH), Hypomineralized Second Primary Molar (HSPM) and Molar Incisor Hypomineralization (MIH): A Narrative Review. *Children* **2021**, *8*, 432. [CrossRef]
37. Zharmagambetova, A.; Tuleutayeva, S.; Akhmetova, S.; Zharmagambetov, A. MICROBIOLOGICAL ASPECTS OF THE ORTHODONTIC TREATMENT. *Georgian Med. News* **2017**, *264*, 39–43.
38. Bartlett, D.; Ganss, C.; Lussi, A. Basic Erosive Wear Examination (BEWE): A new scoring system for scientific and clinical needs. *Clin. Oral Investig.* **2008**, *12* (Suppl. 1), S65–S68. [CrossRef]

MDPI AG
Grosspeteranlage 5
4052 Basel
Switzerland
Tel.: +41 61 683 77 34

Biomedicines Editorial Office
E-mail: biomedicines@mdpi.com
www.mdpi.com/journal/biomedicines

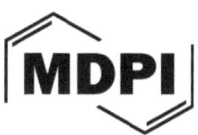

Disclaimer/Publisher's Note: The statements, opinions and data contained in all publications are solely those of the individual author(s) and contributor(s) and not of MDPI and/or the editor(s). MDPI and/or the editor(s) disclaim responsibility for any injury to people or property resulting from any ideas, methods, instructions or products referred to in the content.

www.ingramcontent.com/pod-product-compliance
Lightning Source LLC
LaVergne TN
LVHW072325090526
838202LV00019B/2353